OSTEOPOROSIS

OSTEOPOROSIS Has Been Endorsed by

American Geriatrics Society

The American Geriatrics Society is a nationwide, not-for-profit association of health care providers dedicated to improving the health and well-being of all older adults by developing, implementing, and advocating programs in patient care, research, professional and public education, and public policy.

For information on the AGS please visit www.americangeriatrics.org.

American Society for Bone and Mineral Research

The American Society for Bone and Mineral Research is a professional scientific and medical society established to promote excellence in bone and mineral research, to foster integration of basic and clinical science, and to facilitate the translation of that science to health care and clinical practice.

For information on the ASBMR please visit www.asbmr.org.

OSTEOPOROSIS

AN EVIDENCE-BASED GUIDE TO PREVENTION AND MANAGEMENT

EDITORS

STEVEN R. CUMMINGS, MD

FELICIA COSMAN, MD

SOPHIE A. JAMAL, MD, FRCP(C)

WOMEN'S HEALTH SERIES EDITOR

PAMELA CHARNEY, MD, FACP

AMERICAN COLLEGE OF PHYSICIANS
PHILADELPHIA

Clinical Consultant: David R. Goldmann, MD
Acquisitions Editor: Mary K. Ruff
Manager, Book Publishing: David Myers
Developmental Editor: Vicki Hoenigke
Production Supervisor: Allan S. Kleinberg
Production Editor: Karen C. Nolan
Editorial Coordinator: Alicia Dillihay
Interior and Cover Design: Patrick Whelan
Index: Nelle Garrecht

Manufactured in the United States of America
Composition by UB Communications
Printing/binding by McNaughton & Gunn

American College of Physicians (ACP) became an imprint of the American College of Physicians—American Society of Internal Medicine in July 1998.

Library of Congress Cataloging-in-Publication Data

Osteoporosis: An Evidence-Based Guide to Prevention and Management
    [edited by] Steven R. Cummings, Felicia Cosman, Sophie A. Jamal.
      p. ; cm. — (ACP women's health series)
    Includes bibliographical references and index.
    ISBN 0-943126-95-9
    1. Osteoporosis. I. Cummings, Steven R. II. Cosman, Felicia, 1958- III. Jamal, Sophie (Sophie A.), 1966- IV. Series.
    [DNLM: 1. Osteoporosis—diagnosis. 2. Osteoporosis—therapy. WE 250 O85114 2001]
    RC931.O73 O745 2001
    616.7'16—dc21

                                    2001022189

The authors have exerted reasonable efforts to ensure that drug selection and dosage set forth in this volume are in accord with current recommendations and practice at the time of publication. In view of ongoing research, occasional changes in government regulations, and the constant flow of information relating to drug therapy and drug reactions, the reader is urged to check the package insert for each drug for any change in indications and dosage and for added warnings and precautions. This care is particularly important when the recommended agent is a new or infrequently used drug. ACP–ASIM is not responsible for any accident or injury resulting from the use of this publication.

For a catalogue of publications available from ACP–ASIM, contact:

Customer Service Center
American College of Physicians–American Society of Internal Medicine
190 N. Independence Mall West
Philadelphia, PA 19106-1572
215-351-2600; 800-523-1546, ext. 2600

Visit our Web site at www. acponline.org

02 03 04 05 06/9 8 7 6 5 4 3 2 1

Editors

Steven R. Cummings, MD
Professor of Medicine, Epidemiology & Biostatistics
Director, UCSF Coordinating Center
University of California, San Francisco
San Francisco, California

Felicia Cosman, MD
Associate Professor of Clinical Medicine
Columbia University
New York, New York;
Endocrinologist
Helen Hayes Hospital
Regional Bone Center
West Haverstraw, New York

Sophie A. Jamal, MD, FRCP(C)
Postdoctoral Fellow
Osteoporosis Research
University of Toronto
Sunnybrook and Women's College Health Sciences Centre
Toronto, Ontario, Canada

Women's Health Series Editor

Pamela Charney, MD, FACP
Clinical Professor of Medicine
Clinical Associate Professor of Obstetrics & Gynecology and Women's Health
Albert Einstein College of Medicine
Bronx, New York;
Program Director
Internal Medicine Residency
Norwalk Hospital
Norwalk, Connecticut

Contributors

Dennis Black, PhD
Professor
Department of Epidemiology and
  Biostatistics
University of California, San Francisco
San Francisco, California

Jane Cauley, DrPH
Professor of Epidemiology
Department of Epidemiology
University of Pittsburgh Graduate School
  of Public Health
Pittsburgh, Pennsylvania

Jackie A. Clowes, MBChB, MRCP
University of Sheffield
Bone Metabolism Group
Northern General Hospital
Sheffield, England

Felicia Cosman, MD
Associate Professor of Clinical Medicine
Columbia University
New York, New York;
Endocrinologist
Helen Hayes Hospital
Regional Bone Center
West Haverstraw, New York

Steven R. Cummings, MD
Professor of Medicine, Epidemiology
  & Biostatistics
Director, UCSF Coordinating Center
University of California, San Francisco
San Francisco, California

**Richard Eastell, MD, FRCP(UK,
  Edinburgh, Ireland), FRCPath,
  FMedSci**
Director, Division of Clinical Sciences
  (North)
University of Sheffield Clinical Sciences
  Centre
Northern General Hospital
Sheffield, England

Gail A. Greendale, MD
Associate Professor of Medicine and
  Obstetrics & Gynecology
Research Director, Iris Cantor UCLA
  Women's Health Center
UCLA School of Medicine
Division of Geriatrics
Los Angeles, California

Marc C. Hochberg, MD, MPH
Professor of Medicine and Epidemiology
  & Preventive Medicine
Head, Division of Rheumatology and
  Clinical Immunology
Department of Medicine
University of Maryland School of
  Medicine
Baltimore, Maryland

Sophie A. Jamal, MD, FRCP(C)
Postdoctoral Fellow
Osteoporosis Research
University of Toronto
Sunnybrook and Women's College
  Health Sciences Centre
Toronto, Ontario, Canada

Sundeep Khosla, MD
Professor of Medicine
Department of Endocrinology
Mayo Medical School
Mayo Clinic
Rochester, Minnesota

Robert Lindsay, MBChB, PhD, FRCP
Professor of Clinical Medicine
Columbia University
New York, New York;
Chief, Internal Medicine
Helen Hayes Hospital
Regional Bone Center
West Haverstraw, New York

Robert Marcus, MD
Professor Emeritus
Stanford University
Stanford, California;
Medical Advisor
US Affiliate
Eli Lilly & Company
Indianapolis, Indiana

Michael Nevitt, PhD, MPH
Professor
Department of Epidemiology and
    Biostatistics
University of California, San Francisco
San Francisco, California

Jeri Nieves, PhD
Department of Epidemiology
Columbia University
New York, New York;
Clinical Research Center
Helen Hayes Hospital
West Haverstraw, New York

Ian R. Reid, MD, FRACP
Department of Medicine
University of Auckland
Auckland, New Zealand

Stuart L. Silverman, MD, FACP, FACR
Clinical Professor of Medicine and
    Rheumatology
UCLA School of Medicine
Cedars-Sinai Medical Center
WLA VA Health System;
President, ClinTrials Network
Medical Director, OMC Clinical Research
    Center
Beverly Hills, California

Fiona Wu, FRACP
Department of Medicine
University of Auckland
Auckland, New Zealand

Foreword

Osteoporosis is a common clinical problem associated with substantial disability. Until relatively recently, osteoporosis was viewed as an inevitable part of aging and was typically diagnosed only after a serious complication such as fracture. At the beginning of the 21st century, however, the paradigm has shifted dramatically. We can now diagnose patients at high risk before a fracture occurs with easily performed noninvasive tests that estimate bone mass. We can treat these patients with new, safe, and effective drugs whose efficacy has been proven in carefully conducted clinical trials to reduce the risk of fracture to a clinically meaningful degree. In addition, the role of good nutrition, including calcium and vitamin D, and the value of exercise in the prevention and management of osteoporosis are now better understood.

Doctors Cummings, Cosman, and Jamal have assembled an outstanding array of world experts who review the latest evidence in the realms of bone biology, epidemiology, bone mass measurement, and pharmacologic treatment, offering both scientific content and extensive clinical experience. *Osteoporosis* is a splendid text that offers a comprehensive and up-to-date understanding of this disease and its management while providing important practical guidelines for the clinician.

Given the already high and ever-increasing prevalence of osteoporosis in our society, the task of prevention and management will clearly be placed mainly in the hands of the primary care physician. This book will be a tremendous help to those clinicians who accept that challenge.

Ethel S. Siris, MD
Madeline C. Stabile Professor of Clinical Medicine
Columbia University College of Physicians and Surgeons;
Director, Toni Stabile Osteoporosis Center
Columbia Presbyterian Medical Center
New York, New York

Preface

Fractures often produce pain and disability, occasionally even death. Fortunately, within the last decade rapid, noninvasive tests have become widely available. These allow us to predict the risk of fracture in individuals and therefore to identify patients who require medical management. Also within the last decade a number of medications have been developed that can reduce the risk of fracture. Medical evidence has confirmed that many fractures and their complications are preventable. It is well within the realm of the primary care physician, and in fact should be a mandate of primary care, to clinically assess the risk of fracture, recommend bone mineral density testing where appropriate, and provide treatment when necessary.

Osteoporosis presents the latest information on diagnosis, prevention, and therapy in a concise form that practitioners can use to make judgments about the value of tests and treatments. In addition, an entire section of clinical cases guides the physician in the management of common presentations that arise in practice.

Though much has been learned about osteoporosis, our knowledge of its management remains incomplete. Physicians must often make decisions based on experience and an understanding of the biology and epidemiology of the disease. Additionally, as with other chronic diseases, one must make long-term treatment decisions based on short-term data. We, the editors of this book, a general internist/epidemiologist (Steve Cummings) and two endocrinologists (Felicia Cosman and Sophie Jamal), are practicing physicians who also conduct research in osteoporosis. We are fortunate to have authors who are internationally recognized experts on this disease. Most have extensive clinical experience that they bring to the translating of evidence into practice and who are therefore able to fill the gaps in evidence with seasoned judgment. We are grateful for the effort and intelligence that all the authors have contributed to *Osteoporosis*.

We thank the American College of Physicians-American Society of Internal Medicine for the invitation to edit this book. We are also indebted to Ms. Peggy McDavid, who helped with its organization and production. Finally, we thank our families for their support and patience.

Steven R. Cummings, MD
Felicia Cosman, MD
Sophie A. Jamal, MD

Contents

INTRODUCTION

1. **Bone Biology, Epidemiology, and General Principles** 3
   STEVEN R. CUMMINGS

LABORATORY AND CLINICAL ASSESSMENT OF OSTEOPOROSIS AND FRACTURE RISK

2. **Bone Densitometry and Spine Films** 29
   DENNIS BLACK, MICHAEL NEVITT, AND STEVEN R. CUMMINGS

3. **Markers of Bone Turnover and the Laboratory Evaluation of Secondary Osteoporosis** 59
   JACKIE A. CLOWES AND RICHARD EASTELL

PREVENTION AND TREATMENT

4. **Nutrition** 85
   JERI NIEVES

5. **Physical Activity as a Strategy to Conserve and Improve Bone Mass** 109
   ROBERT MARCUS, SOPHIE A. JAMAL, AND FELICIA COSMAN

6. **Estrogens** 127
   GAIL A. GREENDALE AND JANE CAULEY

7. **Selective Estrogen-Receptor Modulators** 151
   FELICIA COSMAN

8. **Phytoestrogens and DHEA** 169
   SUNDEEP KHOSLA

9. **Bisphosphonates** 181
   MARC C. HOCHBERG

10. **Calcitonin** 197
    STUART L. SILVERMAN

11. **Anabolic Agents** 209
ROBERT LINDSAY

12. **Glucocorticoid-Induced Osteoporosis** 223
IAN R. REID AND FIONA WU

CLINICAL CASES

13. **Clinical Cases** 241
SOPHIE A. JAMAL

SELECTION OF MEDICATIONS AND GUIDELINES FOR FRACTURE PREVENTION

14. **Selection of Medications and Guidelines
for Fracture Prevention** 273
FELICIA COSMAN, SOPHIE A. JAMAL, AND STEVEN R. CUMMINGS

Index 283

Introduction

Chapter 1

Bone Biology, Epidemiology, and General Principles

STEVEN R. CUMMINGS, MD

In this chapter, selected facts and principles from bone biology and epidemiology that have become the foundation for prevention and management of osteoporosis are reviewed.

Bone Biology

Bones are made of protein that is impregnated with crystals of calcium hydroxyapatite (1). They continually undergo remodeling by the coordinated activity of bone cells.

Protein

Ten percent of bone is made of proteins that have several functions. Triple-helix ropes of type I collagen provide the resilient scaffolding that is hardened by the deposition of mineral crystals. Other proteins seed the formation of calcium hydroxyapatite crystals and bind the crystals to the protein foundation. Some proteins allow cells to attach to the surface of bone to initiate replacement of a section with new bone. Other proteins in the matrix of bone act as signals that coordinate the activity of bone cells.

Collagen

Ninety percent of bone protein is type I collagen, the same type of collagen that comprises skin, tendon, dentin, sclera, and the cornea. It is made of two alpha-1 chains that are encoded by the *collA1* gene and one alpha-2 chain that

3

is encoded by the *col1A2* gene. Mutations of these genes cause osteogenesis imperfecta, a rare disease that is characterized by multiple deforming fractures. Some studies have found that common natural variations (polymorphisms) of *col1A1* genes are associated with lower bone density and an increased risk of fractures (2).

All proteins, including collagen, are synthesized and secreted by osteoblasts. Collagen chains form fibrils, and, in turn, these fibrils line up in parallel and are held together by the formation of protein cross-links. (Resorption of collagen by osteoclasts releases cross-links that are measured in chemical assays as markers of the rate of bone resorption, as described in Chapter 3.)

Non-Collagen Proteins (Matrix Proteins)
The remaining 10% of bone protein is made of dozens of diverse types of proteins that have a variety of functions, such as seeding crystal formation, binding calcium crystals, and serving as sites for attachment of bone cells (1). The most abundant protein in the matrix is osteocalcin. Although it is known to bind calcium, its function remains uncertain. Osteocalcin is released into the circulation during both bone formation and bone resorption, and its concentration in serum is commonly measured as a general index of the rate of bone remodeling or "turnover" (see Chapter 3). The bone matrix also contains proteins that stimulate or inhibit the actions of bone cells. For example, bone matrix includes bone morphogenic proteins (BMP) that are potent stimulants of bone formation. It is believed that the release of these factors during bone resorption helps coordinate the activity of bone cells and the process of remodeling.

Mineral

Ninety percent of bone, by weight, is mineral, principally calcium hydroxyapatite, which is composed of calcium, phosphate, and hydroxyl groups (1). Calcium hydroxyapatite forms hexagonal crystals that bind to bone proteins; this accounts for much of the strength and hardness of bone. Pure calcium hydroxyapatite, found in rocks, forms large crystals that are highly resistant to chemical dissolution, but in bones the hydroxyapatite also contains impurities such as magnesium carbonate that cause the crystals in bone to be smaller and easier to dissolve (see below). The mineralization of bone proteins is largely controlled by osteoblasts that actively transport calcium, phosphate, and hydroxyl ions to and from extracellular fluid that surrounds newly formed bone tissue. Bone can also mineralize more slowly as calcium salts in extracellular fluid continue to precipitate. This "passive mineralization" leads bone to gradually become more mineralized with an increasing bone mineral density (BMD) as the bone becomes older (3,4).

Bone Structure

In general, bones have cortical shells surrounding a spongelike network of trabecular bone that is, in turn, surrounded by bone marrow (Fig. 1-1, *A* and *B*).
Osteoporotic bone is characterized by loss and thinning of trabecular bone and
thinning of the cortical shell (Fig. 1-2). Cortical bone is built from *osteons,*
microscopic layered cylinders of bone surrounding a vascular canal. Trabecular
bone is a spongelike latticework of plates and rods of bone coated by *lining cells.*

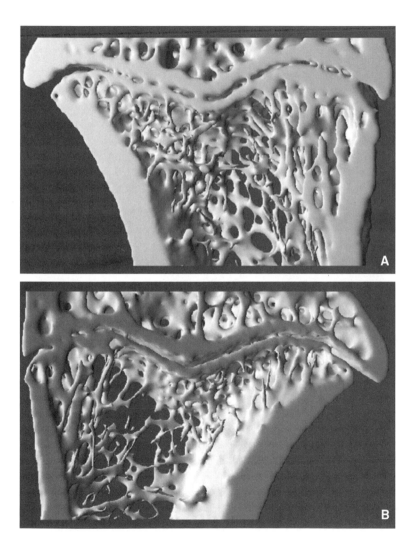

Figure 1-1   *A,* Normal cortical shell and internal trabecular structure. *B,* Thinning of cortical shell and thinning and loss of trabecular structure. (Courtesy of Mary Bouxsein, MD.)

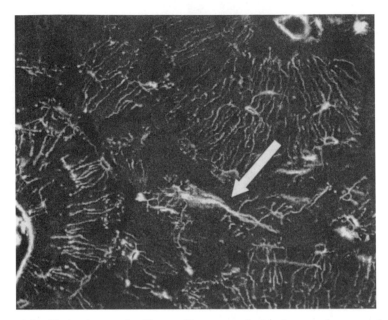

Figure 1-2 Photomicrograph of bone with an area of microdamage. Arrow points to a microscopic crack. (Courtesy of Mitch Schaffler, MD.)

The proportions of cortical and trabecular bone vary greatly, ranging from 70% to 90% in vertebral bodies and the heel, to less than 10% trabecular bone in the midshafts of long bones such as the radius, femoral shaft, and tibia (5,6). The neck of the femur is about 25% trabecular bone, whereas the intertrochanteric region is about 50% to 75% trabecular bone.

Trabecular bone has a much greater surface area and responds more quickly to hormonal changes, such as decline in estrogen concentrations at menopause, increases in parathyroid hormone, or administration of corticosteroids. Thus, bone mass at the lumbar spine, which contains largely trabecular bone, changes faster and to a greater degree than bone mass at sites such as the midradius that are composed mainly of cortical bone (7,8).

Bones provide support against the omnipresent forces of gravity, posture, and movement and protectively encase soft organs, such as the lung and brain, from minor trauma. Like all hard materials used to build bridges or buildings, bones accumulate tiny microscopic fractures, also called *microdamage* or *fatigue damage* (Fig. 1-2). As these tiny fractures accumulate, they can weaken bone (4). The metal shells of airplanes accumulate fatigue damage, mandating that airlines replace them periodically. Instead of replacing our skeletons every few years, vertebrates rely on three types of cells that detect damage, dissolve old damaged bone, and replace it with new bone, a process called *bone remodeling* (Fig. 1-3).

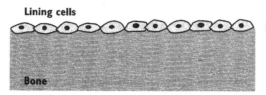

Lining cells

1. Resting Phase
The bone is covered by a protective layer or lining of cells.

Bone

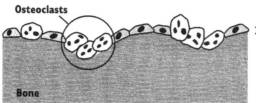

Osteoclasts

2. Resorption
The osteoclasts invade the bone surface, carve it up, and cut out a cavity by dissolving it.

Bone

Cavity made by osteoclasts

3. Resorption Complete
A complete cavity is created in the surface.

Bone

It's like potholes in pavement being formed and repatched.

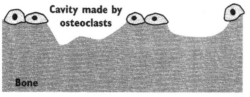

New bone (includes collagen and minerals)   Osteoblasts

4. Formation–Repair
Osteoblasts fill in cavity by building new bone.

Bone

The potholes (bone cavities excavated by the osteoclasts) are filled in with new bone (by the osteoblasts).

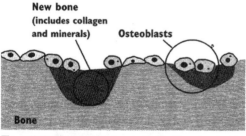

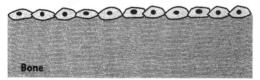

5. Repair Complete
New bone surface has replaced old bone.

Bone

It takes about three weeks for the osteoclasts to dig a pothole (pit in bone) and about three months for the osteoblasts to fill in the pothole with new bone.

Figure 1-3 Normal bone remodeling process. (From Cole RE. Osteoporosis: Unmasking a Silent Thief. Wellpower Publications; 2000; with permission.)

Bone Cells and the Process of Bone Remodeling

Bone remodeling involves three cell types: osteocytes, osteoclasts, and osteoblasts (9).

Osteocytes are spidery cells whose nuclei and main cell bodies live in lacunae inside the bone (Fig. 1-4) (10). Osteocytes communicate with each other and the surface of bone by way of microscopic channels that end in pores on the surface of the bone (canaliculi). Like neurons, osteocytes detect stresses in bone and transmit signals to other bone cells. For example, they detect microdamage and (in a way that has not yet been determined) signals to the surface of bones that (along with other signals) control the process of bone remodeling. Osteocytes originate from osteoblasts (bone-forming cells) that remain trapped in bone after it is formed and mineralized.

Osteoclasts, members of the monocyte-macrophate line of cells, are cells that act to dissolve and reabsorb bone (11). When activated, osteoclasts attach to the surface of bone as integrins on the cell membrane stick to matrix proteins that have been exposed on the surface of the bone. Osteoclasts, which generally fuse to form large multi-nucleated cells, form a skirt (the *ruffled border*) that sticks to matrix proteins on the surface of bone. This creates a

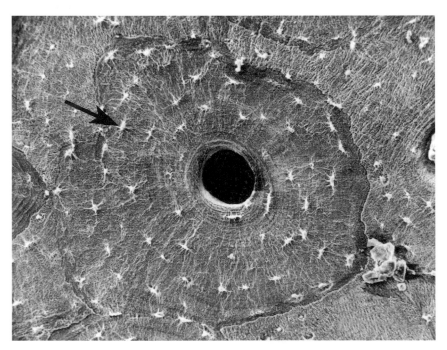

Figure 1-4   Osteon with osteocytes (*arrow*) and networks of canaliculi. (Courtesy of Gastone Marotti, MD.)

pocket under the osteoclast that the osteoclast fills with hydrochloric acid and proteolytic enzymes that dissolve the mineral and protein of the bone beneath it. Osteoclasts may eat away trabecular plates and rods (Fig. 1-5) and can resorb particularly aggressively when estrogen levels drop after oopherectomy or natural menopause or during immobilization. If the rod or plate is thin enough, these aggressive osteoclasts may perforate or disconnect the structure (Fig. 1-6) and irreversibly weaken that section of the bone. Osteoclasts also work in groups that tunnel into cortical bone (which can lead to a "scalloped" or ragged appearance along the endocortical surface when seen on a radiograph).

Osteoblasts, which come from the same precursor cell line as fibroblasts and adipocytes, form bone by producing and secreting collagen and other proteins of the bone matrix that assemble themselves (12). As soon as osteoblasts lay down the protein skeleton, calcium and hydroxyapatite begin to crystallize around the fibrils of collagen, and the bone begins to "mineralize." As osteoblasts synthesize bone proteins, they also make a form of alkaline phosphatase, and some of the proteins they produce, such as osteocalcin, are released into blood where they can be measured to provide an indication of

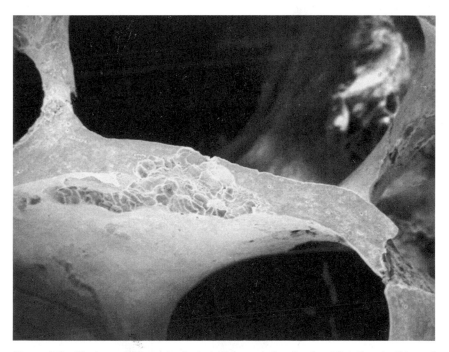

Figure 1-5 Electron micrograph of a trabecular rod showing focal "moth-eaten" loss of bone, with nearly complete loss of connection. This erosion results from osteoclastic bone resorption. (Courtesy of David Dempster, MD.)

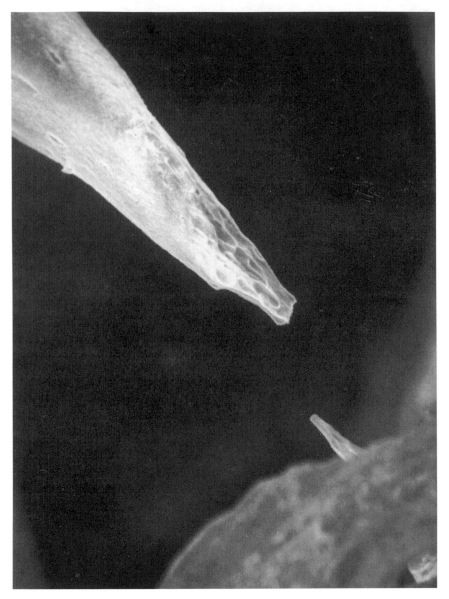

Figure 1-6   Electron micrograph of osteoporotic bone showing complete loss of connection of a trabecular rod caused by osteoclast-mediated bone resorption. (Courtesy of David Dempster, MD.)

the rate of bone formation (see Chapter 3). Osteoblasts contain receptors for hormones, such as estrogen, and are believed to generate the first signals that initiate bone remodeling.

In the normal process of bone remodeling, the activity of osteoclasts and osteoblasts are linked through chemical signals so that resorption of one microscopic section of bone is followed by formation of new bone in that spot (Fig. 1-3). One cycle of remodeling (from the start of osteoclast-mediated bone resorption to the time the osteoblasts finish replacing old bone with new bone proteins) takes from 3 to 8 months (6,13,14). Besides renewing the skeleton, remodeling is one of the carefully balanced systems that serve to maintain concentrations of calcium, phosphate, acid, and base in the circulation. For example, very small decreases in serum calcium stimulate the secretion of parathyroid hormone (PTH), which quickly stimulates bone resorption which in turn releases calcium into the circulation to restore normal calcium concentrations. Exercise, calcium, and vitamin D supplementation, and all of the drugs that reduce the risk of fractures, act by influencing bone remodeling in ways that are described in later chapters of this book.

How Bone Changes with Growth, Aging, and Menopause

Bone is formed as children grow. This process accelerates during puberty and slows and stops in parallel with linear growth (15). Bone continues to add mass and density after linear growth stops so that the total amount of bone reaches a "peak" when in the twenties or early thirties. This process is determined largely by genetic factors (the identities of which are not yet known) that also dictate that men will be larger and have larger bones than women and that blacks will have larger bones with more mass than do whites or Asians. The formation of bone is also influenced by hormonal and environmental factors. For example, delayed menarche or prolonged periods of low estrogen (as happens during anorexia nervosa or extreme exercise accompanied by amenorrhea) in teenage girls causes failure to achieve the full genetic potential of bone mass or bone loss. As noted in later chapters, increasing exercise and calcium intake also increases bone mass to some degree during the years that bones are forming (see Chapters 4 and 5).

The process of bone remodeling during adulthood results in a very slow loss of bone as early as the third and fourth decades of life (Fig. 1-7). Some longitudinal studies have found that bone density in women begins to decline a few years before the cessation of menses (16). It is not known whether bone mass can be increased to an important degree during normal adulthood.

On average, women lose bone even more rapidly around and for a few years after menopause. Studies using standard methods, such as dual x-ray absorptiometry, have determined that, on average, women lose 1% to 3% of their bone density per year for about 3 to 5 years after their last menstrual period; the rate is faster in the trabecular bone of the spine (17,18). Estrogen inhibits bone resorption, and the drop in estrogen during menopause leads to

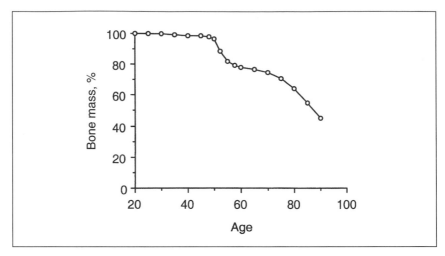

Figure 1-7   Percent of bone mass during a woman's adult life.

more aggressive bone resorption and faster bone loss during the perimenopausal years.

When several years have elapsed since menopause, the rate of bone loss in the hip slows down then begins to accelerate again after age 70, reaching 1% or 2% per year in women older than 80 years of age (Fig. 1-7) (19,20). The causes of the slowing after menopause and acceleration of bone loss in elderly women are not known. (The amount of mineral in the spine tends to increase a little after age 65 because of the development and progression of degenerative arthritis, as noted in Chapter 2.) These general patterns are probably similar for women of all races; however, the magnitude of change is likely to vary by racial group and different regions of the world, although no comparative studies have been reported for non-white women or women outside North America and Europe.

Men also gradually lose bone as they age, but having no acute menopause, there seems to be no accelerated period of bone loss (21). Exactly how much bone men lose during various decades has not yet been worked out by longitudinal studies.

Bones also grow wider with aging (22). While bone is resorbed from the interior, or endosteal, surface of bones, it is slowly added to the outer, or periosteal, surface of bones. Bones that have wider outer diameters are stronger (from common experience, for the same amount of material, wide pipes are stronger than narrow ones). However, the increase in diameter of bones only partially compensates for the decline in the total mass of bone, so that the strength of bone declines with age despite small, favorable changes in geometry.

Epidemiology of Fractures and Fracture Risk

Osteoporosis is a serious concern because it predisposes to fractures that cause pain, disability, and, occasionally, premature death. The epidemiology of fractures is complicated because each type of fracture has its own pattern that varies with age, gender, and regions of the world (23). To simplify this diversity, it helps to focus on the most common and severe types of fractures: vertebral fractures, hip fractures, wrist fractures, and "others." Vertebral fractures have several special characteristics, and, therefore, it is often useful to classify fractures as either vertebral or non-spine fractures. Following are some general principles about the epidemiology of osteoporotic fractures.

Almost All Fractures Are Related to Low Bone Mass
It used to be said that hip, spine, and wrist fractures were *osteoporotic*, implying that other fractures were not. However, prospective studies have since shown that almost all fractures are osteoporotic, inasmuch as the chance of suffering the fracture increases as bone density decreases (24). The only exceptions to this principle appear to be fractures of the skull, fingers, and toes. Fractures that occur as a result of trauma, such as motor vehicle accidents, are not usually considered osteoporotic. However, the limited evidence available indicates that the risk of *traumatic* fractures increases with reductions in bone mass (25).

Women Have a Greater Risk of Fractures Than Men
For most types of fractures and in most regions of the world, women have a greater risk of fracture than do men (Figs. 1-8 and 1-9) (23). In general, after age 50, white women have risks of hip and spine fracture that are about 2 to 3 times greater than those for men (26,27). This is probably due to the fact that women have smaller bones and tend to have lower bone density as they age. Because women, on average, live a few years longer than do men, the lifetime risk of hip and vertebral fractures in women is approximately 3 to 5 times greater than that of men. There are, however, important caveats. In populations such as China, in which the overall risk of fractures is low, men and women have similar rates of hip and non-spine fractures, and, in fact, men have slightly higher risks—for reasons that are not understood (28).

Risk for Most Types of Fractures Increases with Age
The incidence of both vertebral and non-spine fractures rises rapidly after about age 50 in women and men (Figs. 1-8 and 1-9) (23). The rise is most dramatic for fractures of the spine beginning at age 50 and of the hip after age 65. Thus, prevention of fractures will generally produce the greatest benefits over the short run for the oldest patients, whereas relatively young patients—

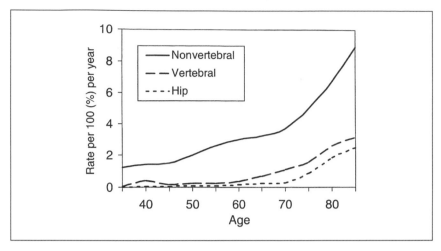

Figure 1-8 Incidence of nonvertebral fractures (including hip fractures), vertebral fractures, and hip fractures in white women. (From Melton LJ, 3rd, Crowson CS, O'Fallon WM. Fracture incidence in Olmsted County, Minnesota: comparison of urban with rural rates and changes in urban rates over time. Osteoporos Int. 1999;9:29–37; with permission.)

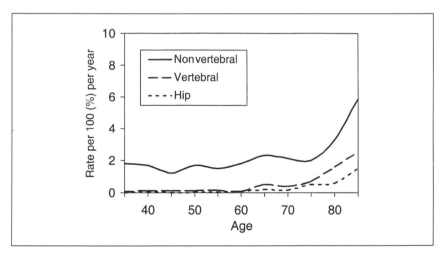

Figure 1-9 Incidence of nonvertebral fractures (including hip fractures), vertebral fractures, and hip fractures in white men. (From Melton LJ, 3rd, Crowson CS, O'Fallon WM. Fracture incidence in Olmsted County, Minnesota: comparison of urban with rural rates and changes in urban rates over time. Osteoporos Int. 1999;9:29–37; with permission.)

in their 50s—have very low risks of fracture during the next 5 years. Part of this increased risk with aging is due to the loss of bone and deterioration of the quality of bone with age, and the risk of falling also increases with age, and the quality of bone deteriorates with age. Consequently, two women who have exactly the same bone density, a woman at age 50 and a woman at age 80, have very different risks of most types of fractures. At the same level of BMD, an 80-year-old woman will have a several-fold greater risk of hip fracture than a 50-year-old woman.

The risk of a few types of fractures does not steadily increase with age. For example, the risk of wrist fractures rises rapidly after menopause in women but begins to plateau and even decline after age 65, presumably because very elderly women are less active in ways that would lead to falls that may cause wrist fractures. Furthermore, elderly women fall differently, in part due to declining reflexes and strength, leading to a lesser ability to quickly and strongly extend their arms during a fall (29).

Patients Who Have Had a Fracture Are More Likely to Have Future Fractures
Of course, women who have low bone mass are more likely to suffer one fracture, and the same low bone mass that made the first fracture more likely also predisposes them to other fractures. However, even beyond this fact, a history of a fracture indicates an increased risk of future fractures, regardless of bone mass (30). Consider two 60-year-old women with the same bone mass, one who suffered a fractured clavicle at age 55 and one who has no history of fractures. The woman with a history of fractures has about a 1.5- to 2-fold greater risk of hip and other types of fractures than does the woman without any history (30,31). Thus, a history of fractures is a flag that the patient is predisposed to fractures in ways we cannot yet measure, perhaps an increased risk of falling or weaker bone structure that cannot be measured by densitometry.

Vertebral Fractures Are Very Common, Often Cause Pain and Disability, and Are Usually Unrecognized
In North America, about half of white and Asian women and about one fifth of all white men will develop a vertebral fracture by the ninth decade (32). Rates of vertebral fracture are slightly lower among women living in China than among whites in the United States (33). The risk among Latino and African-American women appears to be substantially lower than among white women (34).

Most vertebral fractures found on radiographs are not clinically recognized (35). However, even those patients who have vertebral fractures without a diagnosis have back pain and difficulties with ordinary daily activities (36).

Vertebral Fractures, with or without Symptoms, Indicate a Very High Risk of Future Fractures
Women with vertebral fractures usually have bone density that qualifies them as "osteoporotic." In addition, vertebral fractures seem to indicate that the patient has more fragile bones so that women with vertebral fractures have about a 4-fold greater risk of suffering future vertebral fractures independent

of bone mass (37). This increased risk extends to other fractures so that women (and probably men) who have a vertebral fracture also have a 1.5- to 2-fold increased risk of other types of fractures, such as hip fractures (38).

From the Point of View of Public Health and Medical Costs, Hip Fracture Is the Most Important Type of Fracture

Five percent to 20% of people will die in the year after the hip fracture, although only a fraction of these deaths can be attributed to the hip fracture (39). Death rates are particularly high after hip fracture for men and black women. About a quarter of women who suffer hip fractures remain in nursing care facilities for at least a year after the fracture. Even among those who were living independently before the fracture, about half who return home require long-term help with normal activities of daily living. Hip fractures account for more than 75% of the costs, much of the disability, and most of the deaths due to osteoporosis (40). Thus, from society's point of view, the most cost-effective practices and policies are those that reduce the risk of hip fracture. However, many patients may fear vertebral fractures more than hip fractures because they dislike the prospect of shrinking and developing kyphosis and may know women who have chronic back pain and other quality-of-life changes as a result of vertebral fractures.

Most Bone Mass and Much of an Individual's Risk of Fractures Are Genetically Determined

There is a large variation in the maximum bone mass achieved early in life. Most of this variation is hereditary (41,42). It is likely that many genes are involved in the determination of bone mass, but just which genes remains to be established. Gender is one of the most important genetic factors controlling bone mass. On average, women have 5% to 10% lower bone mass than do men (43). A family history of fractures indicates an increased risk of fractures, but this seems to be mostly specific to the type of fracture. Specifically, a family history of hip fracture indicates an increased risk of hip fractures, and a family history of wrist fracture indicates an increased risk of wrist fracture (44). This effect is independent of bone mass of the hip; in other words, it appears that determinants of fracture risk, besides bone mass, must also be inherited. It is useful to ask about a woman's family history of fractures to help estimate her risk.

Several Common Risk Factors Are Related to Decreased Bone Mass

Besides the contribution of genetics and gender, the most important factors that account for lower bone mass are older age, lower body weight, and current use of estrogen therapy (45,46). Corticosteroid use causes rapid and substantial bone loss during the first several months of treatment, and bone mass remains suppressed as long as the treatment continues (see Chapter 12). Cigarette smokers tend to have lower bone density, in part because they weigh less than non-smokers (47). Other factors that have sometimes been associated with lower bone density include very late menarche and very early menopause and prolonged periods of premenopausal amennorhea due to extreme physical activity or anorexia nervosa. Hyperparathyroidism has been associated with lower bone density that may improve after parathyroidectomy (48–50). Studies have differed about whether mild to moderate hyperthyroidism causes bone loss (51,52). Many chronic diseases, such as rheumatoid arthritis, inflammatory bowel disease, chronic lung disease, and disorders associated with malabsorption (such as celiac sprue) are also associated with reduced BMD (see Chapter 2). These factors might be considered "etiologic" risk factors for osteoporosis because they cause a reduction in bone mass.

Some Beliefs About Risk Factors for Osteoporosis Are Probably Not True

Many doctors and patients believe that alcohol intake is bad for bones. In fact, most studies have found that modest intake—1 to 3 drinks per day—is associated with a higher bone density and a lower risk of fractures in women (see Chapter 4) (53). Alcoholism, however, has been associated with an increased risk of osteoporosis.

At one time it was believed that pregnancy and breast-feeding increased the risk of osteoporosis. Indeed, there is a transient decrease in bone density during pregnancy and breast-feeding that returns to normal after birth and weaning (54). Very few women suffer fractures during this temporary decrease in bone mass. Large studies have consistently shown that women who have had more children and breast-fed more babies have no increased risk, perhaps even a slightly lower risk of fractures than other women (55). Additionally, the widespread belief that white women who are fair (blonde or light skinned) have an increased fracture risk has not been born out by large studies; within the white race, hair color does not seem to be related to risk of fracture (30).

Several Common Risk Factors Increase the Risk of Fractures in Ways Besides Decreasing Bone Mass

Most types of fractures are more common in women and whites and increase with age and lower bone mass (Figs. 1-8 and 1-9). As noted previously, past history of fractures, especially a vertebral fracture, indicates an increased risk of fractures that is independent of age and bone density. These factors are also the strongest and most consistent risk factors for vertebral fracture. However, each type of fracture has its own unique risk factors. Because of the importance of hip fractures, it is important to recognize the major risk factors for hip fractures besides gender, age, history of fractures, and low bone density. In particular, women who are at increased risk of falling, associated with impaired vision, use of sedative hypnotics, and overall poor health, have an increased risk of hip fractures. In addition, residence in a nursing home, a parental history of hip fracture, low body weight or recent weight loss, and cigarette smoking have been found by most studies to be strong risk factors for hip fracture. In contrast, women who are active and healthy appear to be at increased risk of wrist (Colles') fracture as a result of falling during recreational or daily activities (56). As with many other types of fractures, low bone mass and impaired vision also appear to increase the risk of wrist fractures (47). Use of corticosteroids is an especially strong risk factor for fractures of the spine and ribs, sites that have a high proportion of trabecular bone (see Chapter 12). Although diabetes, especially type 2 diabetes, has not been consistently found to be a risk factor for low bone density, recent studies indicate that diabetes is a very strong risk factor for fractures of the feet, humerus, and hip, but not wrist or vertebrae (57). Therefore, it may be worthwhile to test for diabetes in patients who present with these types of fractures. (The contribution of other diseases and the potential value of searching for other occult conditions in patients with osteoporosis are covered in Chapter 3.)

Fractures Have Serious Health Consequences

Fractures, such as finger fracture, can be a temporary annoyance and an impediment to some activities or devastating with long-lasting impairments of independence and quality of life, as is common with hip fractures. As noted earlier, hip fractures often lead to nursing home placement and loss of independence and death. Many vertebral fractures, even those that are not diagnosed, produce acute severe pain and disability that persists for weeks to months (36). The long-term effects of vertebral fractures have been underestimated: many ultimately result in back pain and limitation of activities. Vertebral fractures cause a loss of height (about 1 cm for each fracture that occurs) and may contribute to the development of kyphosis. The accumulation of multiple vertebral fractures can deform the thorax and seriously restrict pulmonary function. Women who have vertebral fractures also have a greater overall mortality rate than other women do, probably because vertebral fractures may be a sign of poor health or other conditions that carry an increased mortality (58).

General Principles of Prevention and Treatment

"Prevention" and "Treatment" Are Regulatory Terms/The Unified Goal of Patient Care Is to Prevent Fractures

In North America and Europe, regulatory agencies approve drugs for prevention and treatment of osteoporosis, reflecting two different sets of criteria for deciding whether a drug should be approved for marketing. In FDA parlance, a drug is approved for *prevention* of osteoporosis if trials have shown that the drug slows the rate of loss of BMD in women who do not have osteoporosis. (Other conditions must also be met. For example, approval is granted for prevention only if a randomized trial also shows at least a favorable trend toward reducing the risk of vertebral fractures.) The FDA approves a drug for *treatment* of osteoporosis if at least one trial has shown that the drug reduces the risk of vertebral deformities assessed on spine radiographs. Although this distinction is important to the approval and marketing of drugs, it is less useful and sometimes confusing in clinical practice, because the main goal of all treatment is prevention of fractures.

Exercise, Calcium, Vitamin D, and Modification of Risk Factors Form the Foundation of Fracture Prevention

Regular exercise should be promoted to all adults because it has many benefits besides sustaining bone mass and reducing the risk of fractures (see Chapter 5). Discussions about osteoporosis present another opportunity to recommend and reinforce lifelong habits of regular exercise. There is a consensus that adequate intake of calcium is beneficial to maintaining bone mass, and there is evidence that the combination of calcium and vitamin D reduces the risk of fractures in elderly women and men and in those with osteoporosis (see Chapter 4). These first steps can be recommended to all patients, regardless of their risk of fractures.

As noted earlier, factors that increase the risk of fractures can be eliminated or modified. Specifically, it has been estimated that quitting smoking, successfully treating impaired visual acuity (by providing correct eye wear or treating cataracts), or stopping the use of sedative hypnotics may each decrease the risk of hip fractures by 30% to 40% (59).

Limit Drug Treatment to Those Who Are Most Likely to Benefit from a Reduced Risk of Fractures

Detailed guidelines about selecting patients for various approved drug treatments for fracture prevention are provided in Chapter 14. Here is the main principle: patients with the highest risk of fractures are the ones who are most likely to benefit from drug treatments. It is important to focus on "absolute" risk of fractures in patients more than on relative risk. For example, it is more useful to know that a patient has a 20% risk of suffering a vertebral fracture in the next 5 years than to know that, because of a risk factor, a patient has a 2.0 relative risk of fracture. We believe that risk of hip, vertebral, and non-spine fractures during the next 5 to 10 years are, perhaps, the most useful ways to understand and educate patients about their risk of fracture and potential benefits of treatment. Tables estimating 5-year risks of fracture based on age and BMD are found in Chapter 2.

In general, patients with vertebral fractures and bone density values defined as osteoporosis—two of the strongest risk factors for fracture—will have greater benefits than other patients. Furthermore, trials have found that approved drugs reduce the risk of fractures in these patients. Therefore, the U.S. National Osteoporosis Foundation Guidelines recommend drug treatment for all patients who have vertebral or hip fractures or osteoporosis on measurement of hip or spine BMD (see Chapter 14). Because the risk of most fractures, especially hip fractures, rises with aging, older patients will generally obtain more immediate benefits from treatment than will younger patients.

Look Selectively for "Secondary" Osteoporosis

Most osteoporosis is caused by natural variations in genetic and hormonal factors and aging. This is often referred to as *primary osteoporosis*. *Secondary osteoporosis* refers to low bone density or vertebral fractures that occur at least partly as a result of disease, such as hyperthyroidism, or drug treatment, such as use of corticosteroids (see Chapter 3). There has been very little systematic study of the prevalence of secondary causes of osteoporosis or the value of testing for these conditions, and there is no evidence that it is valuable to screen all women who have low bone density for uncommon diseases; evaluations should be done selectively. In general, it is believed that men with osteoporosis are more likely to have it because of coexisting diseases or drugs, and that the chance of finding secondary causes increases as the severity of osteoporosis increases. An approach to evaluating patients for secondary osteoporosis is described in Chapter 3.

Monitoring the Effectiveness of Treatment

The goal of all clinical care of osteoporosis is to reduce the risk of fractures and their consequences. In a sense, successful treatment to reduce the risk of fractures means that nothing happens. Patients and doctors often look to changes in bone density and levels of markers of bone turnover for reassurance that treatment is working. However, indices are imperfect, and a drug may be reducing the risk of fractures even if the bone density has not improved or seems to be declining; this is reviewed in Chapter 3 and particularly in discussion of Case 6 in Chapter 13. These surrogate measurements of response to therapy are reviewed in Chapters 2 and 3.

Current approved drug treatments are antiresorptive agents, such as bisphosphonates, estrogens, selective estrogen receptor modulators, and calcitonin, which mainly slow the rate of bone loss and may transiently increase bone density during the first few years of use while areas of bone resorption are filled by new bone. The goal is to keep a patient's risk of fractures as low as possible with existing therapy by continuing treatments, probably indefinitely. This strategy may change as agents become available that substantially increase bone mass and restore the microscopic architecture of bone. PTH is the first such agent for the treatment of osteoporosis (see Chapter 11).

Application of Practices and Guidelines Across Various Countries, Regions, and Ethnic Groups

Physicians in North America generally have greater availability of effective drugs, bone density testing, and laboratory tests for bone turnover and secondary causes of osteoporosis than do physicians in other regions of the world, especially developing nations of Asia, the Middle East, and Latin America.

In general, when resources are very limited, it is rational to first use tests and treatments on those who have the greatest absolute risk of fractures. For instance, where densitometry is in very short supply, it may be wise to limit its use to situations in which the result of the test is more likely to have a major impact on treatment decisions and, therefore, to patients who are likely, but not certain, to have bone density values that are low enough to mandate treatment. Additionally, it may be reasonable to limit the use of densitometry to patients who are over age 65 who have had a non-spine fracture or other risk factors for osteoporosis. Densitometry may be unavailable to millions of women, and, in these circumstances, decisions to treat to prevent future fractures may need to be based on the patient's history of fractures and very strong risk factors for fracture, such as very low body weight or chronic use of oral corticosteroids.

When treatments are difficult for patients to obtain or afford, it is important to stress the value of less expensive but effective approaches, such as eliminating risk factors, increasing calcium intake, and regular exercise for sedentary patients. Drug therapies may necessarily be limited to treatment of patients at very high risk, such as those with vertebral or hip fractures.

Additionally, the risk of fractures varies from region to region. Hip fractures are most common in northern Europe, North America, and Hong Kong (23). Women in Latin America or China have risks of hip fractures that are less than one third of the rates observed among white women in the United States. Rates of fractures in southern Europe are substantially lower than those in northern Europe (60). This lower risk means that treatments will, on average, produce lesser benefit for patients in low-risk regions. This may be due to higher levels of bone density among women in low-risk regions, but this has not been established. However, women in China have a much lower risk of hip fractures than women in the United States do, despite having similar average levels of bone density (28,61). Thus, to achieve the same reductions in the risk of hip fractures, the treatment threshold for women in these low-risk regions should be a lower BMD value than that used for women in North America.

Expert groups in Europe and North America have developed somewhat different guidelines for the prevention and treatment of osteoporosis (62). In general, European guidelines tend to be more conservative in the use of testing and drug treatments than U.S. approaches. These differences at least partly represent different philosophies about the use of tests and drugs for prevention of fractures and policies on reimbursement for treatments and tests.

Thus, it is not feasible or rational for countries to adopt practice patterns and guidelines that are developed in the United States: at the very least, they need to be modified to fit the local economy and epidemiology of fractures and philosophies about the use of tests and drug treatments. Resources are also severely limited in some practice settings and for some patients within North America, necessitating a more conservative approach to testing and treatment.

Summary

A small but persistent excess of bone resorption over bone formation leads to a general decrease in bone mass with age. This, combined with an age-related decline in neuromuscular function, leads to an increased risk of most types of fractures. Lifelong regular exercise, adequate calcium intake, and modification of risk factors are the first steps of treatment to prevent fractures. The benefits of drug treatments to reduce the risk of fractures will generally be greater in those who have the greatest risk of fractures. Specifically, patients who have vertebral fractures or osteoporosis according to measurements of bone density of the hip or spine have a high risk of future fractures and are those most likely to benefit from pharmacologic treatments. Approaches to testing and treatment necessarily and rationally differ among regions of the world and practice settings in the United States because of differences in the availability and affordability of these resources and differences in risks of fractures.

REFERENCES

1. **Robbey PG, Boskey AL.** The biochemistry of bone. In: Marcus R (ed). Osteoporosis. San Diego: Academic Press; 1996:95–160.
2. **Uitterlinden AG, Burger H, Huang Q, et al.** Relation of alleles of the collagen type I alpha 1-gene to bone density and the risk of osteoporotic fractures in postmenopausal women. N Engl J Med. 1998;338:1016–1021.
3. **Meunier PJ, Boivin G.** Bone mineral density reflects bone mass but also the degree of mineralization of bone: therapeutic implications. Bone. 1997;21:373–377.

4. **Parfitt AM.** Bone age, mineral density, and fatigue damage. Calcif Tissue Int. 1993;53 (Suppl 1):S82–S85.

5. **Eastell R, Moskilde LI, Hodgson SF, Riggs BL.** Proportion of human vertebral body bone that is cancellous. J Bone Miner Res. 1990;5:1237–1241.

6. **Einhorn TA.** The bone organ system. In: Marcus R (ed). Osteoporosis. San Diego: Academic Press; 1996:3–22.

7. **Laan RF, van Riel PL, van de Putte LB, et al.** Low-dose prednisone induces rapid reversible axial bone loss in patients with rheumatoid arthritis. Ann Intern Med. 1993;119:963–968.

8. **Prior JC, Vigna YM, Wark JD, et al.** Premenopausal ovariectomy-related bone loss: a randomized, double-blind, one-year trial of conjugated estrogen or medroxyprogesterone acetate. J Bone Miner Res. 1997;12:1851–1863.

9. **Rodan GA, Rodan SB.** The cells of bone. In: Riggs BL, Melton LJ (eds). Osteoporosis Etiology, Diagnosis and Management. Philadelphia: Lippincott-Raven; 1995:1–39.

10. **Noble BS, Reeve J.** Osteocyte function, osteocyte death and bone fracture resistance. Mol Cell Endocrinol. 2000;159:7–13.

11. **Teitelbaum SL, Tondravi M, Ross FP.** Osteoclast biology. In: Marcus R (ed). Osteoporosis. San Diego: Academic Press; 1996:61–94.

12. **Ducy P, Schinke T, Karsenty G.** The osteoblast: a sophisticated fibroblast under central surveillance. Science. 2000;289:1501–1504.

13. **Parfitt AM.** The cellular basis of bone remodeling: the quantum concept reexamined in light of recent advances in the cell biology of bone. Calcif Tissue Int. 1984;36:S37–S45.

14. **Dempster D.** Bone remodeling. In: Riggs BL, Melton LJ (eds). Osteoporosis Etiology, Diagnosis and Management, 2nd ed. Philadelphia: Lippincott-Raven; 1995:67–92.

15. **Heaney RP, Matkovic V.** Inadequate peak bone mass. In: Riggs BL, Melton LJ (eds). Osteoporosis Etiology, Diagnosis and Management. Philadelphia: Lippincott-Raven; 1995;115–132.

16. **Riggs BL, Wahner HW, Melton LJ, et al.** Rates of bone loss in the appendicular and axial skeletons of women: evidence of substantial vertebral bone loss before menopause. J Clin Invest. 1986;77:1487–1491.

17. **Nilas L, Christiansen CC.** Rates of bone loss in normal women: evidence of accelerated trabecular bone loss after the menopause. Eur J Clin Invest. 1988;18:529–534.

18. **Recker RR, Lappe J, Davies K, Heaney R.** Characterization of perimenopausal bone loss: a prospective study. J Bone Miner Res. 2000;15:1965–1973.

19. **Greenspan SL, Maitland LA, Myers ER, et al.** Femoral bone loss progresses with age: a longitudinal study in women over age 65. J Bone Miner Res. 1994;9:1959–1965.

20. **Ensrud KE, Palermo L, Black DM, et al.** Hip and calcaneal bone loss increase with advancing age: longitudinal results from the Study of Osteoporotic Fractures. J Bone Min Res. 1995;10:1778–1787.

21. **Orwoll ES, Oviatt SK, McClung MR, et al.** The rate of bone mineral loss in normal men and the effects of calcium and cholecalciferol supplementation. Ann Intern Med. 1990;112:29–34.

22. **Bouxsein ML, Myers ER, Hayes WC.** Biomechanics of age-related fractures. In: Marcus R (ed). Osteoporosis. San Diego: Academic Press; 1996:373–393.

23. **Melton LJ.** Epidemiology of fractures. In: Riggs BL, Melton LJ (eds). Osteoporosis Etiology, Diagnosis and Management, 2nd ed. Philadelphia: Lippincott-Raven; 1995;225–248.

24. **Seeley DG, Browner WS, Nevitt MC, et al.** Which fractures are associated with low appendicular bone mass in elderly women? Ann Intern Med. 1991;115:837–842.

25. **Sanders KM, Pasco JA, Ugoni AM, et al.** The exclusion of high trauma fractures may underestimate the prevalence of bone fragility fractures in the community: the Geelong Osteoporosis Study. J Bone Miner Res. 1998;13:1337–1342.

26. **Orwoll ES (ed).** Osteoporosis in Men. San Diego: Academic Press; 1999.

27. **Lunt M, Felsenberg D, Reeve J, et al.** Bone density variation and its effects on risk of vertebral deformity in men and women studied in thirteen European centers. The EVOS Study. J Bone Miner Res. 1997;12:1883–1894.

28. **Xu L, Lu A, Zhao X, et al.** Very low rates of hip fractures in Beijing, China: The Beijing Osteoporosis Project. Am J Epidemiol. 1996;144:901–907.

29. **Nevitt MC, Cummings SR.** Type of fall and risk of hip and wrist fractures. The Study of Osteoporotic Fractures. J Am Geriatr Soc. 1993;41:909.

30. **Cummings SR, Nevitt MC, Browner WS, et al.** Risk factors for hip fracture in white women. N Engl J Med. 1995;332:767–773.

31. **Melton LJ, Wahner HW, Riggs BL.** Bone density measurement. J Bone Miner Res. 1988;3:ix–x.

32. **Melton LJ, Kan SH, Frye MA, et al.** Epidemiology of vertebral fractures in women. Am J Epidemiol. 1989;129:1000–1011.

33. **Xu L, Cummings SR, Mingwei Q, et al.** Vertebral fractures in Beijing, China. The Beijing Osteoporosis Project. J Bone Min Res. 2000;15:2019–2025.

34. **Villa ML, Nelson L.** Race, ethnicity and osteoporosis. In: Marcus R (ed). Osteoporosis. San Diego: Academic Press; 1996:435.

35. **Cooper C, Atkinson EJ, O'Fallon WM, Melton LJ.** Incidence of clinically diagnosed verterbral fractures: a population-based study in Rochester, Minnesota, 1985–1989. J Bone Miner Res. 1992;7:221–227.

36. **Nevitt M, Ettinger B, Black D, et al.** The association of radiographically detected vertebral fractures with back pain and function: a prospective study. Ann Intern Med. 1998;128:793–800.

37. **Ross PD, Davis JW, Epstein RS, Wasnich RD.** Pre-existing fractures and bone mass predict vertebral fracture incidence in women. Ann Intern Med. 1991;114:919–923.

38. **Black DM, Arden NK, Palermo L, et al.** Prevalent vertebral deformities predict hip fractures and new deformities but not wrist fractures. Study of Osteoporotic Fractures Research Group. JBMR. 1999;14:821–828.

39. **Browner WS, Pressman A, Nevitt MC, Cummings SR.** Mortality following fractures in older women. The Study of Osteoporotic Fractures. Arch Intern Med. 1996;156:521–525.

40. **Ray NF, Chan JK, Thamer M, Melton LJ, III.** Medical expenditures for the treatment of osteoporotic fractures in the United States in 1995. Report from the National Osteoporosis Foundation. J Bone Miner Res. 1997;12:24–35.

41. **Howard GM, Nguyen TV, Harris M, et al.** Genetic and environmental contributions to the association between quantitative ultrasound and bone mineral density measurements: a twin study. J Bone Miner Res. 1998;13:1318–1327.

42. **Slemenda CW, Christian JC, Williams CJ, et al.** Genetic determinants of bone mass in adult women: a reevaluation of the twin model and the potential importance of gene interaction on heritability estimates. J Bone Miner Res. 1991;6:561–567.

43. **Looker AC, Orwoll ES, Johnston CC, et al.** Prevalence of low femoral bone density in older U.S. adults from NHANES III. J Bone Miner Res. 1997;12:1761–1768.

44. **Fox KM, Cummings SR, Powell-Threets K, Stone K.** Family history and risk of osteoporotic fracture. The Study of Osteoporotic Fractures Research Group. Osteop Int. 1998;8:557–562.

45. **Bauer DC, Browner WS, Cauley JA, et al.** Factors associated with appendicular bone mass in older women. Ann Intern Med. 1993;118:657–665.

46. **Orwoll ES, Bauer DC, Vogt TM, Fox KM.** Axial bone mass in older women. Study of Osteoporotic Fractures Research Group. Ann Intern Med. 1996;124:187–196.

47. **Krall EA, Dawson-Hughes B.** Smoking and bone loss among postmenopausal women. J Bone Miner Res. 1991;6:331–338.

48. **Khan A, Bilezikian J.** Primary hyperparathyroidism: pathophysiology and impact on bone. CMAJ. 2000;163:184–187.

49. **Christiansen P, Steiniche T, Brixen K, et al.** Primary hyperparathyroidism: effect of parathyroidectomy on regional bone mineral density in Danish patients: a three-year follow-up study. Bone. 1999;25:589–595.

50. **Silverberg SJ, Jacobs TP, Siris E, et al.** A 10-year prospective study of primary hyperparathyroidism with or without parathyroid surgery. N Engl J Med. 1999;341:1249–1255.

51. **Bauer DC, Nevitt MC, Ettinger B, Stone K.** Low thyrotropin levels are not associated with bone loss in older women: a prospective study. J Clin Endocrinol Metab. 1997;82:2931–2936.

52. **Franklyn JA, Betteridge J, Daykin J, et al.** Long-term thyroxine treatment and bone mineral density. Lancet. 1992;340:9–13.

53. **Ganry O, Baudoin C, Fardellone P.** Effect of alcohol intake on bone mineral density in elderly women: The EPIDOS Study. Am J Epidemiol. 2000;151:773–780.

54. **Sowers M, Crutchfield M, Jannausch M, et al.** A prospective evaluation of bone mineral change in pregnancy. Obstet Gynecol. 1991;77:841–845.

55. **Fox KM, Sherwin R, Scott JC, et al.** Reproductive correlates of bone mass in elderly women. Study of Osteoporotic Fractures Research Group. J Bone Miner Res. 1993;8:901–908.

56. **Kelsey JL, Browner WS, Seeley DG, et al.** Risk factors for fractures of the distal forearm and proximal humerus. Am J Epidemiol. 1992;135:477–489.

57. **Schwartz AV, Sellmeyer DE, Ensrud KE, et al.** Older women with diabetes have an increased risk of fracture: a prospective study. J Clin Endocrinol Metab. 2001;86:32–38.

58. **Kado DM, Browner WS, Palermo L, et al.** Vertebral fractures and mortality in older women: a prospective study. Arch Intern Med. 1999;159:1215–1220.

59. **Cummings SR.** Treatable and untreatable risk factors for hip fracture. Bone. 1996;18(Suppl 3):165S–167S.

60. **Lyritis GP.** Epidemiology of hip fracture. The MEDOS Study. Mediterranean Osteoporosis Study. Osteoporos Int. 1996;6 (Suppl 3):11–15.

61. **Lau EMC, Lee JK, Suriwongpaisal P, et al.** The incidence of hip fracture in four Asian countries. The Asian Osteoporosis Study (AOS). Osteoporos Int. 2001;12:239–243.

62. **Kanis JA, Delmas P, Burckhardt P, et al.** Guidelines for diagnosis and management of osteoporosis. Osteoporos Int. 1997;7:390–406.

Laboratory and Clinical Assessment of Osteoporosis and Fracture Risk

CHAPTER 2

Bone Densitometry
and Spine Films

DENNIS BLACK, PHD
MICHAEL NEVITT, PHD, MPH
STEVEN R. CUMMINGS, MD

Osteoporosis is defined as low bone mass and fragility of bone (1). Measurement of bone mass with bone densitometry has become a common and useful test for estimating a patient's risk of fractures, diagnosing osteoporosis, and making decisions about treatment. In this chapter, common methods of measuring bone mass and the clinical uses of bone mass measurements are reviewed.

The occurrence of a vertebral fracture is generally a sign of skeletal fragility, indicating that the patient has a high risk of fractures regardless of her bone mass. Presence of vertebral fractures alone in postmenopausal women or in older men is usually sufficient to establish a diagnosis of osteoporosis and to warrant treatment. Vertebral fractures must be diagnosed using spine radiographs. In this chapter, the use of spine radiographs for the diagnosis of vertebral fractures is reviewed.

Bone Densitometry

Bone is a three-dimensional structure made of proteins and calcium hydroxyapatite. X-ray or radiation-based methods, such as dual and single x-ray absorptiometry, measure the amount of the calcium mineral. Characteristics of bone can also be assessed using ultrasound. The amount or density of mineral in bone and the ultrasonic properties account for as much as 70% to 90% of the strength of bones tested under laboratory conditions (2–4).

Terminology

Bone Mass, Bone Density, and Bone Mineral Density

Many terms are used to describe the amount and density of a bone; these are summarized in Table 2-1. *Bone mass* refers to the amount of bone in the skeleton or in one location. No technology, however, produces a measurement called "bone mass." *Bone mineral content* (BMC) is the amount of mineral in a section of the skeleton. *Bone density* and *bone mineral density* (BMD) refer to mineral content per unit of area or volume. Quantitative computed tomography (QCT) scans measure the average concentration of mineral in a defined volume, and the result is often called *volumetric bone density*. Most techniques, such as dual x-ray absorptiometry, assess the amount of mineral (or BMC) in a two-dimensional projection and divide the result by the area. This is sometimes called *areal density*. In clinical practice (and in this book), the result is simply referred to as the patient's bone density or BMD.

Areal density can sometimes be misleading because it is influenced by the size of the bone. This is illustrated in Figure 2-1. If two bones of different size have exactly the same density, the larger bone will have a greater BMD than the small one. In clinical practice, this means that standard methods, such as dual energy x-ray absorptiometry (DXA), will tend to somewhat underestimate the true bone density of very small patients and overestimate the true bone density of large patients. Nevertheless, BMD has proven to be a clinically useful term in patients of all sizes.

T Scores and Z Scores

Different bones contain different amounts of mineral so that the normal amount of bone mass (gram or milligram) and bone density (g or mg/unit area or volume) differ from site to site. Two terms, *T score* and *Z score*, are commonly used to report bone densitometry results. Both of these rely on a standard deviation (SD) for the measurement. SD represents the normal variability in a measurement in a population: the distance between the 5th and 95th percentile of a group covers about 4 SDs. For hip and spine BMD, 1 SD corresponds to about 10% to 15% of the mean value.

A Z score is the number of SDs below (minus) or above (plus) the mean BMD value for people of the same age. A Z score of 0 means that the patient has a value that is exactly at the mean for his or her age. A Z score of –2.0 means that the patient has a BMD at that site, by that method, that is 2 SDs below the mean value of others who are the same age.

In contrast, a T score is the number of SDs below the mean value of BMD for young (20- to 30-year-old) adults. A T score of 0 means that the patient has a BMD value that is exactly at the mean for young adults. A T score of –2.5

Table 2-1   Common Terms Used in Bone Densitometry

Bone mass
A nonspecific term that refers to the amount of bone tissue. This may refer to the total amount of protein and mineral, or to the amount of mineral in the whole skeleton or in a particular segment of bone.

Bone mineral content
The amount of mineral measured in a defined section of bone. *Total body bone mineral content* refers to the mineral content of the whole skeleton.

Bone density or bone mineral density
The average concentration of mineral in a two- or three-dimensional image or average concentration in a defined section of bone. This term is also used to refer to the results of all types of bone densitometry.

Areal bone density
The bone mineral content divided by the area of the image of a bone projected in two dimensions. This is the type of "bone density" that is produced by dual and single energy x-ray absorptiometry.

Volumetric bone density
The bone mineral content of a section of bone divided by the volume of that section. This type of bone density is produced by quantitative computed tomographic (QCT) scans.

Trabecular bone density
The mineral density of a section of bone that contains only or largely trabecular bone.

Microfracture or microdamage
Cracks in bone that remain localized to a very small place in a bone. These are not detected by standard radiographs but by special microscopic techniques in bone samples.

T score
The difference between the value for an individual and the mean value of a group of young (usually 20–30 year old) adults of the same gender. Both the mean value and the size of a standard deviation of the measurement vary between techniques and between sites of measurement.

Z score
The difference between the mean value of the individual and a group of people of the same gender and same age.

Osteoporosis
Defined by a Working Group of the World Health Organization as a T score of at least –2.5 (also called *densitometric osteoporosis* to distinguish this from a diagnosis of osteoporosis made on the basis of the presence of a vertebral fracture on x-ray).

Osteopenia
A term coined by the World Health Organization to refer to T scores between –1.0 and –2.5.

Bone ultrasound attenuation
A slope of the line connecting the amount of attenuation of sound energy across a spectrum of sound frequencies.

Speed of sound
The fastest rate of transmission of a specific frequency of sound through a defined section of bone.

Coefficient of variation
A measurement of reproducibility defined as the standard deviation of repeated measurements divided by the mean value for the measurement in the group tested, expressed as a percent.

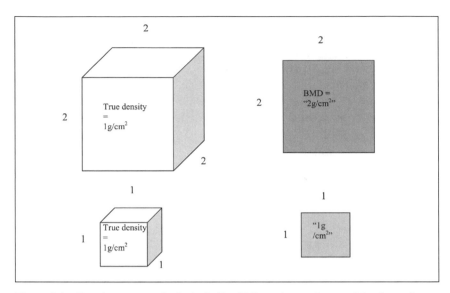

Figure 2-1 Densitometry methods, including DXA, project an image of the three-dimensional bone onto a two-dimensional plane. Assume that two bones have exactly the same true density: 1 g/cm³. A bone measuring 1 cm on a side will contain 1 g of mineral projected onto a 1 cm² square, so its real bone mineral density (BMD) would be 1 g/cm² (*left*). The larger bone, measuring 2 cm × 2 cm × 2 cm, will contain 8 g of mineral projected on a 2 cm × 2 cm square with an area = 4 cm². Thus, the larger bone will artifactually appear to have a much greater density: 2 g/cm² (*right*).

means that the patient has a BMD value at that site, by that method, that is 2.5 SDs below the average value found in healthy 20- to 30-year-old adults.

For young adults, Z and T scores will be similar. Because BMD declines with age at all sites, after about age 30, T scores are lower than Z scores, and the difference increases with age. For example, at age 50, a woman who has a normal femoral neck BMD for her age will have a Z score of 0 and a T score of –0.7 (using Hologic systems). At age 80, a woman with a normal femoral neck BMD (Z score = 0) will have a T score of –2.3. This reflects the fact that normal elders have lower bone density than normal young adults do.

Every measurement and manufacturer has its own unique normal values. In addition, the amount and density of bone varies from bone to bone in normal people (the correlation between two different bones in the same person is about 0.6) (5). Therefore, it is common for patients to have somewhat different T scores and Z scores if BMD is measured at several different skeletal sites.

Normal values of BMD vary between women and men, and among the various races (see Chapter 1). In general, black and Latino patients have higher BMD than whites (6). Asians tend to have slightly lower BMD than whites owing mainly to their smaller body sizes. Densitometers report T and Z scores that are specific to the patient's gender, and some report scores also specific to race. This approach allows the clinician to assess whether the patient has normal BMD in accordance with same. However, this approach can be confusing. For example, because normal white men have higher BMD than normal white women, a man with a T score of −2.5 has a higher BMD than a white woman who has a T score of −2.5 (7). The man will also have a lower risk of fracture. The same applies to BMD values for non-white women who normally have higher BMD than white women. This has led to controversy about whether the diagnosis of "osteoporosis" should be based on comparisons of BMD with normal values for one's own race and gender, or to some standard value for all adults that represents a certain risk of fractures.

Techniques for Assessing Bone Mass

A number of technologies can be used to assess bone mass, including DXA and single energy x-ray absorptiometry (SXA), quantitative ultrasound (QUS) of bone, quantitative computed tomography (QCT), and radiographic absorptiometry (RA). Table 2-2 summarizes the pertinent characteristics of commonly used tests; these methods have also been reviewed in detail by Eddy et al (8). Accuracy error is an estimate of the error in measuring the actual amount of bone mineral per unit volume. Precision error is the ability of the measurement to yield similar values over repeated assessments. Note that the precision of a measurement depends on the specific operator and machine; therefore, precision error of measurements made in a local hospital or in a specialist's office may be different, and sometimes a little poorer, than the precision listed in Table 2-2 (or advertised by the manufacturer). The radiation doses are quite low for all techniques and, with the exception of QCT, are much less than a patient gets from a mammogram or chest radiogram (8).

Dual Energy X-Ray Absorptiometry (DXA)

DXA is an accurate and precise technique that can be used to measure bone density at many skeletal sites (Table 2-2). Table model ("standard") DXA machines can measure BMC; BMC in the hip, spine, radius, and calcaneus; or the total amount of mineral in the whole skeleton. Patients remain clothed and are carefully positioned on a table for a scan that requires only a few minutes and produces a printed report.

Hip BMD
Hip DXA is considered the "gold standard" by many experts (including the authors of this chapter) for assessing risk of fracture and making a diagnosis of

Table 2-2   Summary of Techniques for Assessment of Bone Mass

	Site/Scan Time (minutes)	Accuracy Error (%)	Precision Error (%)	Radiation Exposure (millirem)
Peripheral DXA (pDXA)	Radius, calcaneus 5–15 min	3–8	1–3	~1
Single energy x-ray absorptiometry (SXA)	↓	↓	↓	↓
Dual x-ray absorptiometry (DXA or DEXA)	Spine, hip, radius, calcaneus, whole body 5–10 min	3–9	1–2	~1–5
Quantitative computed tomography (QCT)	Spine, hip, radius 10–30 min	5–15	2–4	~50
Radiographic absorptiometry (RA)	Hands 5–10 min	5–10	5–10	~5
Radiogrammetry ultrasound	Calcaneus, tibia 5–10 min		3–4	0

Adapted from Grampp S, Genant HK, Mathur A, et al. Comparisons of noninvasive bone mineral measurements classification. J Bone Miner Res. 1997;12:697–711; Eddy D, Johnston C, Cummings SR, et al. Osteoporosis: review of the evidence for prevention, diagnosis, treatment and cost-effective analysis. Osteoporos Int. 1998;8:S7–S80.

osteoporosis. Hip DXA is a stronger predictor of hip fracture than BMD of other sites and predicts the risk of all fractures as well as or better than other measurements (Table 2-3) (9,10). BMD of the hip is not affected by degenerative arthritis of the hip.

BMD of the hip actually refers to the femoral neck (the most extensively studied) or the total hip (which has slightly better precision than femoral neck BMD). These two measurements are highly correlated. For technical reasons, most patients will have slightly lower T scores of the femoral neck than of the total hip.

Spine BMD

Spine BMD measures the lumbar vertebrae, L1 through L4, in a posteroanterior projection. Because the spine has more trabecular bone than other sites, spine BMD is more sensitive to the effects of hormones and drugs. Spine BMD tends to be a little more precise than hip DXA (Table 2-2), so some physicians prefer to use spine BMD to monitor the effects of corticosteroid treatment and drug treatments.

Spine BMD reflects the mineral content of the whole lumbar spinal column, including the vertebral bodies, the posterior elements, and the facet joints, and also incorporates calcium in the overlying abdominal aorta. Therefore,

Table 2-3   Comparison of Ability of Various Bone Mass Measurements to Predict Fracture Risk*

Fracture Site	BMD Measurement Site			
	Forearm	Lumbar Spine	Calcaneus	Femoral Neck
Wrist	1.8	1.6	1.8	1.6
Vertebrae	1.6	2.0	NA	1.9
Hip	1.6	1.3	1.8	2.6

* Numbers indicate relative increase in fracture risk per standard deviation decrease in the measurement. (Adapted from Eddy D, Johnston C, Cummings SR, et al. Osteoporosis: review of the evidence for prevention, diagnosis, treatment, and cost-effectiveness analysis. Osteoporos Int. 1998;8:S7- S80.)

spine BMD is artifactually increased by degenerative arthritis and aortic calcification, both of which become increasingly common and severe after age 65. For this reason, spine BMD tends to increase after about age 65, rather than decrease as seen in other BMD measurements (11,12). Therefore, unless there are specific reasons for measuring spine BMD, such as treatment with corticosteroids, spine BMD should not be ordered for adults who are over age 65 or in those with known spinal degenerative arthritis.

Spine DXA measurement can be artifactually increased if one or more of the vertebral bodies included in the measurement is fractured or affected by local changes owing to degenerative arthritis; well-trained densitometry operators generally note and exclude fractured vertebral bodies from the results, but fractures and localized arthritic changes (such as spurring) can be missed. An unusual step-up in BMD from one level to the next and then a step-down in BMD can be a clue that a vertebral fracture or localized arthritis may be artifactually increasing the average spine BMD. Excluding the involved vertebrae from the analysis will produce a more accurate estimate of spine BMD.

Peripheral DXA (pDXA)
Smaller devices use DXA to measure bone density in the forearm. The distal radius is generally used because it contains both trabecular and cortical bone. Because they are small and relatively inexpensive devices, they can be more widely available in physicians' offices than standard DXA. A pDXA test generally costs less than DXA of the hip or spine.

Single Energy X-Ray Absorptiometry (SXA)

This technique involves the use of a single energy x-ray beam to obtain estimates of bone mass at the radius and the heel. SXA is performed with relatively small devices that are easily moved. SXA and pDXA share essentially the same characteristics, advantages, and disadvantages.

Quantitative Computed Tomography (QCT)

QCT of the spine is available on standard CT units. Techniques for QCT of the hip are being developed. A device is also available for performing QCT at the wrist, also known as peripheral QCT (pQCT). QCT is unique among current techniques in that it provides the ability to assess three-dimensional bone density (g/cm^3), and it permits separate measure of trabecular bone density that is more sensitive to the effects of hormones and drug treatments. QCT can also provide other details about bone structure including cortical width and density in specific subregions. Case-control studies suggest that QCT of the spine may be more strongly associated with risk of vertebral fractures than spine DXA is (13–15).

Measurements Based on Hand Radiographs

Several techniques are available for assessing bone mass from radiographs. Radiographic absorptiometry usually assesses the density of proximal pha-langes using a tapered wedge of aluminum, which allows standardization of density measurement (16). In this approach, the film is generally sent to a processing center for computer analysis.

Radiogrammetry measures the width of the cortex of the phalanges (and sometimes of the radius) on standard radiographs of the hand and wrist. Because density is not measured, no aluminum wedge is needed. These di-mensions can be measured manually with calipers, but computerized systems have been developed to automatically assess cortical measurements from films. This can be done locally without centralized processing.

Besides the use of x-ray film and the need for computer processing, this method shares most of the characteristics, advantages, and disadvantages of pDXA and SXA (Table 2-2).

Quantitative Ultrasound

Ultrasound densitometry assesses the speed of sound or the pattern of absorp-tion of different wavelengths of sound, called broadband ultrasound attenuation (BUA), or a combination of these parameters (17). This measurement involves no radiation (Table 2-2). Instruments are currently available that measure ul-trasound in the calcaneus (the most extensively studied), the tibia, and the radius. Ultrasound measurements are correlated with bone strength *in vitro* (2). The modest correlation ($r = \sim 0.4$ to 0.6) between ultrasound and BMD by densitometry has led some to present the possibility that ultrasound may assess a property of bone structure besides the amount of mineral in the bone, but its ability to predict fractures resembles that of pDXA, SXA, and other peripheral measurements of bone density (18,19). The precision of ultrasound of the calcaneus is somewhat poorer than that of DXA, SXA, and RA (Table 2-2).

Clinical Uses of Densitometry

Prediction of Fracture Risk

Prospective studies have established that fracture risk increases with age (9,10,18). This relationship is stronger for some types of fractures (e.g., hip and vertebral fractures) than for others (e.g., fractures of the ankle) (Figs. 2-2

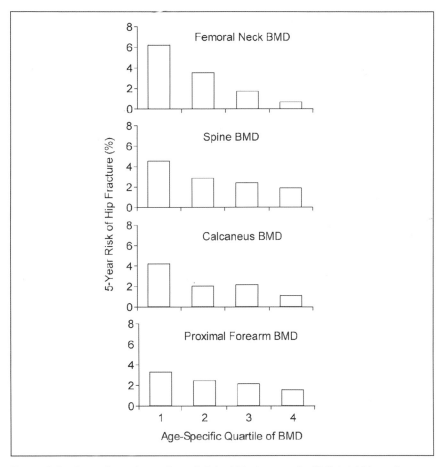

Figure 2-2   Age-adjusted quartile and risk of hip fracture for DXA total hip, spine, spa wrist, spa calcaneus for women aged 65 years or older. (Unpublished data from the Study of Osteoporotic Fractures.)

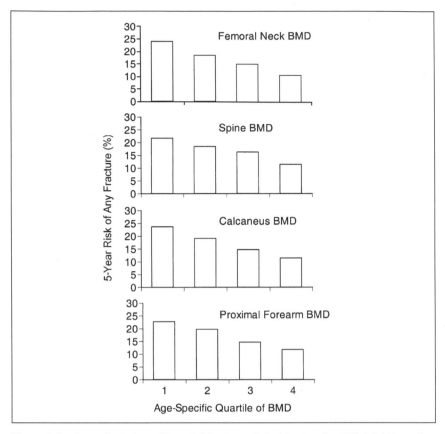

Figure 2-3 Age-adjusted quartile and risk of any clinical fracture for DXA total hip, spine, spa wrist, and spa calcaneus in women aged 65 years or older. (Unpublished data from the Study of Osteoporotic Fractures.)

and 2-3). The relationship is also stronger for some types of measurements than for others (Table 2-3). There is no "fracture threshold" or cutpoint below which fracture risk abruptly increases (Figs. 2-2 and 2-3). Therefore, BMD is best thought of as having a continuous gradient of risk, analogous to blood pressure where higher blood pressure means higher risk of stroke.

The relationship between BMD and fracture risk is customarily quantified by the "relative risk per standard deviation decrease in BMD." For example, a relative risk/standard deviation (RR/SD) of 1.5 means that a woman with a BMD that is 1 SD below the mean for her age has a 50% higher fracture risk than a woman with a BMD that is average for her age. It is important to note that these values are multiplicative. For example, consider a BMD test that carries a 2.0-fold relative risk of fracture per SD and the fact that patients who have average BMDs (Z score of 0) are known to have a 10% risk of fracture during the next 5 years.

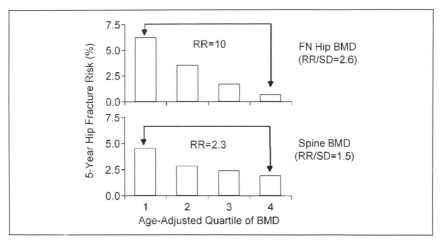

Figure 2-4   Comparison of the hip fracture risk between age-adjusted quartiles at the hip and spine. (Unpublished data from the Study of Osteoporotic Fractures.)

If a patient's BMD is 1 SD below that mean (Z score = –1.0), the patient's risk of fracture is about 20% per 5 years. If her BMD is 2 SD below (Z score = –2.0), then the risk is 2.0 times 2.0, or 4.0-fold higher, or about 40% during the next 5 years. Therefore, relatively modest differences between the values of RR per SD translate into large differences in the predictive accuracy of BMD measurements.

For example, spine BMD predicts hip fracture with an accuracy of about 1.4 to 1.6 RR per SD compared with 2.6 per SD for hip BMD. Note that in Figure 2-4 the increase in hip fracture risk from the lowest to the highest quartile for hip BMD is about 10 compared with only 2.3 for the spine. Therefore, the advantage of hip BMD is substantially greater than suggested by the relatively small difference between 1.5 and 2.6.

Prediction of Various Types of Fractures

One might expect that a BMD measurement at a specific site would be most predictive of fractures at that site. This is true for hip BMD and hip fractures (Table 2-3) but not for other types of measurements and other types of fractures (9,10). Hip and spine BMD have similar value for predicting vertebral fracture. All BMD sites have similar value for predicting "all fractures" (9).

Estimating Fracture Risk from Bone Mineral Density, Age, and Risk Factors

BMD can be used in conjunction with age and other risk factors to determine risk of fracture. In general, women with osteoporosis (T score less than or

Table 2-4   Estimated Five-Year Risk (%) of Various Types of Fractures for White Women at Various Ages and Femoral Neck T Scores

Age*	Femoral Neck BMD T Score							
	−3.5	−3.0	−2.5	−2.0	−1.5	−1.0	−0.5	0.0
Any Low Trauma Fracture (Excluding Vertebral Fracture)								
50	15	12	10	9	7	6	5	4
60	19	16	14	12	10	8	7	6
70	25	21	18	16	13	11	9	8
80	32	28	24	20	17	15	12	10
Vertebral Fracture								
50	5	3	2.4	1.8	1.3	0.9	0.7	0.5
60	8	6	4	3	2.2	1.6	1.2	0.9
70	13	10	7	5	4	3	2	1.5
80	22	16	12	9	7	5	4	3
Hip Fracture								
50	1.5	0.9	0.5	0.3	0.2	0.1	0.1	<0.1
60	3.2	1.9	1.2	0.7	0.4	0.3	0.2	0.1
70	7	4	2.5	1.5	0.9	0.6	0.3	0.2
80	13	9	5	3	2	1.2	0.7	0.4

* These values were derived from the Study of Osteoporotic Fractures (SOF) using Hologic QDR 1000 densitometers and the NHANES 1995 as reference data. SOF BMD measurements were performed on a cohort of women over age 67. A logistic model was fit using age and femoral neck BMD as predictors. Data for women age 60 and below are shown in italics and should be viewed cautiously because these are derived by extrapolation using the model fit to women over age 67.

equal to −2.5 at the hip) are considered "high risk." Table 2-4 and Figure 2-5 show the 5-year risk of hip fracture as a function of age and femoral neck BMD; Figure 2-6 shows the 5-year risk as a function of age and total spine BMD.

Because risk of fracture continues for life and increases with age, some women and physicians like to take the long view of "lifetime risk" of fractures (20). Table 2-5 shows the lifetime hip fracture risk as a function of age and femoral neck BMD. Of note is that for the same level of BMD, lifetime risk of hip fracture varies only slightly with age because the risk of hip fracture and mortality rates rise with aging.

As described in Chapter 1, other risk factors, including history of postmenopausal fracture, presence of vertebral fracture, and family history of hip fracture, are also predictive of hip fracture, independent of BMD, and are therefore useful adjuncts to BMD in assessing risk of fracture.

Diagnosing Osteoporosis

In 1992, the World Health Organization defined *osteoporosis* as a T score of −2.5 or lower at any site of measurement (21). This cut-off is rather arbitrary.

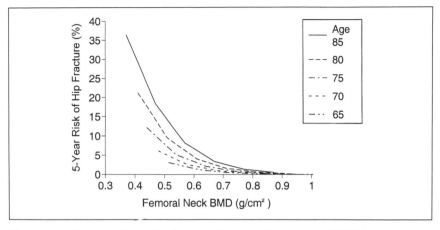

Figure 2-5   Five-year risk of hip fracture, by age and femoral neck BMD. (Unpublished data from the Study of Osteoporotic Fractures.)

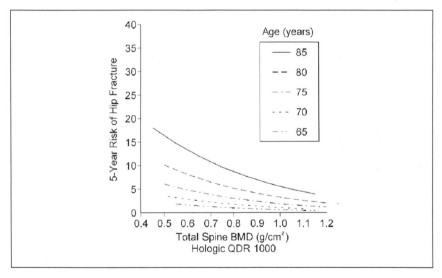

Figure 2-6   Five-year risk of hip fracture, by age and total spine BMD. (Unpublished data from the Study of Osteoporotic Fractures.)

It was designed to compare the prevalence of osteoporosis in different countries, not to aid in the care of individual patients. The diagnosis of "osteoporosis" based on BMD can be confusing because, if multiple sites are measured, patients will often have "osteoporosis" at one site and not another. Therefore, many experts (including the authors) prefer to make a diagnosis of "osteoporosis" when the T score at the femoral neck, total hip, or spine is less than or equal to –2.5.

Table 2-5   Lifetime Risk (%) of Hip Fracture for White Women at Various Ages and Femoral Neck T Scores

Age*	Femoral Neck BMD T Score							
	–3.5	–3.0	–2.5	–2.0	–1.5	–1.0	–0.5	0.0
50	49	41	33	27	21	16	13	10
60	47	40	33	27	21	17	13	10
70	46	39	33	27	21	17	13	10
80	41	35	30	24	20	16	12	10

* These estimated lifetime risks of hip fracture are calculated from statistical models using parameters described by Eddy et al (8) and BMD reference data from NHANES (6). These models are subject to several unverifiable assumptions, and therefore the risks should be viewed cautiously. The femoral neck T score values are derived from the Study of Osteoporotic Fractures (9) and are valid for Hologic densitometers.

Patients are sometimes unnecessarily distressed by receiving a report that they have osteopenia. Osteopenia is neither cause for alarm nor reason to start treatment. Many experts have stopped using the term to describe BMD results. *Osteopenia* was defined by a WHO conference as a bone density T score between –1.0 and –2.5 (21). The upper end of range, T score = –1.0, was decided, largely arbitrarily, to indicate women whose bone density was below normal for young adults. About half of all postmenopausal women have a bone density value in this range, and most normal women over age 65 could be labeled as having osteopenia. This term is often distressing to patients, but they should be reassured that they do not have a disease. Recommendations about treatment should be based on considerations of risk of fractures and potential benefits of treatment at various levels of BMD (Table 2-4 and Chapter 14).

Medical Evaluation

BMD might be valuable in deciding whether an individual patient should undergo an evaluation for unusual "secondary" causes of osteoporosis (see Chapter 3). This area has received virtually no systematic study, so the approach depends on expert and personal opinion. Because BMD declines with age, most experts believe that decisions about whether to look for unusual causes of osteoporosis should be based on comparisons with other patients of the same age; in other words, evaluations may be worthwhile only when a patient's Z score is low (less than –2 or –3) regardless of T score (see Chapter 3).

BMD can help determine whether a fracture is due to osteoporosis. For example, BMD may be valuable when a relatively young patient or a man suffers a fracture. It can be helpful if a patient has a vertebral fracture in a location, such as T5, that would be unusual for osteoporosis (see the clinical cases in Chapter 13). Although there is no evidence about this point, it is reasonable to believe that the higher the BMD, the greater is the chance that another process, such as trauma or cancer, caused the fracture.

Drug Treatments

Decisions about treatment involve more considerations than the value of bone density or risk of fracture and should include potential benefits and costs of the specific therapy. Recently, the National Osteoporosis Foundation defined treatment guidelines for individuals based on T scores of the femoral neck (8). These recommendations were based largely on evidence from randomized trials about the effectiveness of treatments to prevent fractures. These guidelines also considered the cost-effectiveness of treatments. Recommendations, based in part on the NOF Guidelines, are presented in Chapter 14.

In general, trials have found that pharmacologic treatments have reduced the risk of fracture among women who have osteoporosis, defined as T score at the femoral neck or, in some trials, at the spine. Women who have higher levels of bone density have a lower fracture risk, and treatment of those individuals may be less effective for preventing nonspine fractures (see Chapters 9 and 14). Guidelines presented in Chapter 14 suggest pharmacologic treatment to reduce the risk of fracture for women with a hip or spine BMD T score below –2.5 and perhaps below –2.0 if the patient has one or more strong risk factors for fracture.

Who Should Have a Bone Density Measurement?

Like any other test, BMD may be worthwhile when there is a reasonable chance that it will influence decisions about treatment or the extent of clinical evaluation of the patient. The authors adapted Table 2-6 from the analysis sponsored by the National Osteoporosis Foundation (8).

Men and Non-White Women

Because of the paucity of data and lower risk of fractures for men and non-white women, guidelines have not yet been developed for when to measure BMD in these patients. However, some groups of men and non-white women will have a substantially increased risk of having very low bone density and an increased risk of fractures: those with vertebral fractures and those who are receiving chronic oral corticosteroid therapy. It is also reasonable to test men and non-white women who have had adulthood fractures with minimal trauma and those who have chronic medical conditions, such as hyperparathyroidism, that may substantially increase the risk of osteoporosis (see Case 3 in Chapter 13).

Table 2-6   Guidelines for Measuring Bone Mineral Density in White Women for Assessing Risk of Fracture and Making Treatment Decisions

The decision to test for BMD should be based on an individual's risk profile, and testing is never indicated unless the results are likely to influence a treatment decision. BMD testing is recommended for:
1. Postmenopausal women aged 65 years and older regardless of additional risk factors. (This recommendation includes women aged 65 years and older who have been taking osteoporosis therapy and have not previously had a BMD test.)
2. Postmenopausal women under age 65 years with one or more additional risk factors for osteoporosis.*
3. Postmenopausal women who have had a fracture of any type as an adult.

* Risk factors include parental history of hip fracture, current cigarette smoking, a body weight < 125 lb, use of (or plans to use) oral corticosteroids longer than 3 months, or serious chronic illnesses known to increase fracture risk.

Patients in Long-Term Care

Patients in long-term care facilities have a very high (2% to 6% per year) risk of hip fractures (22). One survey of white women in Maryland nursing homes found that 64% of women aged 65 to 74 years and 86% of those over 85 years of age had T scores of less than –2.5 in the forearm (23). Therefore, measuring BMD in these women would identify many cases of osteoporosis. However, there may be practical difficulties of moving patients to DXA scanners. Although almost all patients in long-term care would qualify for BMD testing under various guidelines, it is also reasonable to consider pharmacologic treatment for such patients without testing BMD. Note, however, that a recent study found that risedronate did not substantially decrease the risk of hip fracture among women aged 80 or older who had an increased risk of hip fractures on the basis of risk factors alone (24). In contrast, there was a 39% reduction among women under age 80 who had a femoral neck BMD T score that was less than or equal to –3.0. Therefore, it may also be reasonable to measure nursing home residents' hip BMD, when it is feasible, to help make decisions about use of bisphosphonate therapy.

Which Site(s) Should Be Measured?

Because hip BMD is the best predictor of hip fracture, hip BMD may be particularly useful in women over age 65 because risk of hip fracture rises rapidly after age 65. Hip DXA scans typically report BMD for several subregions of the hip, the femoral neck, the trocanter, Ward's triangle (a 1 cm^2 region selected by BMD software as the lowest value in the femoral neck), and total hip BMD that includes all subregions. These results are highly correlated and have similar predictive value for fractures. The femoral neck and total hip measurements have been the most extensively studied. Therefore, for simplicity and consistency with guidelines, it is recommended that femoral neck or total hip be the primary site for estimating fracture risk and making a diagnosis of osteoporosis.

As noted earlier in this chapter, spine BMD should generally not be used to assess fracture risk after about the age 65, because arthritis and aortic calcification tend to artifactually increase spine BMD (11). Spine BMD has traditionally been used more commonly than hip BMD for risk assessment in 45- to 60-year-old women. Spine and hip BMD seem to have similar predictive value for fractures that occur commonly in this age group (such as wrist fractures rather than hip fractures) (10).

Peripheral versus Central DXA

PDXA and ultrasound are less expensive and more widely available in some areas than standard DXA. PDXA predicts risk of fracture and is reasonably precise for following treatments. However, peripheral densitometry does not predict fractures as accurately as hip DXA, and treatments produce smaller changes in pDXA than in spine or hip BMD.

Measurements of bone density in the forehand, heal, or hand are sometimes used as an initial screening test to determine which patients should have measurements taken of the hip or spine. There is a general correlation of peripheral measurements with hip and spine BMD: women with low peripheral values tend to have low hip and spine values and vice versa. It is likely that a woman with a very low T score value (below –3) on a peripheral measurement will have a hip BMD T score below –2.5. Conversely, a woman with a high normal peripheral BMD T score (greater than 0) is unlikely to have a hip BMD T score below –2.5. However, the specific relationships between peripheral BMD and hip or spine BMD vary dramatically by site and type of peripheral measurement, and age and data are not available to quantify the likelihood of low hip BMD for a given value of peripheral BMD. In general, a woman with a very high peripheral BMD T score (above 0 or +1) is extremely unlikely to have low BMD at the hip and therefore may not require central DXA. However, in all other cases, it is recommended that hip BMD be used as the definitive diagnostic tool.

How Many Measurements Should Be Taken?

Most densitometry services that perform DXA routinely measure and report BMD at both the hip and the spine, generally at the same price as one measurement. Although it is instinctive to believe that "more is better," sometimes there are advantages to measuring just one site, because the two results may appear to be in conflict, which could prove confusing to patients and clinicians. Measurement of two sites increases the chance that one site will be low. However, if only one of two sites is low enough to warrant starting treatment, it may not be clear which measurement should be used to make the decision. Two considerations might help. First, because hip BMD is a stronger predictor of hip fracture and less likely to be influenced by arthritis and artifacts, if hip and spine BMD differ (especially if the spine BMD T score is higher), then decisions should be based on hip BMD. Second, if a patient has only one low value, her general risk of fracture is probably less than if both sites were low.

As noted previously, elderly patients tend to have higher T scores of the spine than of the hip because spine DXA, but not hip DXA, is influenced by arthritic changes and aortic calcification. This usually accounts for a T score for spine BMD that is higher than that for hip BMD in an elderly patient. On occasion, a patient will have a spine BMD score that is substantially lower than her hip BMD score. This may occur with use of corticosteroids or with Cushing's disease, but it usually has no clinical explanation. Many experts believe that patients who have a spine BMD T score that is below –2.5, but a higher hip BMD, should, nevertheless, be regarded as indicating osteoporosis.

If hip or spine BMD has been measured, there is generally no advantage to also obtaining another measurement of peripheral BMD, such as BMD of the radius.

Is an Ultrasound Measurement Also Necessary?

Ultrasound has been shown to predict hip fractures even after statistical adjustment for BMD (18,19). This means that adding an ultrasound measurement to a measurement of BMD of the hip might improve the prediction of hip fracture. However, the amount of information that is added is relatively small and hard to discern without computer-assisted analysis of the results; therefore, in practical terms, it is probably not worth adding another measurement of bone ultrasound if BMD of the hip is already known.

Monitoring

Patient Receiving Treatment

Although bone densitometry is commonly used to monitor the effectiveness of treatments such as bisphosphonates, the interpretation of such measurements can be confusing. One goal of monitoring is to determine whether a patient is responding to treatment. This is difficult because "responding" is not the same as "gaining BMD." A patient who loses BMD—for example, 3%—during treatment may well have lost more (e.g., 5% to 6%) without treatment. They are really responding despite the report that they are losing BMD. Results of BMD can also be misleading for other reasons. Patients who lose BMD during the first period of treatment usually regain much of that BMD during the next period (Table 2-7) (25). This is due to "regression to the mean," meaning that unusual results of measurements (such as loss of BMD on a treatment that usually causes an increase) are probably due to imperceptible errors in one of the measurements. An uncommon error is usually absent from a third measurement, meaning that the extreme loss or gain eventually returns toward the averages expected for patients taking that treatment.

In addition, even women who are taking their medication who seem to lose BMD during the first period of monitoring probably benefit from reductions in risk of fracture, as do women who gain BMD during treatment (25a). Therefore, treatments should not be changed because the patient appears to lose BMD during the first period of monitoring (regardless of whether the time between the measurements is 1 year, 2 years, or longer).

It is possible that three or four BMD measurements taken over several years will improve the ability to determine whether a patient is improving or maintaining BMD to a desirable degree. However, the benefits of initiating a medical evaluation for causes of suboptimal response or of switching or adding a second drug are not known.

Many clinicians believe that monitoring a therapy improves adherence. There are no data that address this question directly, but most problems with

Table 2-7   Change in Total Hip Bone Density During Year One Compared with the Probability of Gaining Bone and the Mean Percentage Gain in Bone During the Second Year of Treatment with Alendronate

Percent Change in BMD During Year 1	N (%) Who Gained During Year 2	Mean % Gain During Year 2
<–4 (loss)	34 (92%)	4.8 (2.7, 6.9)*
–4 to –2	75 (74%)	1.8 (1.1, 2.4)
–2 to 0	274 (79%)	1.7 (1.4, 2.0)
0 to +2	557 (70%)	1.0 (0.9, 1.2)
+2 to +4	493 (65%)	0.8 (0.6, 1.0)
+4 to +6	244 (60%)	0.5 (0.2, 0.7)
+6 to +8	69 (52%)	0.1 (–0.4, 0.5)
>+8 (gain)	22 (36%)	–1.0 (–1.9, –0.1)

* 95% confidence intervals in parentheses.
From Cummings SR, Palermo L, Browner W, et al. Monitoring osteoporosis therapy with bone densitometry: misleading changes and regression to the mean. Fracture Intervention Trial Research Group. JAMA. 2000;283:1318–21; with permission.

adherence happen within the first 3 months of starting treatment so that BMD done 1 or 2 years into treatment is not likely to have much impact on adherence. Monitoring bone density should not replace periodic discussions with individual patients about problems they may have had with adherence and practical solutions to staying with effective treatment.

If BMD were used to monitor the effects of treatment, the ideal measurement site would show the greatest ratio of change during treatment to precision of the measurement. The spine is often favored for monitoring, especially for patients receiving steroids, because treatments generally produce greater changes in the spine than in other sites, and the spine is as precise, or nearly as precise, as other measurements. Because of the uncertain value of monitoring, it may not be worthwhile to obtain different or additional measurements of bone density before starting treatment that is mainly for the purpose of monitoring treatment.

Clinical considerations about monitoring the effects of treatment with BMD are also discussed in Case 4 in Chapter 13.

Patients Not Receiving Treatment

The best approach to following up BMD in patients who are not being treated is uncertain. The same phenomenon of regression to the mean is seen in patients who are receiving treatment and those who are not being treated. If a patient seems to have a large decrease in bone density while not being treated, her bone density will usually increase during the next period of monitoring, even without treatment (25). Some believe that bone loss that is sustained over more than two periods of measurement and beyond the level attributable to error in the measurement (more than a cumulative 5% over 2 years of measurement) may warrant treatment to prevent bone loss.

Patients whose BMD values are not low enough to make drug treatment worthwhile will eventually lose bone, and repeat measurement of BMD should be considered. The repeat measurement should be made when there is a reasonable chance that the patient will have a BMD value that is near the level at which pharmacologic treatment might be started. The timing of the repeat measurement depends on the current BMD: the lower the value and the closer to a threshold at which treatment would be started, the sooner the BMD measurement should be repeated. It is also helpful to know the average rate of bone loss expected for the patient's age. For example, on average, women who are at least 5 years postmenopausal lose bone at less than 0.5% per year. Therefore, it will generally take more than 10 years for a postmenopausal woman whose T score is –1.0 to develop a BMD T score of –2.0 or lower. Weight loss or development of clinical conditions that cause bone loss may prompt earlier remeasurement of BMD. Average rates of bone loss are more rapid (1% to 3% per year) within the first 3 to 5 years of menopause and in patients who recently started steroid therapy. Measurements should be repeated sooner in these patients.

Assessment of Vertebral Fractures

Vertebral fractures are often asymptomatic or not diagnosed. The diagnosis of a vertebral fracture requires lateral radiographs of both the thoracic and the lumbar spine. Severe vertebral fractures are usually clear on radiograph, but sometimes, especially for "mild" deformities in the vertebral body, the diagnosis can be uncertain, and even experts may disagree. Nevertheless, because vertebral fractures are so common and are a sentinel sign of osteoporosis that should be treated, it is important to recognize vertebral fractures. In this section, the prevalence and importance of vertebral fractures, indications for radiographs, and interpretation of radiographs are reviewed.

Vertebral fractures are very common in older women. They are found on radiographs in 5% to 10% of white women at age 55, rising to 30% to 40% by age 80 (26,27). Statistically, in white women, the risk of developing a vertebral fracture on radiograph is 0.5% per year at age 55 and 2% to 3% per year at age 80 (28). Data from population-based surveys demonstrate that only about one third of the vertebral fractures seen on spine radiographs come to clinical attention (28). However, even fractures that are found only on radiograph are associated with an increased chance of having caused the patient back pain and difficulty in activities that involve movements of the back, such as putting on shoes and socks or getting into and out of a car (29,30).

As noted in Chapter 1, the finding of a vertebral fracture on radiograph signals that the patient has a 4-fold increased risk of having another vertebral fracture, a 2-fold increased risk of a subsequent hip fracture, and a 50% greater risk of nonvertebral fractures compared with women without a fracture (31,32). This increase in risk is in addition to risk of fracture related to the patient's bone density (31). A postmenopausal woman with a vertebral fracture has a high enough risk of other fractures that pharmacologic treatment is worthwhile (see Chapter 14).

When Should Spine Radiographs Be Ordered?

The value of screening all older women for vertebral fracture has not been studied. However, finding that a patient has a vertebral fracture, even if it is asymptomatic, substantially increases estimates of her risk of fracture; this generally means that pharmacologic treatment is warranted to reduce her risk of future fractures (see Chapter 14).

In general lateral radiographs of the thoracic and lumbar spine should be ordered in any patient in whom a vertebral fracture is suspected clinically (Table 2-8). Clinical suspicion is heightened by new or worsening back pain, height loss, and exaggerated thoracic kyphosis.

Back pain is the most common symptom of vertebral fractures, but many other conditions cause this very common symptom. Back pain should trigger an order for a spine film in patients who have a reasonably high risk of vertebral fracture and clinical symptoms and signs suggesting that vertebral fracture is a likely cause of the pain. The features of back pain that make finding a vertebral fracture more likely have not been well studied. It is believed that acute back pain that is on or very near the spinal column and localized to a region the size of just one or two vertebral bodies is more likely to be caused by an acute vertebral fracture than is diffuse or laterally located back pain. Generally, films should be taken in postmenopausal women who have new or worsened back pain and in patients who are taking oral corticosteroids who develop new or worsened back pain. However, other causes of low back pain are very common, and vertebral fractures are rare in otherwise healthy young adults. These patients do not warrant spine films for the purpose of identifying vertebral fractures.

A vertebral fracture causes, on average, approximately 1 cm loss of height (33). However, after about age 50, women and men tend to slowly lose height as a result of other poorly understood processes of drying of intervertebral discs and loss of muscle tone in the back. The chance of finding a vertebral fracture increases with the degree of height loss. It has been noted that patients who have lost more than 2 inches (4 cm) from their peak height in young adulthood have a relatively high prevalence of vertebral fracture, and it may be worthwhile to obtain a lateral spine radiograph (34).

Vertebral fractures may alter the anatomy of the spine. The resulting lordosis, kyphosis, or strains on the supporting structures of the back may also lead to low back pain or diffuse pain that is not localized to the affected vertebral fracture. Kyphosis is a common manifestation of multiple vertebral fractures, especially "wedge-type" fractures. The presence of notable kyphosis, especially with a history of recurrent or chronic back pain, should prompt an order for

Table 2-8   When to Take Lateral Spine Films to Look for Vertebral Fracture

- New or worsened midline back pain in:
  Women or men with osteoporosis by BMD or previous spine fracture
  Patients taking oral corticosteroid therapy
  Older (≥ 55 years) postmenopausal women
- Patients who have lost ≥ 2 inches in height since about age 24
- Patients who have developed prominent thoracic kyphosis
- Spine DXA scan suggests the presence of a vertebral fracture

lateral spine radiographs. However, many patients with kyphosis, even prominent kyphosis, do not have vertebral fractures.

Types and Locations of Vertebral Fractures

Vertebral fractures are most common in the midthoracic region, around T7, owing to the biomechanical stresses induced by natural curvature of the thoracic spine. Fractures also commonly occur at T12 and L1, the junction of the immobile thoracic and mobile lumbar spine, presumably owing to biomechanical stresses induced by different movements of the rib cage and abdomen. Wedge, crush, and endplate are types of vertebral deformities that take their names from compression of different parts of the vertebral body. *Endplate* fractures are characterized by indentation or discontinuity that is limited to the central area of the endplate (Fig. 2-7); *wedge* refers to compression of the anterior edge primarily (Fig. 2-8); *crush* refers to flattening of the whole vertebral body (Fig. 2-9). These types of fractures may also be associated with distinct patterns of biomechanical stresses in the spine. Wedge fractures predominate in the midthoracic area and T–L junction, whereas endplate fractures are most common in the lumbar spine. All types of fractures are associated with height loss and back pain, but there is some evidence that lumbar fractures are associated with greater back pain and disability (35). In general, however, the risk of future fractures and the efficacy of antiresorptive therapy in preventing fractures do not appear to differ by the location or type of an existing fracture (36).

Vertebral fractures incurred by the patient at a young age owing to sports or occupational trauma may be less likely to signal osteoporosis. However, the age of onset of a vertebral fracture cannot usually be determined by the appearance of the vertebral fracture on a standard radiograph. Among patients who have had a vertebral fracture that is incidentally found on radiograph, especially in young or middle aged patients and in men, there is an increased chance that the vertebral fracture is due to previous severe trauma that the patient may not recall. In these cases, a measurement of bone density may help determine the odds that the vertebral fracture is traumatic. Most atraumatic vertebral fractures in postmenopausal women occur in patients whose spine or hip BMD is below a T score of –2.0 (27) There is no evidence that variation in the degree or type of trauma associated with a vertebral fracture in older women has any important implications for risk of future fractures or the value of treatment to prevent additional fractures.

Interpreting Spine Radiographs

Vertebral radiographs should be obtained using a standard protocol that allows optimal visualization of the vertebral body contours (37). The radiologic

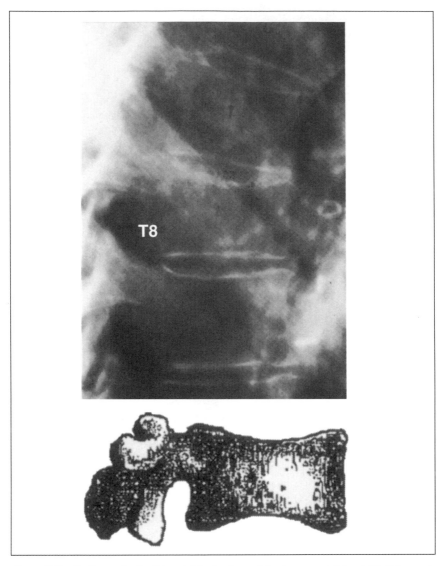

Figure 2-7   Radiograph of mild endplate fracture of the lower endplate of T8. It is manifest by slight indentation and irregularity and loss of continuity of the endplate. Below this photograph is an idealized drawing of a moderately severe endplate fracture.

diagnosis of a vertebral fracture is based on loss of height of the vertebral body or a break in the continuity of the cortical shell of a vertebral body (Fig. 2-7). Radiologists usually agree about the presence of severe vertebral fractures, when judged qualitatively on spine radiographs. Radiologists may disagree about whether some mildly deformed vertebrae represent vertebral fractures

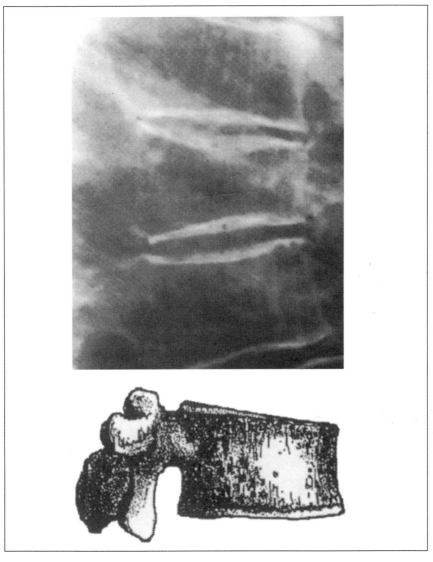

Figure 2-8 Lateral radiograph and drawing of a moderately severe wedge fracture. The posterior margin of the vertebral body is unaffected; the anterior margin is decreased more than the middle portion of the body.

or other artifacts. In these cases, it may be valuable to obtain a measurement of bone density. Fractures that are due to osteoporosis should be distinguished by radiologic evaluation from other deformities that affect the vertebral body, including Scheuerman's disease, juvenile kyphosis, and hypertrophic lipping. Schmorl's nodes (Fig. 2-10), which are caused by protrusions of the

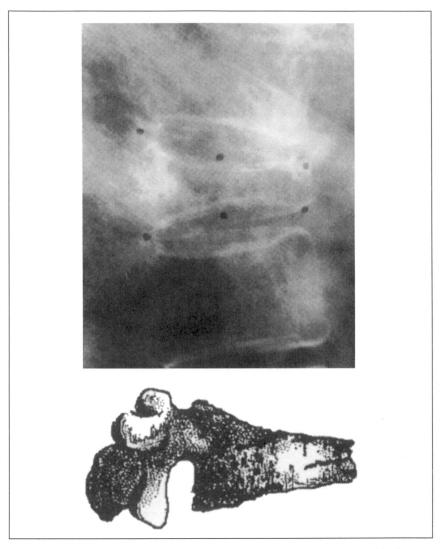

Figure 2-9   Lateral spine radiograph and drawing of a severe crush fracture. The fracture has caused a loss of height of the posterior margin of the vertebral body. There has been a severe loss of height of the anterior and middle portion of the vertebral body.

intervertebral disk into the vertebral body, are common in osteoporosis, although not pathognomonic of the condition (37).

One approach to assessing vertebral fractures, called the "semiquantitative" approach, estimates the severity of vertebral fractures on a scale from mild (1) to severe (3). This approach is commonly used in research (38). The diagnosis of vertebral fractures can also be based on, or confirmed by, measurement of

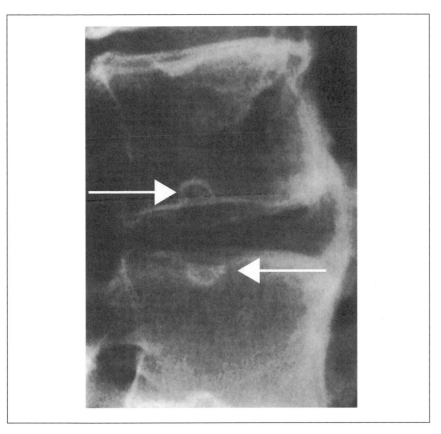

Figure 2-10   Schmorl's node (in the center of the circle outlined by arrows): a discrete semicircular indentation of the endplate.

the anterior, middle, and posterior heights of the vertebral body ("morphometry"). A decrease of 20% or at least 4 mm in any height from one film to the next is a reasonably reliable indicator that a vertebral fracture has occurred (38). If there are no previous films for comparison, a 25% decrease in vertebral height compared with adjacent vertebrae is indicative of a vertebral fracture. Complex computer algorithms can be used to refine this approach and to identify mild fractures, but these algorithms have been used mainly in research settings.

Identifying Vertebral Fractures on DXA Scans of the Spine

Some DXA devices obtain a lateral image of the entire spine for identifying potential vertebral fractures based on morphometry. This technique, known as morphometric x-ray absorptiometry (MXA), has several practical advantages, including a very low radiation dose, lower cost because no radiographic film is needed, and the convenience of performing the assessment at the same time as a BMD examination. Although this technique is not ready for routine use in primary care practice, early validation studies are promising. In general, this technique detects nearly all severe fractures but misses some moderate ones that can be seen on a radiograph. Overlying structures and tissues degrade image quality in the upper thoracic spine, but fractures are uncommon in this area and usually occur in conjunction with fractures lower in the spine. This technique has promise for use in screening for vertebral fractures. If an MXA scan is normal, then a radiograph would probably not be worthwhile, but if the scan suggests that a fracture may be present, a radiograph would be needed to confirm the diagnosis.

Summary

It is worthwhile to measure bone density in postmenopausal women who are at increased risk of fracture and who would consider pharmacologic treatment to reduce their risk. Such women include white women aged 65 and older and postmenopausal women younger than 65 who have a strong risk factor, such as a history of fracture. Bone density at the hip is often the preferred site, especially for older women, because it predicts hip fracture more strongly than do measurements at other sites. Pharmacologic treatment is generally recommended for women with osteoporosis, defined as a T score of less than –2.5 at the hip or spine and for all patients who have a vertebral fracture, regardless of whether the fracture is symptomatic.

Most vertebral fractures escape clinical diagnosis. However, a vertebral fracture signals a high risk of future fractures. Thus, physicians should consider ordering lateral spine films in patients at increased risk of vertebral fractures (such as those taking corticosteroids) who develop back pain suggestive of vertebral fracture.

REFERENCES

1. **Peck WA, Burckhardt P, Christiansen C, et al.** Consensus Development Conference: Diagnosis, prophylaxis, and treatment of osteoporosis. Am J Med. 1993; 94:646–650.

2. **Bouxsein ML, Courtney AC, Hayes WC.** Ultrasound and densitometry of the calcaneus correlate with the failure loads of cadaveric femurs. Calcif Tissue Int. 1995; 56:99–103.

3. **Courtney A, Wachtel E, Myers E, Hayes W.** Age-related reduction in the strength of the femur tested in a fall-loading configuration. J Bone Joint Surg. 1995;77:387–395.

4. **Link TM, Majumdar S, Lin JC, et al.** Assessment of trabecular structure using high resolution CT images and texture analysis. J Comput Assist Tomogr. 1998;22:15–24.

5. **Grampp S, Genant HK, Mathur A, et al.** Comparisons of noninvasive bone mineral measurements in assessing age-related loss, fracture discrimination, and diagnostic classification. J Bone Miner Res. 1997;12:697–711.

6. **Looker AC, Orwoll ES, Johnston CC Jr, et al.** Prevalence of low femoral bone density in older U.S. adults from NHANES III. J Bone Miner Res. 1997; 12:1769–1771.

7. **Orwoll E.** Assessing bone density in men. J Bone Miner Res. 200;15:1867–1870.

8. **Eddy D, Johnston C, Cummings SR, et al.** Osteoporosis: review of the evidence for prevention, diagnosis, and treatment and cost-effectiveness analysis. Osteoporos Int. 1998;8(Suppl 4): S7–S80.

9. **Cummings SR, Black DM, Nevitt MC, et al.** Bone density at various sites for prediction of hip fractures. Lancet. 1993;341:72–75.

10. **Marshall D, Johnell O, Wedel H.** Meta-analysis of how well measure of bone mineral density predict occurrence of osteoporosis fractures. Br Med J. 1996;312:1254–1259.

11. **Steiger P, Cummings SR, Black DM, et al.** Age-related decrements in bone mineral density in women over 65. J Bone Miner Res. 1992;7:625–632.

12. **Ensrud KE, Palermo L, Black DM, et al.** Hip and calcaneal bone loss increase with advancing age: longitudinal results from the Study of Osteoporotic Fractures. J Bone Miner Res. 1995;10:1778–1787.

13. **Lang TF, Li J, Harris ST, et al.** Assessment of vertebral bone mineral density using volumetric quantitative CT. J Comput Assist Tomogr. 1999;23:130–137.

14. **Grampp S, Genant HK, Mathur A, et al.** Comparisons of noninvasive bone mineral measurements in assessing age-related loss, fracture discrimination, and diagnostic classification. J Bone Miner Res. 1997;12:697–711.

15. **Jergas M, Breitenseher M, et al.** Estimates of volumetric density from projectional estimates improve the discriminatory capacity of dual x-ray absorptiometry. J Bone Miner Res. 1995;10:1101–1110.

16. **Yang S-O, Hagiwara S, Engelke K.** Radiographic absorptiometry for bone mineral measurement of the phalanges: precision and accuracy study. Radiology. 1994;192: 857–859.

17. **Kaufman JJ, Einhorn TA.** Ultrasound assessment of bone. J Bone Miner Res. 1993;8:517–525.

18. **Bauer DC, Gluer CC, Cauley JA, et al.** Broadband ultrasound attenuation predicts fractures strongly and independently of densitometry in older women: a prospective study. Study of Osteoporotic Fractures Research Group. Arch Intern Med. 1997;157: 629–634.

19. **Schott AM, Weill-Engerer S, Hans D, et al.** Ultrasound discriminates patients with hip fracture equally as well as dual energy x-ray absorptiometry and independently of bone mineral density. J Bone Miner Res. 1995;10:243–249.

20. **Melton LJ, Kan SH, Wahner HW, et al.** Lifetime fracture risk: an approach to hip fracture risk assessment based on bone mineral density and age. J Clin Epidemiol. 1988;41:985–994.

21. **Kanis JA, Melton LJ, Christiansen C, et al.** The diagnosis of osteoporosis. J Bone Miner Res. 1994; 9:1137–1141.

22. **Ooms ME, Vlasman P, Lips P, et al.** The incidence of hip fractures in independent and institutionalized elderly people. Osteoporos Int. 1994;4:6–10.

23. **Zimmerman SI, Girman CJ, Buie VC, et al.** The prevalence of osteoporosis in nursing home residents. Osteoporos Int. 1999;9:151–157.

24. **McClung MR, Guesens P, Miller P, et al.** Effect of risedronate on the risk of hip fracture in elderly women. N Engl J Med. 2001; 344:333–340.

25. **Cummings SR, Palermo L, Browner W, et al.** Monitoring osteoporosis therapy with bone densitometry: Misleading changes and regression to the man. Fracture Intervention Trial Research Group. JAMA. 2000;283:1318–1321.

25a. **Chapurlat RD, Palermo L, Ramsay P, Cummings SR.** Are non-responders responding? Risk of fracture of those who lose bone with alendronate. Results from FIT. J Biomed Mater Res. 2001 (In Press).

26. **O'Neill TW, Felsenberg D, Varlow J, et al.** The prevalence of vertebral deformity in European men and women. The European Vertebral Osteoporosis Study. J Bone Miner Res. 1996;11:1010–1018.

27. **Melton LJ, Kan SH, Frye MA, et al.** Epidemiology of vertebral fractures in women. Am J Epidemiol. 1989;129:1000–1011.

28. **Cooper C, Atkinson EJ, O'Fallon WM, et al.** Incidence of clinically diagnosed vertebral fractures. A population-based study in Rochester, Minnesota, 1985–1999. J Bone Miner Res. 1992;7:221–227.

29. **Ettinger B, Black DM, Nevitt MC, et al.** Contribution of vertebral deformities to chronic back pain and disability. J Bone Miner Res. 1992;7:449–455.

30. **Nevitt MC, Ettinger B, Black DM, et al.** The association of radiographically detected vertebral fractures with back pain and function. A prospective study. Ann Intern Med. 1998;128:793–800.

31. **Ross PD, Davis JW, Epstein RS, et al.** Pre-existing fracture and bone mass predict vertebral fracture incidence in women. Ann Intern Med. 1991;114:919–923.

32. **Black DM, Arden NK, Palermo L, et al.** Prevalent vertebral deformities predict hip fractures and new deformities but not wrist fractures. Study of Osteoporotic Fractures Research Group. J Bone Miner Res. 1999;14:821–828.

33. **Huang C, Ross PD, Lydick E, et al.** Contributions of vertebral fractures to stature loss among elderly Japanese-American women in Hawaii. J Bone Miner Res. 1996; 11:408–411.

34. **Ismail AA, Cooper C, Felsenberg D, et al.** Number and type of vertebral deformities: epidemiological characteristics and relation to back pain and height loss. European Vertebral Osteoporosis Study Group. Osteoporos Int. 1999;9:206–213.

35. **Cockerill W, Ismail AA, Cooper C, et al.** Does location of vertebral deformity within the spine influence back pain and disability? European Vertebral Osteoporosis Study Group. Ann Rheum Dis. 2000;59:368–371.

36. **Nevitt MC, Ross PD, Palermo L, et al.** Association of prevalent vertebral fractures, bone density, and alendronate treatment with incident vertebral fractures: effect of number and spinal location of fractures. The Fracture Intervention Trial Research Group. Bone. 1999;25:613–619.

37. **Genant HK, Jergas M, Van Kuijk C (eds).** Vertebral fracture in osteoporosis. Sebastopol: Radiology Research and Education Foundation; 1995.

38. **Genant HK, Jergas M, Palermo L, et al.** Comparison of semiquantitative visual and quantitative morphometric assessment of prevalent and incident vertebral fractures in osteoporosis. J Bone Miner Res. 1996;11:984–999.

CHAPTER 3

Markers of Bone Turnover and the Laboratory Evaluation of Secondary Osteoporosis

JACKIE A. CLOWES, MBChB
RICHARD EASTELL, MD

Key Points

- Selective use of laboratory tests can help in the care of patients with osteoporosis.

- Markers of bone turnover can be used for several purposes, including predicting future rate of bone loss, predicting risk of osteoporotic fractures, and monitoring response to treatment.

- Bone turnover markers cannot be used to diagnose osteoporosis.

- Osteoporosis due to medical conditions such as Cushing's disease is termed *secondary osteoporosis*.

- Up to 20% of women and 64% of men presenting to specialists or metabolic bone clinics with osteoporosis have diseases linked to osteoporosis.

- Most women with osteoporosis who are seen by primary care physicians are likely to have *primary osteoporosis*.

Cont'd.

> • Laboratory tests can help identify many causes of secondry osteo-
>   porosis and are especially valuable when the underlying condi-
>   tion results in a change in patient management.
>
> • There is no clear evidence on what criteria should prompt inves-
>   tigation for secondary osteoporosis or which laboratory tests are
>   worthwhile.

Selective use of laboratory tests can assist in the care of patients with osteo-porosis. Bone turnover can be assessed by laboratory tests that measure bone formation and bone resorption. These tests may have value in predicting bone loss, predicting osteoporotic fractures, identifying individual patients most likely to respond to drug treatments for osteoporosis, and monitoring patients' responses to treatment. Osteoporosis caused by a medical condition, such as Cushing's disease, is termed "secondary osteoporosis." Laboratory test-ing can help identify many causes of secondary osteoporosis. This is especially valuable when the underlying condition can be treated, leading to an improve-ment in bone density with a reduction in the risk of osteoporotic fractures. This chapter addresses the clinical role of laboratory tests for estimating rates of bone turnover and the identification of secondary causes of osteoporosis.

Biochemical Markers of Bone Turnover

Bone Remodeling

Bone is constantly undergoing remodeling through a process of bone resorp-tion that is coupled with the process of bone formation (see Chapter 1). Markers of bone turnover reflect whole-body bone remodeling, are noninva-sive and relatively inexpensive, and therefore have largely replaced invasive and expensive methods such as bone biopsy for estimating rates of bone re-modeling. Bone turnover markers represent either the enzymes involved in bone formation (generated by osteoblasts) and resorption (generated by os-teoclasts) or the formation and degradation products of bone matrix metabo-lism (primarily type I collagen). Many of the bone resorption markers can be measured in both serum and urine, but bone formation markers can cur-rently only be measured in serum or plasma (Table 3-1).

Bone resorption decreases rapidly a few days after the initiation of an anti-resorptive treatment such as estrogen and reaches a nadir after a few weeks. The changes in bone formation are slower, starting after a few weeks and

Table 3-1   Bone Turnover Markers

Bone Marker	Characteristics	Sample Urine (U) Serum (S)	Storage Required	Total Co-efficient of Variation (CV$_T$)	Least Significant Change (LSC)
Bone Formation Markers					
Total alkaline phosphatase (total ALP)	Tissue nonspecific isoenzymes	S	−70°C	6–11	16–30
Bone-specific alkaline phosphatase (bone ALP)	Bone isoform associated with osteoblast activity	S	−70°C	7–9	18–26
Osteocalcin (OC)	Non-collagenous bone matrix protein synthesized by osteoblasts	S	−70°C	7–27	20–64
Procollagen type I C pro-peptide (PICP)	Propeptide released during maturation of type I collagen	S	−20°C	9–10	24–26
Procollagen type I N pro-peptide (PINP)	Propeptide released during maturation of type I collagen	S	−20°C	8	21
Bone Resorption Markers					
Urine calcium (Ca)	Product of bone resorption	U	−20°C	33–45	91–126
Hydroxyproline (Hyp)	Product of type I collagen degradation	U	−20°C	18–41	50–147
Pyridinoline (PYD) (HPLC)	Free and peptide-bound collagen crosslinks	U	−20°C	10–26	28–58
Free PYD (immunoactive)	Free collagen crosslinks	U	−20°C	10–27	28–76
Deoxypyridinoline (DPD) (HPLC)	Free and peptide-bound collagen crosslinks	U	−20°C	12–63	34–174
Free (DPD) (immunoactive)	Free collagen crosslinks	U	−20°C	9–20	26–54
Type I collagen telopeptide:					
N-terminal (NTX)	All peptide bound forms of type I collagen	U S	−20°C −70°C	16–33 17–21	43–92 47–59
C-terminal (CTX)		U S	−20°C −70°C	48 12–21	133 33–58
C-terminal generated by MMPs (ICTP or CTX-MMP)		S	−20°C	10	27
Hydroxylysine (Hyl)	Amino acid product of type I collagen degradation	U	−20°C	10	27
Tartrate-resistant acid phosphatase (TRAP)	Osteoclastic enzyme	S	−70°C	11	31

reaching a plateau after several months. Drugs that stimulate de novo bone formation, such as parathyroid hormone or fluoride, cause markers of bone formation to increase within days of administration.

Markers of Bone Formation

The markers of bone formation include the enzyme bone-specific alkaline phosphatase (bone ALP), osteocalcin (OC), a small non-collagenous protein, and fragments of type I collagen: procollagen type I C propeptide (PICP) and procollagen type I N propeptide (PINP). ALP is found in various tissues including liver, kidney, and bone. After synthesis, ALP undergoes different degrees of glycosylation, which enables bone-specific ALP (bone ALP) produced by osteoblasts to be quantified separately from ALP of hepatic origin. Although bone ALP immunoassays have a high specificity, there remains a 15% to 20% cross-reactivity with liver ALP.

OC (or bone gla-protein) is synthesized by osteoblasts and subsequently modified by a vitamin K–dependent reaction. It represents 1% of the organic bone matrix where it binds to hydroxyapatite crystals. Although its precise function remains unclear, it appears to relate to osteoblast synthetic activity and bone remodeling. In most patients, OC reflects total bone turnover, both resorption and formation. OC is rapidly degraded in serum into different fragments. Difficulties comparing results between studies arise because of the heterogeneity in OC fragments, the different types of assays, and the instability of the OC molecule.

Osteoblasts secrete type I procollagen. Subsequent cleavage of large fragments from the carboxy and amino terminal ends result in the formation of mature type I collagen and the production of the PICP and PINP fragments. PICP correlates weakly with bone formation rate by histomorphometry, with a significant contribution from type I collagen synthesis in tissues besides bone. PINP appears to exist in intact trimeric and smaller monomeric forms. Assays detecting both forms of PINP show variable sensitivity, specificity, and responsiveness to bone turnover in different models but are more promising than intact PICP.

Markers of Bone Resorption

The markers of bone resorption are clinically more useful and include the pyridinium crosslinks of type I collagen (DPD and PYD) and the telopeptides of type I collagen (NTX and CTX) (Fig. 3-1). PYD and DPD are pyridinium crosslinks that are formed between neighboring mature collagen molecules during the extracellular maturation of collagen fibrils. They are not reused after collagen degradation and are excreted in urine as peptide-bound (60%) and free (40%) forms. PYD is present in many skeletal tissues, including

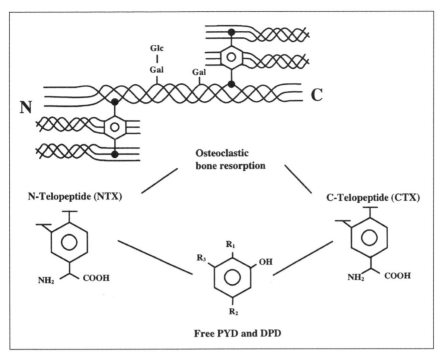

Figure 3-1   Type 1 collagen is broken down by osteoclasts to release telopeptides (NTX, CTX) and pyridinoline (PYD, DPD) breakdown products as markers of bone resorption.

cartilage, bone, ligaments, and skeletal muscle, whereas DPD occurs only in bone and dentin. DPD is a more specific marker of bone resorption. In postmenopausal osteoporosis, urinary DPD correlates with the rate of bone resorption that is estimated by bone biopsy and calcium kinetics.

The type I collagen telopeptides are small peptides that contain PYD and DPD groups that have been isolated in both urine and serum. They are called N-terminal telopeptide of type I collagen (NTX) and C-terminal telopeptide of type I collagen (CTX). Both NTX and CTX show a significant response to antiresorptive therapy and are currently considered the best indices of bone resorption. Several other types of bone markers are used less frequently in clinical practice (Table 3-1) (1,2).

Use and Interpretation of Bone Turnover Markers

Markers of bone turnover can be used for several purposes: 1) predicting the future rate of bone loss, 2) predicting the risk of osteoporotic fractures, and 3) monitoring response to treatment. Bone turnover markers cannot be used to diagnose osteoporosis. Studies to date demonstrate that bone turnover markers have been most helpful in attempting to monitor response to treatment. These studies are reviewed in the following sections.

Predicting Rate of Postmenopausal Bone Loss

At menopause, there is an increase in bone turnover, and bone is resorbed faster than it is formed. This results in an increased rate of bone loss leading to low bone density and an increased fracture risk. In general, women who have the highest rates of bone resorption tend to have higher rates of bone loss (3). However, the ability of bone turnover markers that are measured at baseline to predict the subsequent change in bone mineral density has been variable even in large prospective studies (Table 3-2) (2). For example, one study found that women whose markers of bone resorption were above the median had a 56% to 72% chance of bone loss at the hip greater than 1.1% per year (4). However, about half of those with values that are below the median bone marker value also lost bone at the faster rate. In another large prospective study, postmenopausal women with markers of bone resorption above the upper limit of the premenopausal range had a 35% to 56% chance

Table 3-2   Predicting Rate of Postmenopausal Bone Loss

Bone Marker	Correlation (r) of Baseline Bone Marker with Change in Bone Mineral Density		
	Spine BMD	Hip BMD	Wrist BMD
Bone Formation Markers			
Bone specific alkaline phosphatase (bone ALP)	+ 0.03 to + 0.11	+ 0.05 to + 0.19	− 0.11
Osteocalcin (OC)	− 0.21 to + 0.03	− 0.03 to + 0.12	− 0.19 to − 0.59
Serum N-terminal propeptide of type I collagen (PINP)			− 0.03
Serum C-terminal propeptide of type I collagen (PICP)	− 0.47 to + 0.09	+ 0.04	+ 0.02
Bone Resorption Markers			
Urine deoxypyridinoline (DPD)	− 0.34 to + 0.08	− 0.18 to + 0.13	− 0.46
Urine pyridinoline (PYD)	− 0.45 to + 0.08	0.00 to + 0.09	− 0.34
Urine CTX	+ 0.23	+ 0.05 to + 0.08	− 0.61 to − 0.14
Serum CTX			− 0.17
Urine NTX	+ 0.20	+ 0.11 to + 0.15	− 0.19
Urine hydroxyproline (Hyp)	+ 0.15		− 0.45 to − 0.44

Modified from Looker AC, Bauer D, Chesnut III CH, et al. Clinical use of biochemical markers of bone remodelling: current status and future directions. Osteoporos Int. 2000;11:467–480.

of bone loss at the forearm of greater than 0.9% per year, whereas 16% to 36% of women with normal levels of markers lost bone at that rate (5).

The use of markers to predict long-term bone loss would be a valuable way to identify high-risk patients. However, to be clinically useful, markers should be proven to accurately predict bone loss in individual patients at the important fracture sites of the hip and spine (6).

Predicting Fracture Risk

Biochemical markers of bone resorption appear to predict the risk of hip fractures in elderly women independently of bone density. Increased bone resorption may increase fracture risk by increasing the rate of bone loss by disrupting trabecular connectivity or by increasing the number of remodeling sites that could act as areas of weakness and enable fracture propagation. Most studies have found that women with a high level of bone resorption have about a 1.5- to 3-fold increased risk of hip or non-spine fractures. The combination of a marker of bone resorption and a measurement of BMD seems to predict hip fracture better than either test alone. For example, in the EPIDOS study, 16% of subjects had both a low BMD (T score < –2.5) and an elevated urinary CTX (T score > 2 SD mean premenopausal women). In these subjects, there was a 4-fold increased risk of hip fracture compared with a 2-fold increased risk for either a low BMD or a high urinary CTX (7).

The evidence for bone formation markers as predictors of fracture is less consistent (Table 3-3). In one study, OC and bone ALP were not predictive of hip fracture; however, two other studies reported up to a 2-fold increase in fracture risk in women with high levels of bone ALP. Other studies have shown that undercarboxylated OC is associated with a 2-fold increase in hip fracture risk (8,9).

Predicting Response to Treatment

Results of bone markers taken before starting a treatment do not appear to be valuable predictors of an individual patient's chance of responding to treatment. It is also not clear if patients with high bone turnover are more likely to gain bone during treatment. There are currently no data demonstrating the baseline level of a marker before treatment can predict whether treatment will prevent fractures.

Monitoring Response to Treatment

In groups of people in trials, treatments that reduce bone turnover improve BMD. These studies have found a modest correlation ($r = -0.2$ to 0.4) between decreases in various markers of bone turnover and improvements in bone density during treatment.

Table 3-3   Prospective Studies of Bone Turnover Markers and Fracture Risk

Bone Marker	Referent Criteria	Age-Adjusted Relative Risk of Hip Fracture (Confidence Interval)	Age-Adjusted Relative Risk of Incident Vertebral Fracture (Confidence Interval)	Age-Adjusted Relative Risk of Nonspine Fracture (Confidence Interval)
Bone Formation Markers				
Bone specific alkaline phosphatase (bone ALP)	Below upper limit of premenopausal	1.1 (0.7–1.7)		
	Below median	1.0 (0.4–2.5)		1.1 (0.7–1.7)
	Per SD increase	1.1 (0.7–1.7)	1.1 (0.7–1.7)	
	Per SD increase		1.5 (1.1–2.1)	
Osteocalcin (OC)	Below upper limit of premenopausal	1.0 (0.7–1.6)		
	Below median	0.3 (0.1–1.0)		1.1 (0.7–1.7)
	Per SD increase	1.1 (0.9–1.3)	1.0 (0.8–1.3)	
Undercarboxylated osteocalcin (ucOC)	Below upper limit of premenopausal	1.8 (1.0–3.0)		
	Below upper limit of premenopausal	3.1 (1.7–6.0)		
Serum propeptide of type I collagen (PICP)	Per SD increase			0.6 ($p = 0.02$)
Bone Resorption Markers				
Urine free deoxy-pyridinoline (DPD) by ELISA	Below upper limit of premenopausal	1.9 (1.1–3.2)		
	Below median	3.9 (1.3–11.9)		1.7 (1.0–2.7)
Urine free DPD by HPLC	Below median	3.4 (1.1–10.6)		
Urine total DPD	Below median	1.4 (0.5–4.0)		1.6 (1.0–2.6)
Urine free pyridi-noline (PYD)	Below median	3.7 (1.2–11.3)		1.2 (0.7–1.9)
Urine total PYD	Below median	2.6 (0.9–7.6)		1.8 (1.1–2.9)
Urine CTX	Below upper limit of premenopausal	2.2 (1.3–3.6)		
Urine NTX	Below upper limit of premenopausal	1.4 (0.9–2.2)		
Serum CTX	Per SD increase	1.0 (0.9–1.3)	1.1 (0.9–1.3)	
Serum cross-linked C-telopeptide (ICTP)	Per SD increase			0.5 ($p = 0.02$)

Modified from Looker AC, Bauer D, Chesnut III CH, et al. Clinical use of biochemical markers of bone remodelling: current status and future directions. Osteoporos Int 2000;11:467–480.

Several studies have found that postmenopausal women with the largest decreases in markers of bone resorption during treatment with alendronate or hormone replacement therapy (HRT) tend to have the greatest increases in BMD. For example, one study (10) found that, among women whose urine NTX level decreased by at least 30% after 6 months of HRT, 89% gained BMD, whereas 41% of women with smaller decreases in NTX still gained BMD. The greatest change in bone markers from baseline to 6 months was associated with the greatest increase in BMD in response to HRT at 1 year. Another study (11) using alendronate demonstrated that a 50% reduction in bone markers at 6 months compared with baseline was predictive of change in BMD. For example, if a woman had a greater than 50% decrease in serum CTX or urine NTX, she had a 78% to 89% chance of gaining BMD at the lumbar spine after 2 years. Among women with changes of less than 50% decrease, in CTX or NTX, 19% to 29% gained BMD.

Many bone specialists and clinicians use markers to help determine whether a patient is responding to treatment. However, changes in markers during treatment need to be interpreted with care. For a measurement to be useful in making decisions about individual patients, it is important to be sure that any change in that measurement is really because of the effects of the treatment and not just variability in the test. Markers of bone turnover, especially those measured in urine, have substantial day-to-day variability (12). A marker may change between 10% and 60% because of normal day-to-day variations in the patient's status and changes in the performance of the test. The large biological variation in bone turnover markers may mask the effects of treatment. This effect is particularly important in the clinical assessment of an individual patient compared with population data obtained in the clinical trial setting (5). A correct interpretation of an individual's response to treatment, using either BMD or bone turnover markers, requires the calculation of a statistically significant change (Table 3-1).

One approach to determine whether the change in the patient's test results has occurred by chance is to compare the results in the patient with the least significant change (LSC) for that test. The LSC is the minimum change that must be seen in an individual patient to be at least 95% sure that the change is "real," that is, not caused by biological and laboratory variations in the measurements (Fig. 3-2) (13). The LSC is approximately 25% for most formation markers and 40% to 65% for most resorption markers (see Table 3-1) (2,14).

Approximately 65% of patients who take estrogen or bisphosphonates such as risedronate or alendronate have changes that are larger than the LSC for bone resorption markers. In contrast, raloxifene and calcitonin typically produce smaller changes in bone resorption, and therefore fewer patients taking these agents will have changes in markers that are larger than the LSC.

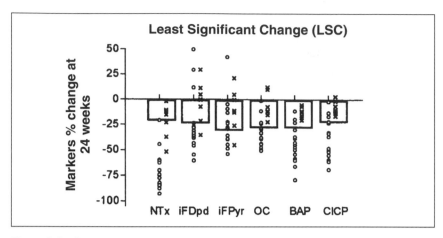

Figure 3-2 Boxes indicate least significant change (LSC). Individuals are shown taking alendronate (○) and calcium (×). The LSC is calculated for duplicate measurements as $2+CV_{ita}$; CV_i is the within subject coefficient of variation; CV_a is the analytical coefficient of variation. Responders are defined below the boxes for LSC. (From Fraser CG, Harris EK. Generation and application of data on biological variation in clinical chemistry. Crit Rev Clin Lab Sci. 1989;27:409–437; with permission.)

In comparison with the large LSC values for markers, the LSC for lumbar spine BMD is 3%, and the LSC for hip BMD is 5%. But even with bisphosphonates, few patients have changes in BMD that are this large during the first year of treatment. Therefore, the percentage change expected for BMD is small compared with the precision error of the measurement (see Chapter 2).

Patients may benefit from substantial reductions in risk of fracture even if they do not have reductions in bone markers or improvements in bone density that are expected or that exceed the LSC (2). Therefore, failure to exceed the LSC in a marker should not, by itself, lead to a change in treatment. However, if a patient has little or no change while taking drugs that are expected to substantially reduce turnover, it is important to carefully check that he or she is taking the medication and, in the case of bisphosphonates, taking it at least 30 minutes before eating or drinking anything but tap water (see Chapter 9); check that there are no secondary causes of osteoporosis.

Monitoring treatment with markers has the advantage that changes in levels can be observed within weeks or months of starting therapy, a time when patients are most likely to discontinue drug treatments (Fig. 3-3) (12,14). The measurement of a marker of bone turnover early in treatment may increase long-term adherence to treatment. Unfortunately, studies determining whether compliance is improved by monitoring treatment have not yet been performed. One recent study noted that a change in bone turnover markers at 6 months could be used to monitor future fracture risk in patients

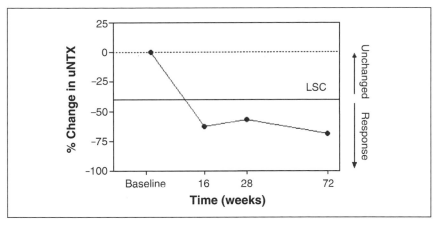

Figure 3-3   Monitoring of bone marker response to antiresorptive agents. The change in bone marker is calculated as the percentage change from baseline. A decrease in bone turnover below the least significant change (LSC) is regarded as a statistically significant response to treatment.

treated with raloxifene therapy. Thus, patients with a 1 SD decrease in OC (8.9 µg/L) or bone ALP (5.5 µg/L) had a 26% and 27% reduction in incident vertebral fracture risk over 3 years. No relationship between the change in BMD and future vertebral fracture risk was identified (15).

If markers are used to monitor a patient's response to antiresorptive therapy, it is important that the specimens are taken at about the same time of day and with the patient in a fasting state. Measuring the marker twice at the start of treatment and twice again at the follow-up visit and comparing the average of these two pairs of measurements can reduce the variability of the test results (Table 3-4). Markers can be used in conjunction with BMD measurements that are made at 1 to 2 years to help determine if a patient is experiencing the changes expected during a particular treatment, but it is not yet clear what patterns of changes in these measurements indicate that the patient is benefiting from treatment or whether the treatment should be changed.

Effect of Biological Variability on the Interpretation of Bone Turnover Marker Results

It is important in the clinical use of bone turnover markers to understand the effect of different sources of biological variability on the interpretation of the results, particularly for an individual patient. Most bone markers have a circadian rhythm with the highest values of bone turnover markers seen in the early morning and the lowest at night, with amplitudes of between ±15% to 30%.

Table 3-4   Practical Considerations in Monitoring Response to Antiresorptive Therapy

Practical Considerations	Current Best Practice		Rationale/Comments
Bone turnover marker	Resorption:	U-NTX, U-CTX, S-CTX, S-NTX, free U-DPD	Consider one resorption and one formation marker
	Formation:	OC, Bone ALP, PINP	
Timing of sample	Serum:	Fasting morning (before 10:00)	Marked circadian variation requires standardized timing of samples
	Urine:	Fasting first or second morning void	Dietary intake may change
Baseline measurement	Urine:	Ideally greater than 1 measurement	Urine markers have a greater variability
	Serum:	Ideally greater than 1 measurement	Multiple samples can reduce variability
Stability	Urine:	Room temperature	Serum markers (particularly OC) are unstable at room temperature
	Serum:	Freeze rapidly	
Sample handling	Avoid hemolysis		For serum samples allow 30 minutes before centrifuging sample
Storage temperature	−20°C		Serum requires long-term (greater than 1 month) storage at −70°C
Follow-up time point for sample measurement (monitoring)	Resorption:	3 months	The nadir for change in resorption markers is 3 months and in formation markers 6 months
	Formation:	6 months	
Treatment goal during monitoring	Change greater than the LSC change for the bone marker Suppress bone marker into the lower half of the premenopausal reference range		Based on association with vertebral fractures

Therefore, it is crucial to control the timing of sample collection. In clinical practice, we currently recommend obtaining a fasting serum sample before 10 a.m. For urinalysis, a fasting first or second void sample with a correction for creatinine is recommended (1). Urine bone resorption markers have a greater day-to-day variability, which may partially arise due to difficulties encountered in obtaining an accurately timed urine sample. To reduce variability, especially for urine samples, it may therefore be useful to obtain more than one measurement before initiating treatment (1). Biological variability also arises from seasonal changes, the effects of growth, aging, gender, and sex hormone status. As a result, local reference ranges are required for each assay at different ages, with different ranges for men and women. Finally, bone markers demonstrate varying stability and require careful sample collection, handling, and storage (Tables 3-1 and 3-4). It is important to note that, even with careful standardization of collection, there is substantial variability in the results in individual patients.

Diseases and treatments that affect bone also influence the levels of markers. Bone turnover markers are generally increased during growth, pregnancy, in metabolic bone diseases (e.g., Paget's, osteomalacia, primary hyperparathyroidism, thyrotoxicosis), and for up to 12 months after a fracture. However, turnover markers may be low during corticosteroid therapy and during antiresorptive therapy.

It would be useful to estimate the net amount of bone being formed by comparing measurements of markers of resorption and formation. Unfortunately, it is not possible to make a direct comparison between results of formation and resorption markers because of marked differences in the sensitivity, specificity, and width of the reference ranges for each assay. Inaccurate conclusions may result if clinicians attempt to calculate an estimation of net excess of resorption over formation (15).

Summary: Using Markers of Bone Turnover in Clinical Practice

It may be useful in some older women to measure a marker of bone resorption to determine whether she has an increased bone turnover because this appears to be another independent risk factor for hip fracture. However, measuring a marker of bone turnover before initiating therapy is not a reliable way to predict whether a patient will have an improvement in bone density during treatment with antiresorptive drugs. Markers are sometimes measured before treatment and then a few weeks to months later to monitor response. The change in marker observed may help to determine whether a patient is responding and adhering to treatment. If markers are used for this purpose, careful attention must be paid to standardized collection of specimens. Some changes in markers may be caused by variability in the markers, and treatment should generally not be altered just because of disappointing changes in a marker.

Laboratory Testing for Secondary Osteoporosis

Who Should Be Evaluated?

The utility of testing for secondary causes of osteoporosis in primary care has not been extensively studied, nor have algorithms for the evaluation of osteoporosis in men or women been systematically developed or evaluated. Therefore, recommendations on which groups of patients to evaluate and which investigations to perform are based on clinical experience and the epidemiology of osteoporosis.

It is important to note that 20% of women and up to 64% of men presenting to specialists or metabolic bone clinics with osteoporosis have diseases that are linked to osteoporosis (16). In primary care, the prevalence of secondary osteoporosis among patients is not known; however, it is likely to be significantly less than that found in secondary care. Furthermore, osteoporosis is common among postmenopausal white and Asian women, so contributing conditions are likely to be identified less frequently in these particular groups. Most women with osteoporosis who are seen by primary care physicians will have primary osteoporosis.

Nevertheless, it is important to perform a focused history and physical examination in patients presenting with osteoporosis, which should concentrate on identifying risk factors for falls and problems relating to the patient's activities of daily living. In addition, secondary causes of osteoporosis should be looked for in patients presenting with unusual clinical features (Table 3-5). Physicians who have limited training and experience in evaluating patients for secondary

Table 3-5   Characteristics That Should Prompt Investigation for Secondary Causes of Osteoporosis

Clinical Presentation and Type of Fracture	No Evaluation Required	Basic Evaluation	Full Evaluation
Wrist, foot, humeral and ankle fractures	All		
Rib fractures (low trauma)			All
Vertebral fractures (low trauma)		All	Men; black and Latino women Any white women under age 50 Vertebral fractures above T4 including the cervical vertebrae
Hip fractures (low trauma)		All	Men; black and Latino women
BMD criteria		Patients with ongoing bone loss ≥ 5% per year, despite therapy)	Consider testing in patients with Z scores ≤ −2.0
Specific clinical symptoms or signs with a low BMD (T score ≤ −1.0) or osteoporotic fractures		Specific investigations based on clinical presentation	

osteoporosis may prefer to refer unusual cases to a local expert in osteoporosis or metabolic bone disease. Even a primary care physician who is comfortable with screening for secondary osteoporosis should consult with an expert about young women or men who have severe osteoporosis or vertebral fractures. These patients probably have a relatively high prevalence of rare diseases, and there may be long-lasting consequences of overlooking a treatable cause.

What Types of Fracture Cases Warrant Evaluation?

Rib and Vertebral Fractures

Rib fractures that happen with little or no trauma suggest pathologies such as Cushing's syndrome, metastatic cancer, or alcoholism. Vertebral fractures that occur with little or no trauma at levels above T4, including cervical vertebrae, are unusual, and a fracture in these vertebrae should prompt an investigation for metastatic cancer or myeloma in all patients, regardless of age. In women and men under age 50, vertebral fractures that occur with little or no trauma are also uncommon, and if osteoporosis is identified, they should be evaluated with a full assessment for secondary causes of osteoporosis (see the section "Which Tests are Worthwhile?" later in this chapter). Even, or especially, if patients with a vertebral fracture have normal or modestly decreased bone density, they should be screened for metastatic cancer and myeloma.

Men have a lower risk of vertebral fractures and are more likely to have a secondary cause of osteoporosis. Alcoholism and cigarette smoking seem to be strong risk factors for clinically diagnosed vertebral fractures in men. These risk factors should be sought and treated in men. Patients who despite therapy sustain two or more vertebral fractures probably warrant a comprehensive laboratory evaluation for all potential causes of secondary osteoporosis.

All patients with a low trauma vertebral fracture warrant basic laboratory evaluation for secondary causes of osteoporosis (see Which Tests Are Worthwhile? below). This is probably sufficient in elderly women (over age 70), with one or two vertebral fractures in common locations (T4 through L4) and a typical appearance on radiograph. In addition, vertebral fractures are quite common in white and Asian elderly women, especially those with low bone density. Therefore, primary osteoporosis is more likely.

Hip Fractures

The risk of hip fractures is increased by many conditions that can be treated, including impaired vision and chronic diseases that cause frailty and impaired mobility. In women with hip fractures, it is reasonable to examine the patient for treatable risk factors and chronic illnesses (see Chapter 13, Case 5) and consider performing a basic laboratory evaluation to screen for more common secondary causes.

Men and black and Latino women have a much lower risk of hip fractures than white women do. More than half of men who suffer hip fractures have a chronic illness that may have contributed to the fracture, most commonly neurologic diseases such as Parkinson's disease or a history of stroke and gastrointestinal diseases such as malabsorption. Therefore, a man (and probably a black or Latino woman) presenting with a hip fracture warrants examination for risk factors and chronic illnesses and probably a "full" laboratory evaluation for secondary osteoporosis.

Wrist, Foot, Ankle, or Humeral Fractures
The occurrence of a common fracture, such as a wrist, foot, ankle, or humeral fracture does not by itself warrant evaluation for pathologic bone disease or secondary causes of osteoporosis.

When Does Low Bone Density Warrant Evaluation?

Z scores are based on comparison of the patient's bone density with the bone density of other patients of the same age. Therefore, in older patients (who commonly have low T scores in comparison with young adults) the Z score is a better guide than the T score to how unusual the patient's bone density is for her (or his) age and gender. By definition, a Z score below –2.0 is found in fewer than 3% of adults and a score below a –3.0 in less than 1%. It is likely that the lower the Z score, the greater is the probability of finding important secondary causes of osteoporosis; thus, it might be worthwhile to perform a basic screening evaluation for common causes of secondary osteoporosis in those with Z scores below –2.0 and a more comprehensive evaluation for the more unusual cases with more extreme osteoporosis (Z scores below –3.0).

Osteoporosis (T score below –2.5 compared with normals of the same gender) is quite common in otherwise healthy older women. The value of a laboratory evaluation for secondary causes of osteoporosis in these patients is currently uncertain. If testing, it is reasonable to screen for general evidence of a chronic disease by asking about changes in weight, bowel habits, or systemic symptoms, and to ask carefully about alcohol abuse. In addition, the clinician may screen for common and potentially treatable causes of low bone density, such as hyperthyroidism and hyperparathyroidism, and perform basic screening laboratory tests. If abnormalities are found, these should be pursued in focused workups for specific secondary causes. For example, a finding of an elevated serum calcium should lead to an evaluation for hyperparathyroidism.

Patients who despite therapy continue to lose bone density that exceeds 5% per year during at least two consecutive periods of monitoring (if bone density is monitored) probably warrant basic screening tests for secondary causes of osteoporosis.

Screening for secondary osteoporosis is probably not worthwhile for women or men who only have osteopenia (bone density T score of −1.0 to −2.5) or with osteoporosis (T score of −2.5) in which the result is within the normal range for their age (Z score above −2.0).

Which Tests Are Worthwhile?

Conditions associated with osteoporosis and specific tests that may be useful to identify these conditions are listed in Tables 3-6 and 3-7. A "basic" screening evaluation should include measurements of calcium levels, renal function, liver function, and thyroid-stimulating hormone, and a complete blood count. In addition, either an erythrocyte sedimentation rate (ESR) (nonspecific) or serum and urine immunoelectrophoresis might be considered for myeloma. If the initial evaluation identifies abnormalities that warrant further investigation, or if there are unusual clinical features suggesting secondary osteoporosis, these abnormalities will help to guide a focused evaluation for specific secondary causes.

A "full" or comprehensive evaluation should include alkaline phosphatase, 24-hour urine calcium (to screen for malabsorption and hypercalciuria), parathyroid hormone (PTH) (primary and secondary hyperparathyroidism), serum and urine immunoelectrophoresis (myeloma), and testosterone and sex hormone binding globulin (SHBG) in all men (hypogonadism) (17). If

Table 3-6   Association Between Clinical Conditions and Risk of Osteoporosis or Fractures*

Clinical Condition	Risk Factor for Osteoporosis	Risk Factor for Fracture
Celiac disease	++	?
Crohn's disease	+	+
Hyperthyroidism	+	+
Hypogonadism males (females)	++ (++)	++ (++)
Hyperparathyroidism	++	+
Myeloma	+	++
Hemochromatosis	+	−
Alcoholic liver disease	+	?
Chronic renal failure	+	−
Cushing's syndrome	+	+
Systemic mastocytosis	+	?

* A strong association is shown by ++, a moderate association by +, inconclusive evidence by ?, and a lack of convincing or insufficient evidence by −.

Table 3-7   Laboratory Tests for the Identification of Secondary Osteoporosis

Basic Investigations	Clinical Condition	Additional Laboratory Tests to Consider
Complete blood count—hemoglobin (Hb)	Malabsorption	PTH 25(OH)D Serum magnesium Phosphate Antigliadin and endomysial antibodies Red cell folate, vitamin B_{12}, ferritin 24-hr urinary calcium
	Myeloma	Bone marrow biopsy Serum and urine protein electrophoresis
Thyroid-stimulating hormone (TSH)	Hyperthyroidism	Thyroxine (T4) Tri-iodothyronine (T3)
Testosterone (T) in men	Hypogonadism	SHBG LH FSH Prolactin
Serum calcium (Ca)	Hyperparathyroidism	PTH
	Malabsorption	Complete blood count PTH 25(OH)D Serum magnesium Phosphate Antigliadin and endomysial antibodies Red cell folate, vitamin B_{12}, ferritin 24-hr urinary calcium
	Osteomalacia	PTH 25(OH)D
Alkaline phosphatase (ALP)	Chronic renal failure	PTH Phosphate
	Osteomalacia	PTH 25(OH)D Serum calcium
Serum and urine protein electrophoresis	Myeloma	Complete blood count Bone marrow biopsy
Liver function—GGT, AST, ALT, ALP	Hemochromatosis	Serum iron Total iron binding capacity (TIBC) Ferritin
	Primary biliary cirrhosis Alcoholic liver disease	Serum immunoglobulins Antimitochondrial antibody, M antibody

Table cont'd.

Table 3-7   Laboratory Tests for the Identification of Secondary Osteoporosis (Cont'd.)

Basic Investigations	Clinical Condition	Additional Laboratory Tests to Consider
Creatinine (Cr)	Chronic renal failure	Alkaline phosphatase PTH Phosphate
24-hour urinary calcium	Malabsorption	Complete blood count PTH 25(OH)D Serum magnesium Phosphate Antigliadin and endomysial antibodies Red cell folate, vitamin B_{12}, ferritin
	Osteomalacia	Fasting urinary calcium PTH 25(OH)D Serum calcium Alkaline phosphatase
	Hyperparathyroidism	PTH Serum calcium
	Idiopathic hypercalciuria	

PTH, parathyroid hormone; 25(OH)D, 25-hydroxyvitamin D; SHBG, sex hormone binding globulin; LH, luteinizing hormone; FSH, follicle-stimulating hormone; γGT, gamma glutamyl-transferase; AST, aspartate aminotransferase; ALT, alanine aminotransferase.

specifically indicated on clinical assessment or previous laboratory tests, rare cases may require measurement of luteinizing hormone (LH), follicle-stimulating hormone (FSH), prolactin (causes of hypogonadism), ferritin (hemochromatosis), urinary cortisol (Cushing's syndrome), gliadin and endomysial antibodies (celiac), and urinary histamine levels (mastocytosis).

If a secondary cause of osteoporosis is identified, it is worth discussing it with the patient and a local expert in osteoporosis or metabolic bone disease, or arranging for a referral. Management is frequently altered by the identification of specific disease processes, and a more comprehensive evaluation may be required. A discussion of the more common tests follows.

Measurement of Sex Hormones

Testosterone

Testosterone deficiency is found in 30% of osteoporotic men and is believed to be a risk factor for hip fractures. Testosterone and SHBG should be measured in all male patients with osteoporosis to elucidate the cause of osteoporosis. Many experts recommend treating those who have a low testosterone level with testosterone replacement therapy rather than with antiresorptive therapy. However, the exact testosterone level that is used to define hypogonadism and determine subsequent treatment is controversial. Some believe, however, that testosterone serves mainly as a source of substrate for estradiol in men. It is important to note that the testosterone level is not a useful guide to whether a man will respond to bisphosphonate therapy: alendronate improves bone density to the same degree in men with low or normal testosterone levels.

Estradiol

Estrogen has a powerful influence on the skeleton of women and men (18). In most studies, premature ovarian failure (before 40 years) and an early menopause (between 40 and 45 years) are associated with increased fracture risk and low bone density, irrespective of the cause. Among older women, undetectable levels of estradiol using very sensitive assays (<5 pg/mL) are associated with low bone density and an increased risk of hip and vertebral fracture. It is not clear, however, whether these patients benefit more from prescription of estrogen than from treatment with other antiresorptive drugs and, therefore, routine measurement of estradiol levels in women and men with osteoporosis or fractures is not yet indicated. In addition, the measurement of estradiol in patients on oral or transdermal HRT to assess response is not indicated.

Gonadotropins and Prolactin

The most common cause of osteoporosis is the loss of ovarian function after menopause and the decline in testicular function in aging men. Hypogonadism is divided into hypogonadotropic hypogonadism (or hypothalamopituitary pathology) with decreased LH, FSH or very high prolactin or into hypergonadotropic (primary) hypogonadism with increased LH, FSH, and normal prolactin. Hyperprolactinemia does not cause osteoporosis unless it is also accompanied by hypogonadism. There is no evidence that the degree of elevation of FSH or LH in menopausal women has any value for assessing risk of fracture or response to hormone therapy. Therefore, these tests should not generally be ordered in postmenopausal women. These tests are of value mainly in investigating the cause of hypogonadism in all men or women under age 40 and for confirming menopause in middle-aged women who have had a hysterectomy.

Measurement of Calcium Homeostasis

Serum Calcium

In greater than 90% of cases in primary care, hypercalcemia is caused by primary hyperparathyroidism or, less commonly, malignancy. If serum calcium is elevated on at least two repeated tests, patients should have a measurement of PTH.

24-Hour Urinary Calcium
The 24-hour excretion of calcium is commonly assessed in patients with osteoporosis. However, the relationship between the excretion of calcium in a 24-hour urine collection, bone density, and risk of fractures is not known. A very low urinary calcium (less then 100 mg/day or 2.5 mmol/day) may suggest malabsorption and should prompt further investigations such as PTH, 25-hydroxyvitamin D 25(OH)D, gliadin, and endomysial antibodies. Idiopathic hypercalciuria may be associated with a low bone density, especially in men. Some of these patients may benefit from treatment with a thiazide diuretic. In addition, the most common cause of renal calculi is hypercalciuria. In such patients, it is reasonable to measure a 24-hour urine assessment before prescribing calcium therapy.

Vitamin D Metabolites
The results of studies have found that low levels of active metabolites of vitamin D ($1,25(OH)_2D_3$) or a combination of low $1,25(OH)_2D_3$ and high PTH, indicating secondary hyperparathyroidism, are not consistently important risk factors for hip fracture. There is also no evidence that treatment with calcitriol, or other analogues of vitamin D, will improve bone mass or decrease fracture risk in patients with low levels of $1,25(OH)_2D_3$. Therefore, there is little or no role for measurement of active metabolites of vitamin D in the primary care setting.

Alkaline Phosphatase
Increased levels of total ALP occur most commonly in liver disease and bone disease, including bone metastasis, hyperparathyroidism, Paget's disease, osteomalacia, and fractures. Note that patients with fractures rarely have total ALP levels that are greater than double the normal range. The measurement of bone ALP is of most value if the patient is suspected of having active Paget's disease despite having a normal total ALP or if a metabolic bone disease is suspected in the presence of mildly abnormal liver and biliary function with no obvious cause. In primary care, it is relatively common to find patients who have elevated alkaline phosphatase levels, and no detectable disease. In general, no further evaluation is required in asymptomatic patients with a high ALP after the common causes of metabolic bone disease and hepatobiliary dysfunction have been excluded.

Parathyroid Hormone
A normal serum calcium, reduced 25(OH)D (<12 ng/mL), and increased PTH (>65 pg/mL) are features of vitamin D insufficiency. Most physicians would treat these patients with calcium and vitamin D. There is, however, inconsistent evidence from prospective studies that women with high levels of PTH

and low levels of 25(OH)D have an increased risk of hip fracture or vertebral fracture.

Primary hyperparathyroidism is uncommon (1% or less of elderly patients in primary care settings). However, primary hyperparathyroidism is associated with decreased bone mass that increases after parathyroidectomy, and retrospective studies have suggested an increased risk of vertebral, forearm, and hip fractures. Because treatment of hyperparathyroidism may have other benefits, it is reasonable to measure calcium and PTH concentrations when testing for secondary causes of osteoporosis. An elevated PTH in the presence of renal impairment may suggest renal osteodystrophy and should be discussed with a specialist.

Other Tests

Thyroid-Stimulating Hormone for Hyperthyroidism

Abnormal thyroid-stimulating hormone (TSH) levels are found in about 5% of elderly adults, and treatment of hyperthyroidism or hypothyroidism may have several benefits. A current or previous history of hyperthyroidism has been associated with osteopenia and an 80% increased risk for hip fracture, but it is not certain whether the effects may be reversed with treatment. Studies have differed as to whether patients with a low TSH have more rapid bone loss and a greater risk of fractures. Despite these uncertainties, it seems reasonable to include a measurement of TSH when screening for common secondary causes of osteoporosis. In patients being treated for hypothyroidism or hyperthyroidism, TSH should be maintained within the normal range unless the patient has a thyroid carcinoma.

Protein Electrophoresis for Multiple Myeloma

When myeloma is suspected, serum protein electrophoresis and urine protein electrophoresis should be measured because approximately 15% of patients with myeloma have an isolated Bence Jones protein in urine with a normal serum protein electrophoresis. It is worth testing for myeloma even if the patient does not have lytic lesions that are typical of the disease. Although 60% of patients with myeloma have lytic lesions, approximately 20% have diffuse osteoporosis, and 20% have no radiologic evidence of the disease.

24-Hour Urine Cortisol for Cushing's Syndrome

Several negative 24-hour urine cortisol measurements may be used to exclude Cushing's syndrome, a rare condition. However, the most sensitive test to diagnose Cushing's syndrome is an overnight dexamethasone suppression test. The diagnosis should be considered in patients who have multiple vertebral fractures, especially if there are other features of the disease (hypertension, hypokalemia, diabetes). It may also be worth screening for Cushing's syndrome in men and young patients who have osteoporosis with vertebral fractures.

Gliadin and Endomysial Antibodies for Celiac Disease

Celiac disease is an uncommon disease that leads to malabsorption, which might in turn lead to decreased absorption of vitamin D and calcium, resulting in decreased bone density. It has been suggested that the prevalence of relatively asymptomatic celiac disease may be increased in patients with osteoporosis. It may be worthwhile to measure gliadin and endomysial antibodies as screening tests for celiac disease in young adults with osteoporosis and chronic diarrhea if there is clinical suspicion of malabsorption or in the presence of megaloblastic anemia. There are clinical reports that bone density can improve after patients with celiac disease are treated with a gluten-free diet.

24-Hour Urine Histamine for Systemic Mastocytosis

Systemic mastocytosis is a very rare disease that is classically associated with unusual bone lesions (sclerotic, lytic, or both) and diffuse osteoporosis. It could be considered in very unusual and severe cases of osteoporosis. Elevated tests for 24-hour histamine secretion, or histamine metabolites, must be followed by a bone marrow biopsy to confirm the diagnosis of systemic mastocytosis.

Summary: Screening for Secondary Causes of Osteoporosis

There have been no good-quality studies of the role of laboratory tests in investigating secondary causes of osteoporosis in patients. Low bone density and fractures are very common, especially in white women. However, primary care physicians should consider secondary causes of osteoporosis, particularly among patients who have unusual fractures, very low bone density for their age, vertebral fractures, or recurrent fractures despite adherence to effective drug treatment. In these patients, judicious use of laboratory testing may be useful. Primary care physicians who have limited experience with the evaluation of secondary osteoporosis may wish to refer some or all of these patients to a physician who specializes in osteoporosis or metabolic bone diseases.

REFERENCES

1. **Delmas PD, Eastell R, Garnero P, et al.** The use of biochemical markers of bone turnover in osteoporosis. Osteoporosis Int. 2000;11(Suppl 6):S2–S17.
2. **Looker AC, Bauer D, Chesnut CH III, et al.** Clinical use of biochemical markers of bone remodelling: current status and future directions. Osteoporosis Int. 2000;11:467–480.
3. **Rogers A, Hannon RA, Eastell R.** Biochemical markers as predictors of rates of bone loss after menopause. J Bone Miner Res. 2000;15:1398–1404.

4. **Bauer DC, Sklarin PM, Stone KL, et al.** Biochemical markers of bone turnover and prediction of hip bone loss in older women. The study of osteoporotic fractures. J Bone Miner Res. 1999;14:1404–1410.

5. **Garnero P, Sornay-Rendu E, Duboeuf F, Delmas PD.** Markers of bone turnover predict postmenopausal forearm bone loss over 4 years. The OFELY Study. J Bone Mineral Res. 1999;14:1614–1621.

6. **Blumsohn A, Eastell R.** The performance and utility of biochemical markers of bone turnover: do we know enough to use them in clinical practice? Ann Clin Biochem. 1997;34:449–459.

7. **Garnero P, Dargent-Molina P, Hans D, et al.** Do markers of bone resorption add to bone mineral density and ultrasonographic heel measurement for the prediction of hip fracture in elderly women? The EPIDOS Prospective Study. Osteoporosis Int. 1998;8:563–569.

8. **Szule P, Chapuy MC, Meunier PJ, Delmas PD.** Serum undercarboxylated osteocalcin is a marker of the risk of hip fracture. A three year follow-up study. Bone. 1996;18:487–488.

9. **Vergnaud P, Garnero P, Meunier PJ, et al.** Undercarboxylated osteocalcin measured with a specific immunoassay predicts hip fracture in elderly women. The EPIDOS Study. J Clin Endocrinol Metab. 1997;82:719–724.

10. **Rosen CJ, Chesnut CH, III, Mallinak NJ.** The predictive value of biochemical markers of bone turnover for bone mineral density in early postmenopausal women treated with hormone replacement or calcium supplementation. J Clin Endocrinol Metab. 1991;82:1904–1910.

11. **Ravin P, Clemmesen B, Christiansen C.** Biochemical markers can predict the response in bone mass during alendronate treatment in early postmenopausal women. Alendronate Osteoporosis Prevention Study Group. Bone. 1999;24:237–244.

12. **Hannon R, Blumsohn A, Naylor K, Eastell R.** Response of biochemical markers of bone turnover to hormone replacement therapy: impact of biological variability. J Bone Miner Res. 1998;13:1124–1133.

13. **Fraser CG, Harris EK.** Generation and application of data on biological variation in clinical chemistry. Crit Rev Clin Lab Sci. 1989;27:409–437.

14. **Braga de Castro Machado A, Hannon R, Eastell R.** Monitoring aledronate therapy for osteoporosis. J Bone Miner Res. 1999;14:602–608.

15. **Bjarnason NH, Sarkar S, Duong T, et al.** Six and 12 month changes in bone turnover are related to reduction in vertebral fracture risk during 3 years of raloxifene treatment in postmenopausal osteoporosis. Osteoporos Int. 2001;12:922–930.

16. **Harper KD, Weber TJ.** Secondary osteoporosis. Diagnostic considerations. Endocrinol Metab Clin North Am. 1998;27:325–348.

17. **Meunier PJ, Delmas PD, Eastell R, et al.** Diagnosis and management of osteoporosis in postmenopausal women: clinical guidelines. Clin Ther. 1999;21:1025–1044.

18. **Riggs BL, Khosla S, Melton LJ.** A unitary model for involutional osteoporosis: estrogen deficiency causes both type I and type II osteoporosis in postmenopausal women and contributes to bone loss in aging men. J Bone Miner Res. 1998;13:763–773.

Prevention and Treatment

CHAPTER 4

Nutrition

JERI NIEVES, PhD

Key Points

- Adequate calcium intake needs to be maintained throughout childhood, adolescence, and young adulthood to have a lasting impact on peak bone mass.

- Intakes of 1200 mg calcium and 400 to 600 IU vitamin D are needed in postmenopausal women and in men aged 51 and older.

- Total calcium intakes of at least 1200 mg daily (including calcium supplements, if necessary) can retard bone loss in postmenopausal women, particularly in elderly and late postmenopausal women.

- The recommended daily calcium intake probably maximizes the efficacy of other osteoporosis therapies, and it is advised for patients receiving these treatments.

- Vitamin D given in conjunction with calcium reduces fracture risk in patients with osteoporosis aged 65 years and older.

- Long-term heavy alcohol consumption might increase the risk of hip fracture; however, moderate intake of alcohol may slightly improve bone density and decrease fracture risk.

- Other nutrients such as magnesium and vitamin K might be important to bone health. Five servings per day of fruits and vegetables will meet the required intakes of these and other potentially important nutrients. The value of nutritional supplementation besides calcium and vitamin D has not been proven.

In this chapter, the role of nutrition in the prevention and treatment of osteoporosis is discussed. Because the primary nutrients are calcium and vitamin D, these will be the focus of the chapter. The dietary requirements for most other nutrients involved in bone health can be met by following the guidelines of the USDA, a diet with at least five servings per day of fruits and vegetables, with moderate intakes of meat and additional sources of dietary calcium. A discussion of phytoestrogens can be found in Chapter 8.

Calcium

Metabolism

Calcium is an essential nutrient that is involved in most metabolic processes and provides mechanical rigidity to the bones and teeth. Skeletal status is often equated with calcium nutrition because 99% of the calcium in the body is stored within the skeleton. To maintain normal metabolic activity, serum calcium concentration is maintained within narrow limits (range 2.1 to 2.6 mmol/L), a process controlled by parathyroid hormone, active vitamin D, and, to a lesser extent, calcitonin, with the skeleton acting as a reserve to meet the calcium needs. Calcium balance in the human is determined by intake, absorption, excretion (fecal and urinary), and incidental losses of calcium. Calcium balance is easily offset when obligatory losses of calcium in the bowel, kidney, and skin are not balanced by adequate calcium intake and absorption.

On average, an adult absorbs only 20% to 30% of the calcium in food or pills (1), but there is tremendous variation between people. In postmenopausal women and aging individuals, there is a decrease in active calcium absorption. Unabsorbed dietary calcium is eliminated in the feces; additional calcium may be secreted into the intestine and then excreted. Numerous factors can influence the amount of calcium available for absorption. Very high phosphorus-to-calcium ratios (3:1), oxalates, iron, phytates, caffeine, and vitamin D deficiency may interfere with calcium absorption, whereas lactose and vitamin D can improve absorption. The ways in which nutrients can alter calcium metabolism are shown in Table 4-1. However, in diets that are adequate in calcium intake, these nutrients have minimal effects on calcium retention in the skeleton.

Obligatory urinary calcium losses increase with menopause. Sodium intake is an important determinant of calcium excretion because sodium competes with calcium for reabsorption in the renal tubules. Every 2300 mg of sodium (approximately 1 teaspoon of salt) increases urine excretion by 23 mg of calcium. An additional dietary calcium intake of 230 to 460 mg is needed to compensate for this loss. A high ratio of animal to vegetable protein also

Table 4-1   Effects of Nutrients on Calcium and Bone Metabolism

	Increases Urine Calcium	Decreases Calcium Absorption
High protein	X	
High sodium	X	
Vitamin D deficiency		X
Oxalates (rhubarb, spinach)		X
Phytates (wheat, bran, beans)		X
Iron		X
High caffeine (>4 cups daily)		X

Table 4-2   Food and Nutrition Board Daily Recommended Average Intake for Calcium and Vitamin D

Age (Yr)	Calcium (mg)	Vitamin D (IU)
3–8	800	200
9–17	1300	200
18–50	1000	400
51–70	1200	400
> 70	1200	600

increases urinary calcium excretion, either because of increased urine acidity or because of phosphate and sulfite residues forming complexes with calcium. Both sodium and protein have the greatest effect on calcium excretion when calcium intake is low (2). Calcium loss can also occur through sweating.

Calcium and Bone Mass

Considerable epidemiologic data have been accumulated on the relationship between calcium intake and bone density. Peak bone mass, attained during adolescence, can be maximized by raising calcium intake to the adequate intake levels recommended by the 1997 Food and Nutrition Board (Table 4-2). Higher calcium intakes have been related to higher bone mass in children, young adults, and postmenopausal women in 64 out of 86 observational epidemiologic studies (2).

In children, calcium supplementation increases bone density between 1% and 6% per year in the total body and between 1% and 10% at each skeletal region compared with placebo (3–9), with results dependent on pubertal stage. Similarly, a meta-analysis of calcium intake in premenopausal women concluded that calcium supplementation led to an average increase in bone density at the spine and forearm of 1.1% per year compared with women receiving placebo (10). However, in most studies, the benefit of added calcium on bone mass disappears when supplementation is halted (3,11), although one trial showed a benefit persisting after 3 to 4 years (12). These data suggest that adequate calcium intake must be maintained throughout childhood, adolescence, and young adulthood to have a lasting impact on peak bone mass.

Reviews of 20 studies of postmenopausal women have concluded that calcium supplementation (500 to 2000 mg/day) can decrease bone loss by approximately 1% per year (Table 4-3) (1,13,14). Therefore, calcium supplementation can be effective in retarding bone loss in postmenopausal women. The beneficial effect of calcium intake on bone mass in postmenopausal women may be modified by factors including age, number of years since menopause, baseline calcium intake before supplementation, and, possibly, physical activity level. The greatest benefit of calcium supplementation is likely to be experienced by elderly and late postmenopausal women and in women with low-baseline calcium intakes.

Recommendations for Calcium Intake

The recommended total daily calcium intake changes with age. The current recommended intakes are listed in Table 4-2. These recommended amounts already take into account the influence of other dietary factors (Table 4-1) on calcium balance. The highest daily intakes are required during the adolescent growth period (ages 9 to 18) and after age 50. These calcium intakes can be achieved by dietary modification (three servings per day of calcium-rich foods) in most individuals, the preferred method of increasing calcium intake. Important dietary sources of calcium are dairy products (milk, yogurt, cheese), dark green vegetables, canned fish with bones (but not fish fillets), nuts, and, more recently, fortified foods (including juices, soy and rice milk, waffles, cereals, crackers, and snack foods). The diet of an average American contains only 600 mg of calcium per day, which falls far below the recommended intakes. Daily calcium intakes for individual patients can easily be calculated by following the formula given in Table 4-4. Calcium-fortified foods can add dramatically to total calcium intakes; however, the quantity added varies from 80 to 1000 mg per serving. If an adequate calcium intake is not possible in the diet, a calcium supplement may be required to meet the recommended intakes at any given age (Table 4-5).

How, When, and What Type of Calcium Supplements?

Ingesting a large amount of calcium at one time causes a decrease in the fraction of the calcium that is absorbed. Thus, taking calcium supplements in several smaller doses (less than 500 mg) during the day rather than all at once will increase the proportion of the calcium that is absorbed, but the effect is modest. The preferred time to take most supplements is with meals, because calcium is better absorbed in an acid environment (with the exception of calcium citrate). The rate of bone resorption tends to increase at night, and a few studies have indicated that calcium supplementation taken at night might reduce this nocturnal rise. Currently, there are insufficient data to specifically recommend nighttime administration of supplements.

Calcium carbonate has more calcium per tablet (40%) than some of the other forms of calcium such as calcium citrate (23%). Two studies from the same group indicating that calcium citrate may be more readily absorbed must be confirmed before recommending calcium citrate over less expensive calcium carbonate. Calcium citrate may be a preferred source for patients with achlorhydria or those on acid blockers. Some supplements that are marketed are not well absorbed. Patients should check their supplements to make sure that United States Pharmacopia (USP) is on the label; this ensures the solubility and purity of the preparation. An alternative, if the USP label is not seen, is to test whether the supplement dissolves after 30 minutes in clear vinegar.

Safety of Calcium Supplementation

In most healthy individuals, total calcium intakes up to 2500 mg/day are safe. However, in patients who have a history of kidney stones, 24-hour urine calcium should be measured before increasing calcium intakes because hypercalciuria may be exacerbated at higher intakes. In general, adequate dietary calcium does not increase the risk of calcium oxalate kidney stone formation (the most common); rather, calcium may prevent stones by binding to oxalate in the intestine (15,16).

Calcium supplements can cause gas, abdominal distention, and constipation in some individuals. It has not been proven that one type of supplement causes fewer side effects than other types. However, if a patient has symptoms with one type, it is reasonable to switch to a different preparation.

There has been some concern regarding the lead content of calcium supplements; however, supplements contribute only a small fraction of lead to overall exposure because trace amounts of lead are plentiful in our food and environment. Most of the lead from supplements will not be absorbed because calcium blocks intestinal lead absorption. In addition, if the USP designation is on the label, acceptable lead standards have been met.

In summary, we suggest that the recommended amount of calcium for each age be consumed each day, preferably by dietary sources, but supplements can be used at any age if needed. The dose of calcium supplement

Table 4-3   Summary of 20 Calcium Trials in Postmenopausal Women with Osteoporosis

First Author	Yr	Controls (n)	Treated (n)	Age	YSM	Calcium Source	Dose (mg)	Duration (yr)	Bone	Calcium versus Placebo; Difference in BMD (%)
Recker	1977	20	22	57	9	Milk	792	2	Metacarpal	+0.8
									Distal radius	+0.8
Horsman	1977	18	24	50	5	Tablets	800	2	Metacarpal	+0.6
									Distal ulna	+3.0
									Distal radius	+1.5
Lamke	1978	17	19	60	—	Tablets	1000	1	Femur neck	+4.5
									Femur shaft	+4.1
Smith	1981	26	17	82	—	Tablets	750	3	Mid-radius	+1.2
Recker	1985	14	16	59	—	Milk	1000	2	Metacarpal	−0.0
									Distal radius	−0.0
Ettinger	1987	12	35	57	2	Tablets	1000 o.n.	2	Metacarpal	+1.0
									Distal radius	+0.8
Hansson	1987	25	25	66	—	Tablets	1000	3	Spine	+0.9
Polley	1987	74	40	56	8	Tablets	1000 o.n.	0.75	Distal forearm	+1.5
Polley	1987	(74)	96	—	—	Milk	750	0.75	Distal forearm	+2.0
Riis	1987	11	14	50	19	Tablets	2000	2	Proximal radius	+1.8
									Distal radius	+0.4

Author	Year					Form	Dose		Site	Change
Smith	1989	38	44	55	7	Tablets	1500	4	TBBM	+1.4
									Spine	−0.8
Dawson-Huges	1990	14	53	55	3	Tablets	500	2	Mid-radius	+0.7
									Mid-ulna	+0.8
									Mid-humerus	+1.2
Dawson-Huges	1990	70	105	60	13	Tablets	500	2	Spine	0
									Femoral neck	+0.1
									Distal radius	+0.9
Prince	1991	41	39	57	6	Tablets	1000 o.n	2	Spine	+0.4
									Femoral neck	+0.8
									Distal radius	+0.7
									Distal radius	+1.0
									Mid-radius	+0.6
									Proximal radius	+0.3
Aloia	1994	36	34	52	2	Tablets	1200	3	TBBM	+1.5
									Spine	−0.7
									Distal radius	+0.0
									Femoral neck	+0.0
									Ward's triangle	+0.0
									Trochanter	0

Table cont'd.

Table 4-3   Summary of 20 Calcium Trials in Postmenopausal Women with Osteoporosis (Cont'd.)

First Author	Yr	Controls (n)	Treated (n)	Age	YSM	Calcium Source	Dose (mg)	Duration (yr)	Bone	Calcium versus Placebo Difference in BMD (%)
Chevalley	1994	25	55	72	23	Tablets	800	1.5	Femoral shaft	+1.0
									Femoral neck	+1.2
									Spine	−0.1
Reid	1995	40	38	58	10	Tablets	1000	4	TBBMD	+0.3
									Femoral neck	+0.3
									Ward's triangle	+0.3
									Trochanter	+0.8
									Spine	+0.5
Prince	1995	42	42	63	16	Tablets	1000 o.n.	2	Trochanter	+1.1
									Intertrochanter	+1.0
									Femoral neck	+0.5
									Ankle	+0.8
Prince	1995	(42)	42	63	16	Milk	1000 o.n.	2	Trochanter	+0.8
									Intertrochanter	+0.9
									Femoral neck	+0.5
									Ankle	+1.0
Recker	1996	102	95	73	—	Tablets	1200	4	Mid-forearm	+0.9

YSM, years since menopause; o.n., every night; TBBM, total body bone mineral; TBBMD, total body bone mineral density.
Adapted from Nordin CBE. Calcium and osteoporosis. Review article. Nutrition. 1997;13:664–686.

Table 4-4   Estimating Daily Dietary Calcium Intake

STEP 1: Estimate calcium intake from calcium-rich foods*

Product	No. of Servings/Day		Calcium Content per Serving (mg)		Daily Dietary Calcium (mg)
Milk (8 oz)	_____	×	300	=	_____
Yogurt (8 oz)	_____	×	400	=	_____
Cheese (1 oz)	_____	×	200	=	_____
Fortified foods	_____	×	**	=	_____

STEP 2: Total from above + 250 mg from nondairy sources = Total daily dietary calcium

* About 75% to 80% of the calcium consumed in American diets is from dairy products.
** Calcium content of fortified foods varies.

Table 4-5   Calcium Content of Common Supplements

Brand	Elemental Calcium/ Tablet (mg)	Vitamin D (IU)/Tablet	Notes
Calcium Carbonate			
Caltrate	600	0	Nonchewable
Caltrate Plus	600	200	Nonchewable
Caltrate Plus Chewables	600	200	+Mg, Zn, Cu, Mn, Boron
Caltrate 600 Plus Soy	600	200	+25 mg soy isoflavones
One-A-Day Calcium Plus	500	100	+Mg (50 mg)
Oscal 500	500	0	Tablet or chewable
Oscal 500 +D	500	125	Oyster shell Ca carbonate
Rolaids	220	0	Chewable
Tums			
Regular & Antigas	200	0	All chewables (calcium
EX	300	0	carbonate)
Ultra	400	0	
A500	500	0	
Viactiv	500	100	Chewable with added Vitamin K (40 µg + 50% DV)
Calcium Citrate			
Citracal Liquitab	500	0	
Citracal	200	0	
Citracal Ultradense + D	315	200	
Citracal Plus	250	125	Magnesium and other minerals
GNC Calcium Citrate	250	0	
GNC 250	125	62.5	Calicum citrate malate
Other			
Posture	600	0	Tricalcium phosphate
Posture D	600	125	Tricalcium phosphate
Centrum	162	400	
Centrum Silver	200	400	
Theragram M	40	400	

should be adjusted based on dietary intakes. The primary objective for bone health is to ensure adequate calcium intake. The choice of which supplement to use and the timing of administration should be dictated by individual preferences. Even with antiresorptive therapy, such as with hormone replacement therapy, calcium supplementation appears to improve the efficacy of the treatment on bone mass (17). Therefore, it is suggested that all patients on any osteoporosis therapy should be advised to maintain an adequate calcium intake to maximize the efficacy of these treatments. In people with osteoporosis, calcium alone is not likely to be sufficient, and a medical treatment for osteoporosis should be considered.

Vitamin D

Vitamin D deficiency is associated with osteomalacia (rickets in children), osteoporosis, muscle weakness, and decreased immune function (18). Plasma levels of 25(OH)D have been used to define vitamin D status as low (<100 nmol/L), insufficient (25–50 nmol/L) or deficient (<25 nmol/L). Vitamin D is cutaneously synthesized after exposure to sunlight and is also obtained from the diet as either ergocalciferol or cholecalciferol. There is a marked seasonal variation in the levels of 25(OH)D in whites owing to the strong influence of sunlight on vitamin D status. Vitamin D is hydroxylated in the liver to calcidiol (25(OH)D) and then to the active metabolite calcitriol (1,25(OH$_2$D)) in the kidney. Calcitriol is the most active metabolite of vitamin D, and specific receptors are found in the kidney, intestine, and bone (18). Its primary function is to increase active intestinal calcium absorption.

In younger individuals, vitamin D synthesis in the skin is the primary determinant of serum 25(OH)D levels, especially in the spring and summer. It has been suggested that approximately 15 to 30 minutes per day of sun exposure on the hands and face may be adequate for vitamin D production, although this estimate is not well documented. Elevations in serum parathyroid hormone (PTH) and greater bone loss are often associated with lower levels of 25(OH)D. Vitamin D insufficiency is believed to play a strong role in osteoporosis. The current U.S. recommendation for vitamin D intake in people aged 51 to 70 years is 10 µg/day (400 IU/day); the recommendation for people over age 70 is 15 µg/day (600 IU/day; Table 4-2). However, higher doses of vitamin D (800 IU/day) in the elderly (65 years and over) may actually be required for optimal bone health. Higher vitamin D doses have been shown to reduce fracture risk in this population when given in combination with calcium. Rich sources of vitamin D include fatty fish, fish-liver oils (cod liver oil), and liver. Several foods are also fortified with vitamin D, including milk, margarine, some soy and rice milks, and cereals.

Vitamin D and Bone Mass

There have been several studies of vitamin D supplementation, typically in combination with calcium (500 to 1200 mg/day). Table 4-6 summarizes the bone density results from eight randomized clinical trials of vitamin D supplementation, most of which also include calcium supplementation. The difference between treatment with vitamin D and placebo resulted in average differences of 1.0%, 1.2%, and 0.2%, respectively, for the spine, femoral neck, and forearm.

Calcium, Vitamin D, and Fractures

A review of 16 observational studies assessing hip fracture and calcium intake found that an increase in usual calcium intake of 1 g/day was associated with a 24% reduction in the risk of hip fracture (19). Two randomized, clinical trials, which evaluated calcium supplementation alone, found vertebral fractures reduced by 28% and symptomatic fractures reduced by 70% in the calcium-supplemented group (Table 4-7). Significant reductions in fracture have also been seen in those randomized clinical trials in which calcium was given in conjunction with vitamin D (26% to 54% reduction in hip and nonspine fracture rates, respectively) (20,21). In the one study in which fractures were not reduced, the participants had higher baseline serum 25(OH)D levels, were not given additional calcium, and were given a lower dose of vitamin D (400 IU) (22). None of these studies assessed vertebral compression fractures.

On the basis of the current evidence, in all individuals over the age of 70, vitamin D intakes of at least 600 IU per day (up to 800 IU/day) are recommended, in addition to the calcium requirement of 1200 mg/day. Vitamin D from foods, supplements, or multivitamins can be used to meet the vitamin D requirement.

Protein

Protein intake in the United States and many other industrialized countries is typically 50% over the recommended allowance. An excessive intake of protein, particularly animal protein with high sulfate contents, increases calciuria in normal adults. For example, increasing animal protein from 40 to 80 g/day increases urine calcium by about 20 to 40 mg/day. However, the effect of a high-protein diet on bone mineral density (BMD) is less clear. Several large epidemiologic studies have shown higher protein intakes are associated with higher BMD in some studies (23–25), but with lower BMD in others (26–27). There have been observational studies of postmenopausal women indicating an increase in fracture risk with higher protein intakes (28), especially protein from nondairy animal sources (29), perhaps because of a metabolic acidosis

Table 4-6　Clinical Trials: Vitamin D and Bone Density

Author	Year	Patients	Age (Mean)	Dietary Calcium (mg/day)	Supplemental Calcium (mg/day)	Dose	Duration	Change in Bone Density (% per year) (Vitamin D Compared with Placebo)	
Dawson-Hughes	1997	389	71	600–700	500	700 IU	3 yrs	Fem neck Spine Total body	+1.2 +0.9 +1.2
Ooms	1995	177 vit D 171 placebo	80	868	—	400 IU	2 yrs	Lft fem neck Rt fem neck Distal radius	+1.0 +1.2 −0.4
Ushiroyama	1995	15 vit D 35 control	53 51	N/A	N/A	1 µg (alfacalcidol)	1.5	Fem neck	+1.0
Chapuy	1992	27 vit D 29 placebo	84	511 514	1200 N/A	800 IU	18 mo	Fem neck	+1.0
Dawson-Hughes	1991	124 vit D 125 placebo	62	108 89	810 727	400 IU	12 mo	Spine Total body	+0.7 +0.1
Orwoll	1990	41 vit D 36 placebo	57	1159	1000 N/A	25 µg	3 yrs	Proximal Distal radius Spine	+0.4 +0.3 −0.4
Baeksgaard	1998	240	62	900	1000	560 IU	2	Spine Fem neck Distal radius	+1.6 +1.0 +0.5
Lau	2001	—	—	800	—	200 IU	—	Spine Fem neck Troch Total body	+1.1 +1.8 +0.7 +1.5

Table 4-7   Clinical Trials: Calcium, Vitamin D, and Fractures

Author	Date	Number of Subjects	Subject Age (Yr)	Subject Characteristic	Intervention	Duration of Follow-Up	Results and Comments
Reid	1995	78	58	Healthy volunteers; baseline calcium = 734 mg/day	1000 mg calcium vs placebo	4 years	Symptomatic fractures reduced 70% in the calcium group
Recker	1996	197	73	Healthy volunteers; baseline calcium = 433 mg/day	1200 mg calcium vs placebo	4.3 years	Vertebral fractures incidence reduced by 28%; stronger effect (45% reduction) in women with prior fractures
Lips	1996	2578	75	2570 elderly males; calcium = 868 mg/day	400 IU vit D vs placebo	4 years	Vit D alone led to no reduction in hip or nonvertebral fractures
Komulainen	1998	464	53	Recently postmenopausal; calcium = 800 mg/day	300 IU/d (vit D) vs placebo	5 years	53% reduction in nonvertebral fractures
Chevalley	1995	93	72	82 female, 11 male; baseline calcium = 619 mg/day	800 mg calcium vs placebo (vit D repleted by 300,000 IU single dose)	18 months	31% reduction in vertebral fractures
Chapuy	1994	2303	84	Nursing home elderly females; no serious medical conditions	1200 mg calcium and 800 IU vit D vs double placebo	3 years	27% reduction in hip fractures; 26% reduction in nonvertebral fractures
Dawson-Hughes	1997	389	71	176 men, 213 women	500 mg calcium and 700 IU vit D vs placebo	3 years	54% reduction in nonvertebral fractures

leading to bone titration via resorption (28,30–32). These high protein intakes are particularly harmful in the presence of low calcium (2,33).

Conversely, observational studies of the elderly demonstrate that protein intakes that are lower than recommended can have deleterious effects and are associated with higher hip fracture rates (34–37). In this setting, however, low protein intake may be a marker of poor nutritional status or frailty. In randomized, controlled trials, supplementation with protein reduced the hospital length of stay after hip fracture (38,39). In the elderly, low protein intakes may be related to low IGF-1, poor muscle function, and poor immunity, leading to an increased risk of falling, fractures, and medical complications.

The evidence to date suggests that protein intake should be at the recommended levels (50 to 60 g/day) and that calcium intake be adequate (Table 4-2). In the frail elderly with fractures, it might be advisable to provide a protein supplement.

Phosphorus

Phosphorus intake does not seem to influence skeletal homeostasis within normal ranges of intake (RDA 800 mg/day), although excessive intake, particularly when combined with low calcium intake, may be deleterious (40–42). Foods that are high in phosphorus are milk, milk products, poultry, fish, meat, eggs, grains, legumes, and sodas, with only milk (and milk products) also having high amounts of calcium. In general, the major problem with soda consumption on bone health is that calcium-containing beverages may be omitted in favor of soda, not the phosphorus content itself. Phosphorus deficiency may be a marker of general nutritional inadequacy, as is protein deficiency, and in that regard could lead to an increased risk of fracture. At any age, the ratio of phosphorus to calcium is probably more important than the intake of phosphorus alone.

Salt

As discussed earlier, sodium causes an increase in renal calcium excretion. In observational studies, higher salt intake leads to greater rates of bone resorption in postmenopausal women and greater bone loss. Furthermore, those with low calcium and high salt diets have lower BMD (43–44). It is therefore recommended for both skeletal and cardiovascular health that excessive salt intake be avoided. The American Heart Association recommends that daily salt intake be less than 6 g/day (2400 mg sodium). An adequate intake of calcium allows a more liberal use of sodium in the diet.

Caffeine

Excess caffeine intake may have some detrimental effect on calcium balance by slightly decreasing calcium absorption, but, again, with an adequate intake of calcium, there may be no detrimental effects on bone. In some studies, greater bone loss and higher fracture rates have been associated with high caffeine intake (45–50), although coffee intake may be a problem only in the face of inadequate calcium intake (51) or in association with other detrimental lifestyle factors. The evidence to date would suggest that it is prudent to avoid excessive intakes (>4 cups per day) of caffeinated beverages and to make sure that calcium intake is adequate.

Vitamin K

Vitamin K functions as a cofactor in enzymes involved in the synthesis of blood coagulation factors, and it may be required for bone metabolism, to facilitate carboxylation of proteins such as osteocalcin (which is involved in bone formation), and to reduce urinary calcium excretion (52). Observational studies indicate that women with higher intake and serum levels of vitamin K tend to have higher bone density (53–55), and patients who sustain fractures have been reported to have lower serum vitamin K levels (56–58). Epidemiologic studies have also found that higher vitamin K intake is related to lower fracture incidence (59–61). Furthermore, a high percentage of undercarboxylated serum osteocalcin may be a predictor of fracture risk (52,62). Vitamin K is present in dark green, leafy vegetables, fruits, and vegetable oils with small amounts in dairy products and grains. Vitamin K_2 is found in fermented dairy products, soy products, fish, meat, liver, and egg. The recommended intakes for vitamin K are 80 µg for men and 65 µg for women.

Several small, controlled supplementation studies have found reductions in calcium excretion, bone resorption, and the undercarboxylated fraction of osteocalcin in patients who received vitamin K supplementation. In postmenopausal women with fracture, 1 mg of vitamin K_1 supplementation increased the percent of carboxylated osteocalcin from 55% to 75%. A compound derived from vitamin K (MK4) had a positive effect on BMD in large doses when given to women with osteoporosis (63) and strokes (64). High pharmacologic doses of vitamin K_2 (45 mg) were related to lower rates of bone loss and a lower incidence of fractures in a group of 241 patients (65).

The current evidence is limited to observational studies, studies on intermediate end points, and small studies with bone density and limited fracture data. Based on the current evidence, there are insufficient data to recommend vitamin K supplementation. A healthy diet high in fruits and vegetables ensures that vitamin K intake is adequate for most of the population.

Antagonistic Effect of Warfarin on Vitamin K

Warfarin (Coumadin) competitively inhibits the effect of vitamin K. Antagonism of vitamin K with Coumadin derivatives can result in the undercarboxylation of specific proteins involved in bone metabolism, including osteocalcin, raising concern that using these drugs might increase the risk of fracture. In one cohort study, warfarin use for more than 1 year was an independent predictor of spine and hip fracture (66), but this was not confirmed by another prospective study (67). Concern about osteoporosis should not deter appropriate use of anticoagulants for prevention of thromboembolic disease.

Vitamin C

Vitamin C is an essential cofactor for collagen formation and synthesis of hydroxyproline and hydroxylysine. Rich dietary sources of vitamin C include citrus fruit and juices, peppers, broccoli, tomato products, and green leafy vegetables. The dietary reference intakes for vitamin C are 75 mg/day for adult women and 90 mg/day for adult men. Epidemiologic studies show a positive association between vitamin C and bone mass, and one study (although not another) found that higher vitamin C was associated with fewer fractures; however, there are no randomized clinical trials (68–74). Recommended intakes of five or more servings of fruits and vegetables should supply enough vitamin C for bone health.

Vitamin A

Recommended dietary allowance of vitamin A is 800 µg/day retinol equivalents (RE) for women and 1000 µg RE for men. Excess vitamin A may be detrimental to bone health, with intakes of higher than 1500 µg RE related to a 2-fold increased risk of hip fracture in some but not all studies (75–77a).

Magnesium

Magnesium complexed with adenosine triphosphate takes part in many enzyme reactions, including synthesis of proteins and nucleic acid. The recommended intake for healthy adult men is 420 mg, and for women the recommended intake is 320 mg/day. Because magnesium is present in most foods, particularly vegetables, whole seeds, and bananas, deficiency is rarely seen in healthy people. However, a magnesium supplement may be valuable in the frail elderly with poor diets (78), people with intestinal disease (79), alcoholics, and people taking diuretics or receiving chemotherapy, both of which deplete magnesium. In addition, as calcium supplements sometimes result in constipation, a supplement with magnesium may counteract this effect.

Several small epidemiologic studies have found that higher magnesium intakes are associated with higher BMD in elderly men and women (80,81). There have been only small, controlled clinical trials of magnesium supplementation (79,82) that were primarily effective in magnesium-depleted subjects. There is little evidence that magnesium is needed to prevent osteoporosis in the general population.

Fluoride

Fluoride is an essential trace element that is required for skeletal and dental development. The adequate daily adult intake is 4 mg for men and 3 mg for women. The concentration of fluoride in the soil, water, and many foods varies by geographic region. Major dietary sources include drinking water, tea, coffee, rice, soybeans, spinach, onions, and lettuce. There is no need to add fluoride supplements to an adult diet for skeletal health.

The lower doses of fluoride typically found in drinking water have no effect on bone density or on fractures (83–85). However, excess fluoride ingestion may be detrimental (86). Fluoride as a pharmacologic therapy is discussed in Chapter 11.

Boron

Boron is not an essential nutrient, so there is no recommended intake. A few studies have found that 3 mg daily of boron may have some effect on calcium balance and estrogen metabolism (81,87). Boron is present in several foods such as fruits, vegetables, nuts, eggs, wine, and dried foods.

Alcohol

In both men and women, high intake of alcohol can depress osteoblast function and reduce bone formation. Inebriation may also increase the risk of fall-related injuries, although two to three drinks a day has not been associated with an increased risk of falls. Moderate alcohol intake increases estradiol concentrations and has been associated with higher bone mass in some but not all studies (88–94). However, long-term heavy alcohol consumption may increase the risk of hip fracture (95), whereas regular limited consumption of alcohol 5 days per week significantly reduces the risk of vertebral deformity (RR = 0.65; CI = 0.43–0.99) (96). The possible benefit of moderate alcohol intake on BMD and spine fractures should be evaluated with consideration of the risks and benefits of alcohol on the risk of other diseases. There is no reason to advise patients who drink alcohol in moderate amounts to cut down or stop for reasons of preventing osteoporosis or fractures. The exact upper safe limit of alcohol for maintaining bone health has not been determined. It is extremely important to ask patients about their alcohol intake, recognize alcoholism, and refer patients for treatment.

Other Dietary Factors

In general, good nutrition is as important for skeletal integrity as it is for any other organ system. Wide deviations such as protein malnutrition and starvation, including anorexia nervosa, have marked detrimental effects on bone (97). The importance of dietary variation within normal practice is more difficult to document. The effects of other minor nutrients and trace metals (vitamin B_{12}, folate (71), manganese, zinc, and copper), which have been reported only in observational studies, remain unknown. One controlled trial has shown that a combination of these minerals was able to reduce spinal bone loss in postmenopausal women (98).

Food Groups

Several recent epidemiologic studies have indicated that higher intakes of fruits and vegetables and lower intakes of protein from meat sources leads to improved bone health as assessed by markers of bone turnover and bone density (48,80,99). This could be a result of the higher potassium content, higher pH (basic) diet, or the higher intake of vitamins (vitamins C and K, etc.) associated with fruit and vegetable consumption.

Animal protein can be high in phosphoric and sulfuric acid and can lead to urinary calcium loss. In fact, a high protein-to-potassium ratio is related to greater bone loss in longitudinal studies (100). Avoiding excessive protein intakes (greater than 60 g/day) will improve calcium balance and perhaps overall health. However, low protein intakes may be dangerous, particularly in the frail elderly.

Summary

The nutritional needs for optimizing bone health are met by a diet that provides adequate calcium and vitamin D through dairy or calcium-fortified foods. Foods are a preferred source to maintain calcium balance because other nutrients that might be valuable to bone health are found in high-calcium foods. For people who do not receive an adequate calcium intake from their diet, supplemental calcium can be used. Spreading calcium intake throughout the day increases the total amount of calcium absorbed.

In all individuals over the age of 70, vitamin D intake of at least 600 IU per day (up to 800 IU/day) is recommended for bone health, in addition to the calcium requirement of 1200 mg/day. Vitamin D from foods, supplements, or multivitamins can be used to meet the vitamin D requirement.

In the elderly in whom poor nutritional status is detected (low albumin), or after hip fracture, there may be some benefit from protein supplementation, as well as a multivitamin to ensure the adequacy of other nutrients. Five servings per day of fruits and vegetables will meet the requirements for many nutrients and may contribute to improved skeletal health.

REFERENCES

1. **Nordin BE.** Calcium and osteoporosis. Review Article. Nutrition. 1997;13:664–686.
2. **Heaney RP.** Calcium, dairy products and osteoporosis. J Am Coll Nutr. 2000;19:83S–99S.
3. **Johnston CC, Miller JZ, Slemenda CW, et al .** Calcium supplementation and increases in bone mineral density in children. N Engl J Med. 1992;327:923–987.
4. **Lloyd T, Andon MB, Rollings N, et al.** Calcium supplementation and bone mineral density in adolescent girls. JAMA. 1993;270:841–844.
5. **Lloyd T, Martel JK, Rollings N, et al.** The effect of calcium supplementation and Tanner stage on bone density, content and area in teenage women. Osteoporos Int. 1996;6:276–283.
6. **Lee WT, Leung SS, Leung DM, et al.** A randomized double-blind controlled calcium supplementation trial, and bone and height acquisition in children. Br J Nutr. 1995;74:125–139.
7. **Nowson CA, Green RM, Hopper JL, et al.** A co-twin study of the effect of calcium supplementation on bone density during adolescence. Osteoporos Int. 1997;7:219–225.
8. **Chan GM, Hoffman K, McMurry M.** Effects of dairy products on bone and body composition in pubertal girls. J Pediatr. 1995;126:551–556.
9. **Cadogan J, Eastell R, Jones N, Barker ME.** Milk intake and bone mineral acquisition in adolescent girls. A randomized, controlled intervention trial. Br Med J. 1997;315:1255–1260.
10. **Welten DC, Kemper HCG, Post GB, Van Staveren WA.** A meta-analysis of the effect of calcium intake on bone mass in young and middle-aged females and males. J Nutr. 1995;125:2802.

11. **Lee WT, Leung SS, Leung DM, Cheng JC.** A follow-up study on the effects of calcium-supplement withdrawal and puberty on bone acquisition of children. Am J Clin Nutr. 1996;64:71–77.

12. **Bonjour J-P, Carrié AL, Ferrari S, et al.** Calcium-enriched foods and bone mass growth in prepubertal girls. A randomized, double-blind, placebo-controlled trial. J Clin Invest. 1997;99:1287–1997.

13. **Storm D, Eslin R, Porter ES, et al.** Calcium supplementation prevents seasonal bone loss and changes in biochemical markers of bone turnover in elderly New England women. A randomized placebo-controlled trial. J Clin Endocrinol Metab. 1998;83:3817–3825.

14. **Baeksgaard L, Andersen KP, Hyldstrup L.** Calcium and vitamin D supplementation increases spinal BMD in healthy postmenopausal women. Osteoporos Int. 1998;8:255–260.

15. **Curhan GC, Willett WC, Rimm EB, Stampfer MJ.** A prospective study of dietary calcium and other nutrients and the risk of symptomatic kidney stones. N Engl J Med. 1993;328:833–838.

16. **Curhan GC, Willett WC, Speizer FE, et al.** Comparison of dietary calcium with supplemental calcium and other nutrients as factors affecting the risk for kidney stones in women. Ann Intern Med. 1997;126:497–504.

17. **Nieves JW, Komar L, Cosman F, Lindsay R.** Calcium potentiates the effect of estrogen and calcitonin on bone mass: review and analysis. Am J Clin Nutr. 1998; 67:18–24.

18. **Holick MF.** Vitamin D requirements for humans of all ages: new increased requirements for women and men 50 years and older. Osteoporos Int. 1998;8(Suppl):S24–S29.

19. **Cumming RG, Nevitt MC.** Calcium for prevention of osteoporotic fractures in postmenopausal women. J Bone Miner Res. 1997;12:1321–1329.

20. **Chapuy MC, Arlot ME, Duboeuf F, et al.** Vitamin D and calcium to prevent hip fractures in elderly women. N Engl J Med. 1992;327:1637–1642.

21. **Dawson-Hughes B, Harris SS, Krall EA, Dallal GE.** Effect of calcium and vitamin D supplementation on bone density in men and women 65 years of age or older. N Engl J Med. 1997;337:670–676.

22. **Lips P, Graafmans WC, Ooms ME, et al.** Vitamin D supplementation and fracture incidence in elderly persons. A randomized, placebo-controlled clinical trial. Ann Intern Med. 1996;124:400–406.

23. **Kerstetter JE, Looker AC, Insogna KL.** Low dietary protein and low bone density. Calcif Tissue Int. 2000;616:313.

24. **Munger RG, Cerhan JR, Chiu BC-H.** Prospective study of dietary protein intake and risk of hip fracture in postmenopausal women. Am J Clin Nutr. 1999;69:147–152.

25. **Hannan MT, Tucker K, Dawson-Hughes B, et al.** Effect of dietary protein on bone loss in elderly men and women. The Framingham Osteoporosis Study. J Bone Miner Res. 1997;12(Suppl 1):S151.

26. **Wachman A, Bernstein DS.** Diet and osteoporosis. Lancet. 1998;1:958–959.

27. **Kerstetter JE, Looker AC, Insogna KL.** Low dietary protein and low bone density. Calcif Tissue Int. 2000;66:313.

28. **Abelow BJ, Holford TR, Insogna KL.** Cross-cultural association between dietary animal protein and hip fracture: a hypothesis. Calcif Tissue Int. 1992;50:14–18.

29. **Hu JF, Zhao XH, Parpia B, et al.** Dietary intakes and urinary excretion of calcium and acids. A cross-sectional study of women in China. Am J Clin Nutr. 1993;58:389–406.

30. **Meyer HE, Pedersen JI, Loken EB, Tverdal A.** Dietary factors and the incidence of hip fracture in middle-aged Norwegians. A prospective study. Am J Epidemiol. 1997;145:117–123.

31. **Feskanich D, Weber P, Willett WC, et al.** Vitamin K intake and hip fractures in women. A prospective study. Am J Clin Nutr. 1999;69:74–79.

32. **Wang M-C, Villa ML, Marcus R, Kelsey JL.** Associations of vitamin C, calcium and protein with bone mass in postmenopausal Mexican-American women. Osteoporos Int. 1997;7:533–538.

33. **Orwoll ES.** The effects of dietary protein insufficiency and excess on skeletal health. Bone. 1992;13:343–350.

34. **Munger RG, Cerhan JR, Chiu BC.** Prospective study of dietary protein intake and risk of hip fracture in postmenopausal women. Am J Clin Nutr. 1999;69:147–152.

35. **Johnell O, Gullberg B, Kanis JA, et al.** Risk factors for hip fracture in European women. The MEDOS Study. J Bone Miner Res. 1995;10:1802–1815.

36. **Huang Z, Himes JH, McGovern PG.** Nutrition and subsequent hip fracture risk among a national cohort of white women. Am J Epidemiol. 1996;144:124–134.

37. **Bonjour JP, Schurch MA, Rizzoli R.** Proteins and bone health: older adults. Pathol Biol. 1997;45:57–59.

38. **Schurch M-A, Rizzoli R, Slosman D, et al.** Protein supplements increase serum insulin-like growth factor-I levels and attenuate proximal femur bone loss in patients with recent hip fracture. A randomized, double-blind, placebo-controlled trial. Ann Intern Med. 1998;128:801–809.

39. **Tkatch L, Rapin CH, Rizzoli R, et al.** Benefits of oral protein supplementation in elderly patients with fracture of the proximal femur. J Am Coll Nutr. 1992;11:519–525.

40. **Calvo MS, Kumar R, Heath A III.** Persistently elevated parathyroid hormone secretion and action in young women after four weeks of ingesting high phosphorus, low calcium diets. J Clin Endocrinol Metab. 1990;70:1334–1337.

41. **Heaney RP, Gallagher JC, Johnson CC, et al.** Calcium nutrition and bone health in the elderly. Am J Clin Nutr. 1982;36:986–1013.

42. **Spencer H, Kramer L, Osis D, Norris C.** Effect of phosphorus on the absorption of calcium and on the calcium balance in men. J Nutr. 1978;108:447–457.

43. **Devine A, Criddle RA, Dick IM, et al.** A longitudinal study of the effect of sodium and calcium intakes on regional bone density in postmenopausal women. Am J Clin Nutr. 1995;62:740–745.

44. **Mizushima S, Tsuchida K, Yamori Y.** Preventive nutritional factors in epidemiology: interaction between sodium and calcium. Clin Exp Pharmacol Physiol. 1999;26:573–575.

45. **Hernandez-Avila M, Colditz GA, Stampfer MJ, et al.** Caffeine, moderate alcohol intake, and risk of fractures of the hip and forearm in middle-aged women. Am J Clin Nutr. 1991;54:157–163.

46. **Kiel DP, Felson DT, Hannan MT, et al.** Caffeine and the risk of hip fracture. The Framingham Study. Am J Epidemiol. 1990;132:675–684.

47. **Cummings SR, Nevitt MC, Browner WS, et al.** Risk factors for hip fracture in white women. Study of Osteoporotic Fractures Research Group. N Engl J Med. 1990; 332:767–773.

48. **New SA, Bolton-Smith C, Grubb DA, Reid DM.** Nutritional influences on bone mineral density: a cross-sectional study in premenopausal women. Am J Clin Nutr. 1997;65:1831–1839.

49. **Johansson C, Mellström D, Lerner U, et al.** Coffee drinking: a minor risk factor for bone loss and fractures. Age Ageing. 1992;21:20–26.

50. **Cooper C, Atkinson EJ, Wahner HW, et al.** Is caffeine consumption a risk factor for osteoporosis? J Bone Miner Res. 1992;7:465–471.

51. **Harris SS, Dawson-Hughes B.** Caffeine and bone loss in healthy postmenopausal women. Am J Clin Nutr. 1994;60:573–578.

52. **Booth SL.** Skeletal functions of vitamin K-dependent proteins: not just for clotting anymore. Nutr Rev. 1997;55:282–284.

53. **Vermeer C, Knapen MHJ, Jie K-S G, Grobbee DE.** Physiological importance of extra-hepatic vitamin K-dependent carboxylation reactions. Ann NY Acad Sci. 1992; 669:21–33.

54. **Tamatani M, Morimoto S, Nakajima M, et al.** Participation of decreased circulating levels of vitamin K in bone mineral loss of elderly men. J Bone Miner Res. 1995;10:S248.

55. **Szulc P, Chapuy MC, Meuniere PJ, Delmas PD.** Serum undercarboxylated osteocalcin is a marker of the risk of hip fracture in elderly women. J Clin Invest. 1993; 91:1769–1774.

56. **Hart JP, Shearer MJ, Klenerman L.** Electrochemical detection of depressed circulating levels of vitamin K_1 in osteoporosis. J. Clin Endocrinol Metab. 1985;60:1268–1269.

57. **Hodges SJ, Akesson K, Vergnaud P, et al.** Circulating levels of vitamin K_1 and K_2 decreased in elderly women with hip fracture. J Bone Mineral Res. 1993;8:1241–1245.

58. **Hodges SJ, Pilkington MJ, Stamp T, et al.** Depressed levels of circulating menaquinones in patients with osteoporotic fractures of the spine and femoral neck. Bone. 1991;12:387–389.

59. **Booth Sl, Tucker Kl, Chen H, et al.** Dietary vitamin K intakes are associated with hip fracture but not with bone mineral density in elderly men and women. Am J Clin Nutr. 2000;71:1201–1208.

60. **Feskanich D, Weber P, Willett WC, et al.** Vitamin K intake and hip fractures in women. A prospective study. Am J Clin Nutr. 1999;69:74–79.

61. **Vergnaud P, Garnero P, Meunier PJ, et al.** Undercarboxylated osteocalcin measured with a specific immunoassay predicts hip fracture in elderly women. The EIPDOS Study. J Clin Endocrinol Metab. 1997;82:719–724.

62. **Kohlmeier M, Saupe J, Shearer MJ, et al.** Bone health of adult hemodialysis patients is related to vitamin K status. Kidney Int. 1997;5:1218–1221.

63. **Orimo H, Shiraki M, Tomita A, et al.** Effects of menatetrenone on the bone and calcium metabolism in osteoporosis. A double-blinded placebo-controlled study. J Bone Miner Metab. 1998;16:106–112.

64. **Sato Y, Honda Y, Kuno H, Oizumi K.** Menatetrenone ameliorates osteopenia in disuse-affected limbs of vitamin D- and K-deficient stroke patients. Bone. 1998;23: 291–296.

65. **Shiraki M, Shiraki Y, Aoki C, Miura M.** Vitamin K_2 (menatetrenone) effectively prevents fractures and sustains lumbar bone mineral density in osteoporosis. J Bone Miner Res. 2000;15:515–521.

66. **Caraballo PJ, Heit JA, Atkinson EJ, et al.** Long term use of oral anticoagulants and the risk of fracture. Arch Intern Med. 1999;159:1750–1756.

67. **Jamal SA, Browner WS, Bauer DC, Cummings SR.** Warfarin use and risk for osteoporosis in elderly women. Study of osteoporotic fractures research group. Ann Intern Med. 1998;128:829–832.

68. **Hall SL, Greendale GA.** The relationship of dietary vitamin C intake to bone mineral density. Results from the PEPI study. Calcif Tissue Int. 1998;63:183–189.

69. **Odaland LM, Mason RL, Alexeff AI.** Bone density and dietary findings of 409 Tennessee subjects. I. Bone density considerations. Am J Clin Nutr. 1972;25:905–907.

70. **Sowers MR, Wallace RB, Lemke JH.** Correlates of mid-radius bone density among postmenopausal women. A community study. Am J Clin Nutr. 1985;41:1045–1053.

71. **Freudenheim LJ, Johnson NE, Smith EL.** Relationships between usual nutrient intake and bone-mineral content of women 35–65 years of age: longitudinal and cross-sectional analysis. Am J Clin Nutr. 1986;44:863–876.

72. **Hernandez-Avila M, Stampfer MJ, Ravnikar VA, et al.** Caffeine and other predictors of bone density among pre- and perimenopausal women. Epidemiology. 1993;4:128–134.

73. **Leveille SG, LaCroix AZ, Koepsell TD, et al.** Dietary vitamin C and bone mineral density in postmenopausal women in Washington State, USA. J Epidemiol Community Health. 1997;51:479–485.

74. **Weber P.** The role of vitamins in the prevention of osteoporosis: a brief status report. Int J Vitam Nutr Res. 1999;69:194–197.

75. **Melhus H, Michaelsson K, Kindmark A, et al.** Excessive dietary intake of vitamin A is associated with reduced bone mineral density and increased risk for hip fracture. Ann Intern Med. 1998;129:770–778.

76. **Whiting SJ, Lemke B.** Excess retinol intake may explain the high incidence of osteoporosis in northern Europe. Nutr Rev. 1999;57:192–195.

77. **Sigurdsson G.** Dietary vitamin A intake and risk for hip fracture. Ann Intern Med. 1999;131:392.

77a. **Fesskanich D, Singh V, Willett WC, Colditz GA.** Vitamin A intake and hip fractures among postmenopausal women. JAMA. 2002;287:47–54.

78. **Durlach J, Bac P, Durlach V, et al.** Magnesium status and aging: an update. Magnes Res. 1998;11:25–42.

79. **Rude RK, Olerich M.** Magnesium deficiency: possible role in osteoporosis associated with gluten-sensitive enteropathy. Osteoporos Int. 1996;6:453–461.

80. **Tucker KL, Hannan MT, Chen H, et al.** Potassium, magnesium, and fruit and vegetable intakes are associated with greater bone mineral density in elderly men and women. Am J Clin Nutr. 1999;69:727–736.

81. **Nielsen FH.** Studies on the relationship between boron and magnesium which possibly affects the formation and maintenance of bones. Mag Tr Elem. 1990;9:61–69.

82. **Stendig-Lindberg G, Tepper R, Leichter I.** Trabecular bone density in a two-year controlled trial of perioral magnesium in osteoporosis. Magnes Res. 1993;6:155–163.

83. **Cauley JA, Murphy PA, Riley TJ, et al.** Effects of fluoridated drinking water on bone mass. J Bone Miner Res. 1995;10:1076–1086.

84. **Suarez-Almazor ME, Flowerdew G, Saunders LD, et al.** The fluoridation of drinking water and hip fracture hospitalization rates in two Canadian communities. Am J Public Health. 1993;83:689–693.

85. **Kurltio P, Gustavsson N, Vartiomen T, Pekkanen J.** Exposure to natural fluoride in well water and hip fracture. A cohort analysis. Am J Epidemiol. 1999;150: 817–824.

86. **Riggs BL.** Treatment of osteoporosis with sodium fluoride. An appraisal. J Bone Miner Res. 1984;2:266–393.

87. **Nielsen FH, Hunter CD, Mullen LM, Hunt JR.** Effect of dietary boron on mineral, estrogen, and testosterone metabolism in postmenopausal women. FASEB J. 1987;1:394–397.

88. **Feskanich D, Korrick SA, Greenspan SL, et al.** Moderate alcohol consumption and bone density among postmenopausal women. J Womens Health. 1999;8:65–73.

89. **Felson DT, Zhang Y, Hannan MT, et al.** Alcohol intake and bone mineral density in elderly men and women. The Framingham Study. Am J Epidemiol. 1995;142:485–492.

90. **Holbrook TL, Barrett-Connor E.** A prospective study of alcohol consumption and bone mineral density. Br J Med. 1993;306:1506–1509.

91. **May H, Murphy S, Khaw KT.** Alcohol consumption and bone mineral density in older men. Gerontology. 1995;41:152–158.

92. **Grainge MJ, Coupland CA, Cliffe SJ, et al.** Cigarette smoking, alcohol and caffeine consumption, and bone mineral density in postmenopausal women. The Nottingham EPIC Study Group. Osteoporos Int. 1998;8:355–363.

93. **Gonzales-Calvin JL, Garcia-Sanchez A, Bellot V, et al.** Mineral metabolism, osteoblastic function and bone mass in chronic alcoholism. Alcohol Alcohol. 1993;28: 571–579.

94. **Slemenda CW, Hui SL, Longcope C, Johnston CJ.** Cigarette smoking, obesity, and bone mass. J Bone Miner Res. 1989;4:737–741.

95. **Felson DT, Kiel DP, Anderson JJ, Kannel WB.** Alcohol consumption and hip fractures. The Framingham Study. Am J Epidemiol. 1998;128:1102–1110.

96. **Naves Diaz M, O'Neill TW, Silman AJ.** The influence of alcohol consumption on the risk of vertebral deformity. European Vertebral Osteoporosis Study Group. Osteoporos Int. 1997;7:65–71.

97. **Rigotti NA, Neer RM, Skates SJ, et al.** The clinical course of osteoporosis in anorexia nervosa. JAMA. 1991;265:1133–1137.

98. **Strause L, Saltman P, Smith KT, et al.** Spinal bone loss in postmenopausal women supplemented with calcium and trace minerals. J Nutr. 1994;124:1060–1064.

99. **Frassetto LA, Nash E, Morris RC, Sebastian A.** Comparative effects of potassium chloride and bicarbonate on thiazide-induced reduction in urinary calcium excretion. Kidney Int. 2000;58:748–752.

100. **Sebastian A, Harris ST, Ottaway JH, et al.** Improved mineral balance and skeletal metabolism in postmenopausal women treated with potassium bicarbonate. N Eng J Med. 1994;330:1776–1781.

CHAPTER 5

Physical Activity as a Strategy to Conserve and Improve Bone Mass

ROBERT MARCUS, MD

SOPHIE A. JAMAL, MD

FELICIA COSMAN, MD

Key Points

- Persons who are physically active have higher bone mass and lower rates of hip fracture than do sedentary persons.

- Maintaining physical activity has been associated with a 20% to 60% reduction in the rate of hip fractures.

- Exercise programs for persons with osteoporosis who have already sustained fractures should increase the patient's ability to carry out routine daily activities while minimizing the risk for subsequent fractures.

- The optimal exercise regimen for preventing osteoporosis and fractures is unknown. Patients should be advised to adopt a form of exercise based on their age and health status that is likely to be maintained throughout life.

Physical activity influences both the amount of bone acquired during growth, "peak bone mass," and the subsequent loss of bone. In addition, through its effects on muscle mass, strength, and coordination, physical activity also reduces the risk of falls (1). Therefore, physical activity can reduce the risk of osteoporosis-related fractures through both these mechanisms. In this chapter, the physiology of physical activity on bone and muscle is reviewed, as well as the observational and the randomized controlled trial data of the effects of physical activity on bone mineral density (BMD), falls, and fractures.

Physiology

Effects of Exercise on Bone

The skeleton is a strong, resilient structure that permits resistance against gravitational and other forces while providing structural rigidity for locomotion. To carry out these functions, bone adapts to the loading forces (the amount of force that is applied across the bone) that are placed on it. Habitual loading is the sum of all individual daily loading events, each event characterized by its magnitude, or intensity, and number of repetitions, or cycles. This results in bone gain when habitual loading increases, and in bone loss when loading decreases (2). The relationship between mechanical loading and bone mass is curvilinear, with a much steeper slope at very low levels of loading (Fig. 5-1) (3). Thus, there is substantial loss of bone at extremely low loading, as happens with complete immobilization, weightlessness (such as during space travel), or spinal cord injury. Immobilized patients may lose 40% of their original bone mass in 1 year. Studies indicate that standing upright for as little as 30 minutes each day prevents bone loss. By contrast, increasing the level of exercise among already active people results in only very small gains in bone (on average, 1% per year).

Effects of Exercise on Muscle

More than 90% of hip fractures occur as the immediate consequence of a fall onto the hip. Among the important risk factors for falls, muscle strength is relatively more susceptible to improvement with strength training (4). Aging is associated with muscle atrophy, and with degenerative changes in peripheral nerve and neuromuscular junctions. The resulting muscle weakness is a consistent and strong risk factor for falls (5).

Muscle strength of older men and women responds dramatically to resistance exercise (6,7). Strength gains vary from 30% to more than 100% in various muscle groups (7,8). Training-induced strength gains are initially

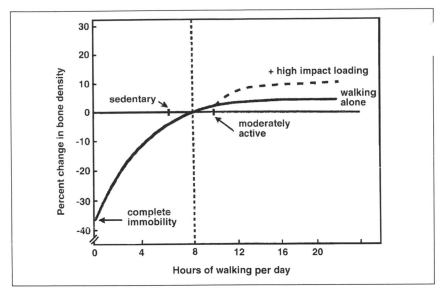

Figure 5-1   The relationship between mechanical loading and bone mass. There is greater gain in bone mass at the lowest levels of activity than at the highest.

rapid but tend to plateau after 12 to 14 weeks, even with progressive increases in training loads (8).

Strength training in young men and women often emphasizes relatively few repetitions with very high loads. This does not seem to be essential for older individuals: a year-long clinical trial comparing low-intensity, high-repetition training and high intensity-low repetition training found that the two approaches produced comparable gains in strength (9,10). Thus, muscle strength can be improved and maintained in older people without high-intensity, and potentially high-risk, training schedules. Further, the gain in muscle strength does not require frequent training. For example, increases in strength and performance in several tasks, such as rising from a chair, improved to a similar degree in older individuals who trained 1, 2, or 3 days each week (10,11). Thus, to attain neuromuscular benefit, most older individuals may best be advised to undertake relatively modest intensity exercise once or twice each week.

Observational Studies

Observational studies demonstrate that people who are physically active have higher bone mass and lower rates of hip fracture than do sedentary individuals (12). However, the benefits of exercise on bone density seem to disappear soon after stopping exercise.

Bone Mass in Athletes

The BMD of trained athletes exceeds that of non-athletic controls for a wide variety of sports. Professional athletes who generate high muscle forces, such as weightlifters, have the highest bone mass (13). Interpretation of these observations is complicated by the fact that elite athletes likely differ from the general population even before the initiation of training. It is important not to lose sight of this issue because one cannot conclude that if the BMD of weightlifters exceeds that of sedentary controls by 20%, the latter would likely experience a 20% gain in BMD should they undertake a weightlifting program.

The effects of exercise on BMD are influenced by many factors, including menstrual status. Several cross-sectional studies demonstrate that amenorrheic women athletes have low bone density and a higher incidence of stress fractures compared with eumenorrheic athletes (14–16). The exception to this may be elite women gymnasts. Although these athletes have a high prevalence of oligomenorrhea and amenorrhea, they actually show higher than predicted BMD at all sites (17). One aspect of gymnastics training may explain this finding: whereas runners load their lumbar vertebrae with approximately three body weights with each step, dismounting from parallel bars or other high-impact gymnastics activities gives vertebral loading of 15 to 20 body weights. Thus, the experience in gymnasts may provide insight to the type of mechanical loads that are the strongest stimuli to bone formation. By contrast, even though collegiate swimmers participate in muscle strength training, they have lower bone mass than do other athletes or even sedentary individuals of similar age (18). Although this may be related to the type of physical activity, elite swimmers spend approximately 25 buoyant hours per week, which is time taken from their possible weight-bearing activity. It may also reflect the fact that successful swimmers have less dense skeletons.

Childhood represents a unique opportunity not only to gain bone density but also to modify skeletal dimensions and architecture in response to mechanical loads. Vigorous exercise during growth years appears to permanently increase the cross-sectional area of the trained region. For example, the dominant forearm of a tennis player has a larger cross-sectional area than does the non-dominant arm (19). As the strength of a bone reflects both its mineral density and size, increases in the dimensions of bone should reduce long-term fracture risk, although BMD eventually decreases.

Bone Mass in Non-Athletes

A critical issue is whether the skeletal benefits enjoyed by elite athletes also extend to the general population. In healthy, normal children and adolescents, observational studies indicate a direct relationship between higher levels of habitual physical activity and higher levels of BMD (20,21). However, the standard measurements of bone density ("areal bone density") used in these studies do not distinguish between increases in density and increases in bone size (because they correct only for two, not three, bone dimensions) (see Chapter 1). Therefore, it is not clear if physical activity increases the dimensions of a bone, its true mineral density, or both.

Another issue in assessing the impact of physical activity on BMD is the fact that most healthy individuals are moderately active. At this level of physical activity, the changes seen in BMD in response to increased activity are small (Fig. 5-1). Therefore, large studies are needed to find significant relationships between physical activity and BMD in these healthy individuals. In adults, some (22–24), but not all (25,26), studies show positive relationships of BMD to levels of physical activity (based either on self-report or as assessed by a pedometer or similar device).

Falls and Fractures

Because physical activity may be a marker of underlying health, it is difficult to interpret the relationship between physical activity and falls in observational studies. However, prospective observational studies suggest a U-shaped relationship such that there is an increased risk of falls among people who are, on one hand, either very frail or sedentary or, on the other hand, extremely active, with a decreased risk of falls among people who engage in moderate physical activity (27–31).

Case-control studies suggest that current or past physical activity (including activity at work, housework, walking, and other recreational activities) is associated with a 20% to 60% reduction in the rate of hip fractures. Most, but not all, prospective studies have found that physical activity is associated with a 30% to 50% reduction in hip fracture risk in both women and men (1). Only a few reports have addressed the relationship of physical activity to the risk of vertebral fractures. Generally, these studies have shown that increased physical activity is associated with a modest reduction of incident vertebral fracture (1).

Randomized Controlled Trials

Bone Mineral Density

A systematic review and meta-analysis of randomized clinical trials of exercise on bone mass in premenopausal and postmenopausal women has been recently published (32). This included 24 studies in postmenopausal women (Table 5-1) and 8 in premenopausal women (Table 5-2). The studies, which

Table 5-1   Characteristics of Randomized Studies of the Effectiveness of Exercise for the Prevention of Bone Loss in Postmenopausal Women

Author	Age (mean)	Intervention	Duration of Exercise Program (months)	No. with Data	Dropout Rate (%)	Compliance Rate (%)*	Measurement Sites	% Difference in BMD†
Bassey (33)	55	"Heel drops"	12	44	30	84	Ultradistal forearm Spine Femoral neck Ward's triangle Trochanter	1.6 2.2 −0.8 −1.0 1.4
Bravo (34)	60	Walking, dancing, stepping up and down, flexibility exercises	12	124	18	?	Spine Femoral neck	1.8 0.8
Chow (35)	56	a) Aerobics b) Aerobics and light resistance training	12	58	17	70	Trunk/upper thighs	a) 5.3 b) 9.1
Ebrahim (36)	67	Brisk walking	24	97	41	100	Spine Femoral neck	−0.1 2.4
Grove (37)	56	Running in place, jumping	12	15	7	83	Spine	7.8
Hatori (38)	57	Walking	7	33	9	?	Spine	2.8
Heikkinen (39)	53	Resistance training	36	69	12	?	Spine Femoral neck	$P > 0.05$ $P < 0.05$
Kerr (40)	58	Resistance training a) Strength b) Endurance	12	46	18	82	Shaft radius Ultradistal radius Femoral neck Ward's triangle Trochanter	a) 1.2 b) 1.1 a) 3.6 b) 0.1 a) 0.4 b) 1.2 a) 1.5 b) 1.0 a) 2.3 b) −0.9

Study						Site	% change
Lau (41)	76	Stepping block	10	50	17	?	Spine	0.6
							Femoral neck	-5.5
							Ward's triangle	-3.6
							Trochanter	-0.1
Lord (42)	72	Strengthening, coordination, balance, and weight-bearing exercise	10.5	138	23	73	Spine	0.7
							Femoral neck	-1.6
							Trochanter	0.0
Lynch (13)	69	Resistance exercise, brisk walking	15	26	?	?	Femoral neck	-1.3
							Trochanter	-1.2
Martin (4)	58	Treadmill	12	55	28	60	Proximal	1.1
							Distal forearm	1.6
							Spine	1.4
McMurdo (15)	65	Weight-bearing exercise	24	92	22	76	Ultradistal forearm	3.7
							Distal forearm	-0.8
							Spine	1.7
Nelson (46)	59	High-intensity strength training	12	39	1	88	Total body	3.2
							Spine	2.8
							Femoral neck	3.4
Notelovitz (47)	45	Resistance weight training	12	20	40	>70	Total body	1.5
							Midshaft radius	4.4
							Spine	6.8
Preisinger (48)	60	Brisk walking and stretching exercises	12–60	146	0	48	Distal wrist	0.6/yr
							Proximal wrist	0.7/yr
Prince (49)	63	Weight-bearing exercise	24	84	?	39	Spine	1.7
							Femoral neck	0.5/yr
							Intertrochanter	0.1/yr
							Trochanter	0.3/yr
							Ultradistal ankle	0.6/yr

Cont'd.

Table 5-1   Characteristics of Randomized Studies of the Effectiveness of Exercise for the Prevention of Bone Loss in Postmenopausal Women (Cont'd.)

Author	Age (mean)	Intervention	Duration of Exercise Program (months)	No. with Data	Dropout Rate (%)	Compliance Rate (%)*	Measurement Sites	% Difference in BMD†
Pruitt (9)	68	Resistance weight training	12	26	35	79	Spine Total hip Femoral neck Ward's triangle	0.8 -0.1 -1.1 2.4
Revel (50)	54	Training of psoas muscles	12	73	6	55	Spine	2.3
Sandler (51)	57	Walking	36	155	?	?	Shaft of forearm	"No effect"
Sinaki (52)	56	Back-strengthening exercises	24	65	4	66	Spine	-0.2/yr
Smidt (53)	56	Resistance exercise program for trunk muscles	12	49	11	?	Spine Trochanter Femoral neck Ward's triangle	0.8 1.0 1.5 -1.2
Svendsen (54)	54	Aerobics and weight training	3	118	2	97	Total body Forearm	0.0 -0.1
Taaffe (10)	68	Leg press with knee extension, knee flexion	12	25	30	79	Spine Middle third of femur	-0.8 2.8

* Compliance rate is the percentage of prescribed exercise sessions that were actually completed.
† Percentage change in bone density in exercise group minus percentage change in bone density in control group. A positive value indicates that subjects in the exercise group lost less bone, on average, than subjects in the control group.

From Wallace BA, Cumming RG. Systematic review of randomized trials of the effect of exercise on bone mass in premenopausal and postmenopausal women. Calcif Tissue Int. 2000;67:10–18; with permission.

lasted on average 1 year, included a wide range of exercise programs, both impact (walking, running, aerobics, dancing, heel drop) and non-impact (resistance training, strength training, weight lifting). In postmenopausal women, the lumbar spine BMD increased by 1.3% per year for impact programs and 1% per year for non-impact programs, compared with control groups. Results among premenopausal women were similar. In postmenopausal women, femoral neck bone mass increased 0.5% per year to 1.4% per year in the impact and non-impact groups, respectively. In premenopausal women, there was no difference in femoral neck BMD among exercise and control groups. However, longer duration studies in this area are needed to assess if and for how long these increases continue. It is possible that exercise may be less effective in people who are habitually physically active (consistent with physiology of exercise on bone described above) (41). Direct comparisons of impact and non-impact training programs are limited, but one study suggests no differences in lumbar spine effects (24).

Falls and Fractures

Data from randomized controlled trials on exercise for fall prevention have been conflicting. Estimates of the risk of falling from each of these studies are illustrated in Figure 5-2. A meta-analysis of fall prevention trials found a modest but significant reduction in the risk of falling (10%) associated with general exercise (such as flexibility, balance, lower-extremity resistance training, and multidisciplinary physical therapy). Of the various modalities, a Tai Chi training program that emphasizes balance resulted in a 40% reduction in the risk of falls (69). This suggests that the exercise does not need to be strenuous. Other but not all randomized controlled trials have also demonstrated a beneficial effect of exercise on falls.

There is only one randomized trial evaluating the effects of exercise on fracture outcomes. In postmenopausal women with prevalent vertebral fractures, back extension exercise resulted in a reduction in the number of new vertebral deformities compared with a control (72).

Exercises for Patients with Vertebral Fractures

Little attention has been devoted to the role of exercise for osteoporotic patients who have already sustained fractures. Frequently, patients and physicians show reluctance to participate in an exercise program because of concerns about additional injury. However, avoidance of activity will aggravate bone loss and place the skeleton at even greater jeopardy. An exercise program should increase a patient's ability to carry out routine daily activities

Table 5-2   Characteristics of Randomized Studies of the Effectiveness of Exercise for the Prevention of Bone Loss in Premenopausal Women

Author	Age (mean)	Intervention	Duration of Exercise Program (months)	No. with Data	Dropout Rate (%)	Compliance Rate (%)*	Measurement Sites	% Difference in BMD†
Bassey (55)	31	Intermittent high-impact exercise	6	27	?	76	Ultradistal forearm	1.1
							Distal radius	0.9
							Spine	-0.4
							Femoral neck	2.1
							Ward's triangle	2.0
							Trochanter	2.9
Blimkie (56)	16	Resistance training	6.5	32	11	?	Total body	0.3
							Spine	1.0
Dornemann (57)	44	High-intensity weightlifting	6	26	26	78	Distal radius	-0.6
							Spine	1.4
							Femoral neck	2.4
Friedlander (58)	29	Aerobics and weight training	24	63	47	61	Spine	1.1
							Femoral neck	2.4
							Trochanter	2.3
							Calcaneus	6.4
Heinonen (59)	39	Jump training and stretching	18	84	14	83	Distal radius	-0.7
							Spine	1.5
							Femoral neck	1.0
							Trochanter	0.6
							Distal femur	1.5
							Patella	0.8
							Proximal tibia	2.6
							Calcaneus	1.8

Study		Exercise					Site	Change†
Lohman (60)	34	Resistance weight training	18	56	46	84	Total body	−0.3
							Radius shaft	0.0
							Spine	1.8
							Femoral neck	1.3
							Ward's triangle	2.6
Sinaki (61)	36	Weightlifting	36	67	30	56	Midshaft radius	−1.2
							Spine	0.4
							Femoral neck	0.2
							Ward's triangle	−0.4
							Trochanter	0.1
Snow-Harter (24)	20	a) Running b) Weight training	8	30	42	a) 97 b) 92	Spine	a) 2.1 b) 2.0
							Femoral neck	a) 0.0 b) 0.0
							Ward's triangle	a) 2.4 b) 0.2
							Trochanter	a) 0.0 b) 1.3

* Compliance rate is the percentage of prescribed exercise sessions that were actually completed.
† Percentage change in bone density in exercise group minus percentage change in bone density in control group. A positive value indicates that subjects in the exercise group lost less bone, on average, than subjects in the control group.

From Wallace BA, Cumming RG. Systematic review of randomized trials of the effect of exercise on bone mass in pre- and postmenopausal women. Calcif Tissue Int. 2000;67:10–18; with permission.

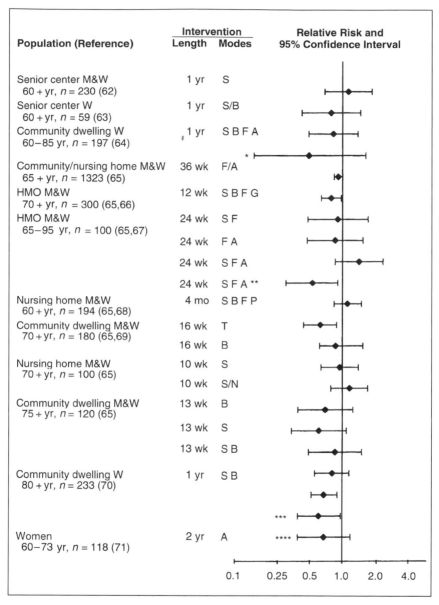

Figure 5-2   Randomized controlled trials of physical activity interventions and falls among older adults. Relative risk (RR) and 95% confidence interval bars (x-axis) associated with interventions (column 3) are compared with control conditions. RR: risk of any fall except *two or more falls, **time to first fall (67), ***first four falls, ****injurious falls. From Gregg EW, Pereira MA, Caspersen CJ. Physical activity, falls, and fractures among older adults: a review of the epidemiologic evidence. J Am Geriatr Soc. 2000; 48:833–893; with permission.

while minimizing the risk for subsequent fracture, and it should lead to a reduction in the risk for falls. For patients with vertebral osteoporosis, activities that place an anterior load on vertebral bodies, such as back flexion exercise, may increase the risk of vertebral fracture. In fact, it is important to educate patients about the potential dangers of lifting in flexion. The force of lifting even modest weights is amplified at the spine. For example, if one lifts a 5-kg weight from a shopping cart using arms that are 50 cm in length, the load is balanced by paraspinous muscles that may be no more than 1 cm long. Therefore, the load on the vertebral body may be magnified 50-fold to a value of 250 kg.

Clinical Recommendations

The optimal exercise regimen for preventing osteoporosis and related fractures is not known. However, any exercise is better than none, and consistent physical activity is likely associated with the greatest long-term benefit. Therefore, patients should be advised to adopt a form of regular exercise that they are likely to maintain throughout life, especially into the late seventh decade and thereafter, when the risk of hip fractures is highest. This may be most successful if patients make exercise a regular part of their weekly schedule and do it with other people to make it a pleasant, and expected, part of their social schedule.

For healthy individuals, a combination of weight-bearing high-impact or low-impact aerobic activity and muscle strengthening (approximately 30 minutes, three times per week) may be ideal for the musculoskeletal and other systemic benefits. For sedentary or frail elderly, a program of walking, low-impact aerobics, or water aerobics, in addition to a muscle strengthening program, is recommended. Specific examples of these types of exercises are listed in Table 5-3. Physicians and patients can learn more about specific exercises from the National Osteoporosis Foundation. Physicians should also consider referring patients to a physical therapist, especially patients who have associated conditions that may limit their ability to participate in an exercise program (for example, patients with osteoarthritis), patients who have been previously sedentary, and patients who are elderly but want to do rigorous activity.

To ensure safety, all previously sedentary older patients without cardiovascular disease should be advised to start with a low-intensity exercise program (for example, strengthening exercises, Tai Chi, or self-paced walking). Patients should be instructed in proper exercise techniques and advised that if chest pain, shortness of breath, or dizziness develops, they should rest. Patients with persistent or recurring symptoms should see their physician. Patients with overt cardiovascular disease require consultation with a cardiologist for risk assessment before starting a moderate exercise program (73).

Table 5-3   Exercise Prescription for Patients*

A   Examples of Weight-Bearing Aerobic Exercise for Healthy Individuals
Brisk walking
Jogging
Dancing
Standard aerobic exercise
Cross-country skiing
Heavy gardening
Racquet sports (squash, tennis, handball)

A   Examples of Weight-Bearing Aerobic Exercise for Sedentary or Frail Elderly Individuals
Walking
Low-impact aerobics
Light gardening

B   Muscle Strengthening (Concentrate on large muscles of the back, shoulder, upper arms, pelvis, hip, and upper legs.)
Weightlifting (tailor to patient's age and conditioning)
Exercise machines (tailor to patient's age and conditioning)
Calisthenics program
Other: Tai Chi, swimming, water aerobics, gardening (may be particularly good for frail elderly patients and patients with other comorbid conditions)

* Choose one from the appropriate "A" category and one from the "B" category.

REFERENCES

1. **Gregg EW, Pereira MA, Caspersen CJ.** Physical activity, falls, and fractures among older adults: a review of the epidemiologic evidence. J Am Geriatr Soc. 2000;48:883–893.

2. **Rubin CT, Lanyon LE.** Dynamic strain similarity in vertebrates: an alternative to allometric limb bone scaling. J Theoret Biol. 1984;107:321–327.

3. **Marcus R.** Mechanisms of skeletal response to exercise. In: Bilezikian JP, Raisz LG, Rodan GA (eds). Principles of Bone Biology. San Diego: Academic Press;1996;1: 1435–1445.

4. **Cummings SR, Nevitt MC, Browner WS, et al.** Risk factors for hip fracture in white women. N Engl J Med. 1995;332:767–773.

5. **Whipple RH, Wolfson LI, Amerman PM.** The relationship of knee and ankle weakness to falls in nursing home residents. J Am Geriatr Soc. 1987;35:13–20.

6. **Frontera W, Meredith C, O'Reilly K, et al.** Strength conditioning in older men: skeletal muscle hypertrophy and improved function. J Appl Physiol. 1988;64:1038–1044.

7. **Charette SL, McEvoy L, Pyka G, et al.** Muscle hypertrophy response to resistance training in older women. J Appl Physiol. 1991;70:1912–1916.

8. **Pyka G, Lindenberger E, Charette S, Marcus R.** Muscle strength and fiber adaptations to a year-long resistance training program in elderly women. J Gerontol. 1994;49: M22–M27.

9. **Pruitt LA, Taaffe DR, Marcus R.** Effects of a one-year high versus low intensity resistance training program on bone mineral density in older women. J Bone Min Res. 1995;10:1788–1795.

10. **Taaffe DR, Pruitt L, Pyka G, et al.** Comparative effects of high- and low-intensity resistance training on thigh muscle strength, fiber area, and tissue composition in elderly women. Clin Physiol. 1996;16:381–392.

11. **Taaffe DR, Duret C, Wheeler S, Marcus R.** Once-weekly resistance exercise improves muscle strength and neuromuscular performance in older adults. J Am Geriatr Soc. 1999;47:1208–1214.

12. **Cumming RG, Nevitt MC, Cummings SR.** Epidemiology of hip fractures. Epidemiol Rev. 1997;19:244–257.

13. **Snow-Harter C, Marcus R.** Exercise, bone mineral density, and osteoporosis. Exercise Sport Sci Rev. 1991;19:351–388.

14. **Drinkwater BL, Nilson K, Chesnut CH III, et al.** Bone mineral content of amenorrheic and eumenorrheic athletes. N Engl J Med. 1984;311:277–281.

15. **Marcus R, Cann C, Madvig P, et al.** Menstrual function and bone mass in elite women distance runners: endocrine and metabolic features. Ann Intern Med. 1985;102:158–163.

16. **Myburgh KH, Bachrach LK, Lewis B, et al.** Low bone mineral density at axial and appendicular sites in amenorrheic athletes. Med Sci Sports Exerc. 1993;25:1197–1202.

17. **Robinson TL, Snow-Harter C, Taaffe DR, et al.** Gymnasts exhibit higher bone mass than runners despite similar prevalence of amenorrhea. J Bone Min Res. 1995;10:26–35.

18. **Taaffe DR, Snow-Harter C, Connolly DA, et al.** Differential effects of swimming versus weight-bearing activity on bone mineral status of eumenorrheic athletes. J Bone Miner Res. 1995;10:586–593.

19. **Haapsalo H, Sievanen H, Kannus P, et al.** Dimensions and estimated mechanical characteristics of the humerus after long-term tennis loading. J Bone Miner Res. 1996;11:864–872.

20. **Slemenda CW, Miller JZ, Hui SL, et al.** Role of physical activity in the development of skeletal mass in children. J Bone Min Res. 1991;6:1227–1233.

21. **Ruiz JC, Mandel C, Garabedian M.** Influence of spontaneous calcium intake and physical exercise on the vertebral and femoral bone mineral density of children and adolescents. J Bone Min Res. 1995;10:675–682.

22. **Recker RR, Davies KM, Hinders SM, et al.** Bone gain in young adult women. JAMA. 1992;268:2403–2408.

23. **Aloia JF, Vaswani AN, Yeh JK, Cohn SH.** Premenopausal bone mass is related to physical activity. Arch Intern Med. 1988;148:121–123.

24. **Snow-Harter C, Bouxsein ML, Lewis BT, et al.** Effects of resistance and endurance exercise on bone mineral status of young women. A randomized exercise intervention trial. J Bone Min Res. 1992;7:761–769.

25. **Sowers MR, Wallace RB, Lemke JH.** Correlates of mid-radius bone density among postmenopausal women. A community study. Am J Clin Nutr. 1985;41:1045–1053.

26. **Mazess RB, Bardin HS.** Bone density in premenopausal women: effects of age, dietary intake, physical activity, smoking, and birth-control pills. Am J Clin Nutr. 1991;53: 132–142.

27. **Tinetti ME, Speechley, Ginter SF.** Risk factors for falls among elderly persons living in the community. N Engl J Med. 1988;319:1701–1707.

28. **Graafmans WC, Ooms ME, Hofsree HMA, et al.** Falls in the elderly. A prospective study of risk factors and risk profiles. Am J Epidemiol. 1996;143:1129–1136.

29. **Sorock GS, Labiner DM.** Peripheral neuromuscular dysfunction and falls in an elderly cohort. Am J Epidemiol. 1992;136:584–591.

30. **O'Loughlin JL, Robitaille Y, Boilvin J, Suissa S.** Incidence of and risk factors for falls and injurious falls among the community-dwelling elderly. Am J Epidemiol. 1993;137:342–354.

31. **Tinetti ME, Doucette J, Claus E, Marottoli R.** Risk factors for serious injury during falls by older persons in the community. J Am Geriatr Soc. 1995;43:1214–1221.

32. **Wallace BA, Cumming RG.** Systematic review of randomized trials of the effect of exercise on bone mass in pre- and postmenopausal women. Calcif Tissue Int. 2000; 67:10–18.

33. **Bassey EJ, Ramsdale SJ.** Weight-bearing exercise and ground reaction forces. A 12-month randomized controlled trial of effects on bone mineral density in healthy postmenopausal women. Bone. 1995;16:469–476.

34. **Bravo G, Gauthier P, Roy PM, et al.** Impact of a 12-month exercise program on the physical and psychological health of osteopenic women. J Am Geriatr Soc. 1996;44: 756–762.

35. **Chow R, Harrison JE, Notarius C.** Effect of two randomised exercise programmes on bone mass of healthy postmenopausal women. BMJ. 1987;295:1441–1444.

36. **Ebrahim S, Thompson PW, Baskaran V, Evans K.** Randomised placebo-controlled trial of brisk walking in the prevention of postmenopausal osteoporosis. Age Ageing. 1997;26:253–260.

37. **Grove KA, Londeree BR.** Bone density in postmenopausal women: high impact vs low impact exercise. Med Sci Sports Exerc. 1992;24:1190–1194.

38. **Hatori M, Hasegawa A, Adachi H, et al.** The effects of walking at the anaerobic threshold level on vertebral bone loss in postmenopausal women. Calcif Tissue Int. 1993;52:411–414.

39. **Heikkinen J, Kyllonen E, Kurttila-Matero E, et al.** HRT and exercise: effects on bone density, muscle strength and lipid metabolism. A placebo-controlled 2-year prospective trial on two estrogen-progestin regimens in healthy postmenopausal women. Maturitas. 1997;26:139–149.

40. **Kerr D, Morton A, Dick I, Prince R.** Exercise effects of bone mass in postmenopausal women are site-specific and load-dependent. J Bone Miner Res. 1996;11: 218–225.

41. **Lau EMC, Woo J, Leung PC, et al.** The effects of calcium supplementation and exercise on bone density in elderly Chinese women. Osteoporos Int. 1992;2:168–173.

42. **Lord SR, Ward JA, Williams P, Zivanovic E.** The effects of a community exercise program on fracture risk factors in older women. Osteoporos Int. 1996;6:361–367.

43. **Lynch P, Judge JO.** Relationship of prolonged resistance training and femur bone density in older women. J Am Geriatr Soc. 1992;40:SA29.

44. **Martin D, Notelovitz M.** Effects of aerobic training on bone mineral density of postmenopausal women. J Bone Miner Res. 1993;8:931–936.

45. **McMurdo MET, Mole PA, Paterson CR.** Controlled trial of weight-bearing exercise in older women. BMJ. 1997;314:569.

46. **Nelson ME, Fiatarone MA, Morganti CM, et al.** Effects of high-intensity strength training on multiple risk factors for osteoporotic fracture. A randomized controlled trial. JAMA 1994;272:1909–1914.

47. **Notelovitz M, Martin D, Tesar R, et al.** Estrogen therapy and variable-resistance weight training increase bone mineral in surgically menopausal women. J Bone Miner Res. 1991;6:583–590.

48. **Preisinger E, Alacamlioglu Y, Pils K, et al.** Therapeutic exercise in the prevention of bone loss. A controlled trial with women after menopause. Am J Phys Rehabil. 1995;74:120–123.

49. **Prince R, Devine A, Dick I, et al.** The effects of calcium supplementation (milk powder or tablets) and exercise on bone density in postmenopausal women. J Bone Miner Res. 1995;10:1068–1075.

50. **Revel M, Mayoux-Benhamou MA, Rabourdin JP, et al.** One-year psoas training can prevent lumbar bone loss in postmenopausal women. A randomized controlled trial. Calcif Tissue Int. 1993;53:307–311.

51. **Sandler RB, Cauley JA, Hom DL, et al.** The effects of walking on the cross-sectional dimensions of the radius in the postmenopausal woman. Calcif Tissue Int. 1987;41:65–69.

52. **Sinaki M, Wahner HW, Offord KP, Hodgson SF.** Efficacy of nonloading exercises in prevention of vertebrae bone loss in postmenopausal women. A controlled trial. Mayo Clin Proc. 1989;64:762–769.

53. **Smidt GL, Lin S, O'Dwyer KD, Blanpied PR.** The effect of high-intensity trunk exercise on bone mineral density of postmenopausal women. Spine. 1992;17:280–285.

54. **Svendsen OL, Hassager C, Christiansen C.** Effect of an energy-restrictive diet, with or without exercise, on lean tissue mass, resting metabolic rate, cardiovascular risk factors, and bone in overweight postmenopausal woman. Am J Med. 1993;95:131–140.

55. **Bassey EJ, Ramsdale SJ.** Increase in femoral bone density in young women following high impact exercise. Osteoporos Int. 1994;4:72–75.

56. **Blimkie CJ, Rice S, Webber CE, et al.** Effects of resistance training on bone mineral content and density in adolescent females. Can J Physiol Pharmacol. 1996;74:1025–1033.

57. **Dornemann TM, McMurray RG, Renner JB, Anderson JJB.** Effects of high-intensity resistance exercise on bone mineral density and muscle strength of 40- to 50-year-old women. J Sports Med Phys Fitness. 1997;37:246–251.

58. **Friedlander AL, Genant HK, Sadowsky S, et al.** A two-year program of aerobics and weight training enhances bone mineral density of young women. J Bone Miner Res. 1995;10:574–585.

59. **Heinonen A, Kannus P, Sievanen H, et al.** Randomised controlled trial of effect of high impact exercise on selected risk factors for osteoporotic fractures. Lancet. 1996;348:1343–1347.

60. **Lohman T, Going S, Parmenter R, et al.** Effects of resistance training on regional and total bone mineral density in premenopausal women. A randomised prospective study. J Bone Miner Res. 1995;10:1015–1024.

61. **Sinaki M, Wahner HW, Bergstrath EJ, et al.** Three-year controlled, randomised trial of the effect of dose-specific loading and strengthening exercise on bone mineral density of spine and femur in nonathletic, physically active women. Bone. 1996;19:233–244.

62. **Reinsch S, MacRae P, Lachenbruch PA, Tobis JS.** Attempts to prevent falls and injury. A prospective community study. Gerontologist. 1992;32:450–456.

63. **McRae PG, Felmer ME, Reinsch S.** A 1-year exercise program for older women: effects on falls, injuries, and physical performance. J Aging Phys Activity. 1994;2:127–142.

64. **Lord SP, Ward JA, Williams P, Strudwick M.** The effect of a 12-month exercise trial on balance, strength, and falls in older women. A randomized controlled trial. J Am Geriatr Soc. 1995;43:1198–1206.

65. **Province MA, Hadley EC, Hornbrook MC, et al.** The effects of exercise on falls in elderly patients. A pre-planned meta-anlaysis of the FICSIT Trials. JAMA. 1995;273: 1341–1347.

66. **Tinetti ME, Baker DJ, McAway G, et al.** A multifactorial intervention to reduce the risk of falling among elderly people living in the community. N Engl J Med. 1994;331: 821–827.

67. **Buchner DM, Cress ME, de Lateur BJ, et al.** The effect of strength and endurance training on gait, balance, fall risk, and health services use in community-living older adults. J Gerontol A Biol Sci Med Sci. 1992;32:450–456.

68. **Mulrow CD, Gerety MB, Kanteen D, et al.** A randomized trial of physical rehabilitation for very frail nursing home residents. JAMA. 1994;271:519–524.

69. **Wolf SL, Barnhart HX, Kumer NG, et al.** Reducing frailty and falls in older persons: an investigation of Tai Chi and computerized balance training. J Am Geriatr Soc. 1996;44:489–497.

70. **Campbell AJ, Robertson MC, Gardner MM, et al.** Randomised controlled trial of a general practice programme of home based exercise to prevent falls in elderly women. Br Med J. 1997;315:1065–1069.

71. **McMurdo MET, Mole PA, Paterson CR.** Controlled trial of weight-bearing exercise in older women in relation to bone density and falls. Br Med J. 1997;314:569.

72. **Sinaki M, Mikkelsen BA.** Postmenopausal spinal osteoporosis: flexion versus extension exercises. Arch Phys Med Rehab. 1984;65:593–596.

73. **Gill TM, Di Pietro L, Krumholz HM.** Role of exercise stress testing and safety monitoring for older persons starting an exercise program. JAMA. 2000;284:342–349.

CHAPTER 6

Estrogens

GAIL A. GREENDALE, MD
JANE CAULEY, DRPH

Key Points

- Five estrogens and two estrogen/progestin fixed combinations are FDA approved for prevention of osteoporosis (prevention of bone loss). Estrogens are not approved for the treatment of osteoporosis (prevention of fractures).

- Randomized placebo-controlled studies demonstrate that all estrogens and estrogen/progestin combinations approved for osteoporosis prevention maintain or improve bone mass density.

- Because almost all studies of estrogen or estrogen/progestin and the prevention of bone loss gave the subjects supplemental calcium, women using hormone replacement therapy (HRT) should have a total (diet plus supplement) daily intake of 1200 mg of elemental calcium.

- Many observational studies find an approximate 50% reduction in risk of osteoporotic fracture among current users of estrogen. However, there have been few trials, and observational studies may overestimate the fracture-protective effect of HRT.

- Estrogens and estrogen/progestin combinations affect numerous symptoms and systems in addition to the skeleton. Before deciding whether to start or continue estrogen for prevention of osteoporosis, providers and patients should also understand and consider the non-skeletal risks and benefits of HRT.

Endogenous estrogens are 18 carbon steroids that are made in female ovaries, the fetal-placental unit, and the male testes. In both genders, the adrenal cortex makes estrone. Estrogens are also produced in fat tissue by the conversion of precursors made by the adrenal cortex. The major endogenous estrogens in non-pregnant women are estradiol, estriol, and estrone.

Many lines of evidence support a role for estrogen in developing and maintaining skeletal integrity. Osteoblasts (1) and osteoclasts (2) have estrogen receptors, and bone turnover increases when estrogen levels fall (3). Estrogen counters the formation of pro-inflammatory cytokines (which promote bone resorption) by bone marrow cells and bone cells (4). Estrogen also has systemic effects (for example, it reduces parathyroid hormone secretion) that influence calcium balance and bone loss (5).

Estrogen has long been the mainstay of therapy for prevention of postmenopausal osteoporosis. Although a number of randomized clinical trials support estrogen's role in maintaining bone mineral density (BMD), most of the data concerning fracture outcomes with hormone replacement therapy (HRT) are from observational studies. In general, these studies have found that fracture rates among estrogen users are lower than those of non-users (6). Estrogen affects many organs other than bone; therefore, the clinician must also consider other risks and benefits when making decisions about prescribing estrogen as preventive therapy. Observational studies find that estrogen use is associated with primary prevention of cardiovascular disease (7). Additionally, an overall beneficial effect of postmenopausal estrogen use is suggested by findings that all-cause mortality in hormone users is 30% to 50% lower than that of non-users (8,9). The consistency, biological plausibility, and benefits of estrogen that are evident in numerous cohort studies of fracture and heart disease prevention have lead to a widespread view that estrogen is beneficial for postmenopausal women. Results of randomized trials designed to determine whether estrogen prevents coronary heart disease (CHD) or fractures are still needed. Evidence about estrogen is in flux, so patients should periodically review with their physicians the potential benefits and risks of estrogen therapy.

Bone Mineral Density

Trials consistently show that estrogens, alone or in combination with progestogens, maintain or modestly increase BMD (10–18). Improvement in BMD is not influenced by concomitant administration of medroxyprogesterone acetate (MPA) or micronized progesterone. Table 6-1 details results from the placebo-controlled randomized trials with BMD outcomes that supported FDA approval of the five formulations of estrogen currently approved for osteoporosis prevention (Table 6-2). In the Postmenopausal Estrogen/Progestin Interventions Trial (PEPI), conjugated equine estrogens (CEE, 0.625 mg) increased spine BMD by about 4% to 5% and hip BMD by about 1.7% at 3 years (19). All other formulations, including esterified estrogens, ethinyl estradiol, the 17ß-estradiol patch, and estrone, produced a similar improvement in BMD (Table 6-1).

In general, the addition of MPA or micronized progesterone has not added to the gains in BMD seen with the doses and types of estrogen used in clinical practice. Some trials suggest that when estrogen is combined with an androgenic progestin (such as norethisterone acetate) BMD may increase more than it does when estrogen is used (19,20). However, these studies have not had an estrogen-only control arm.

Supplemental Calcium with Estrogen and Estrogen-Plus-Progestin Treatments

Because all trials summarized in Table 6-1, with the exception of PEPI, also gave or recommended supplemental calcium, we cannot determine whether calcium independently contributes to the improvement in BMD that is seen with estrogen alone. Therefore, postmenopausal women who are taking estrogen should also have a total (diet plus supplement) intake of 1200 mg of elemental calcium daily (21).

Osteoporotic Fractures

Observational Studies

Many observational studies have reported lower fracture rates in postmenopausal women who take estrogen than in women not receiving this therapy (6,22–25). Examination of the effect of estrogen on wrist fractures alone revealed an approximately 60% reduction in the risk of wrist fracture (22,24,26). The relative risk of vertebral fractures among estrogen users was also reduced by approximately 40% (24). Several studies have reported a 20% to 50% reduction in the risk of hip fracture among older women using estrogen (22,23,27). A meta-analysis of observational data estimated a 25% decrease in the risk of hip fracture among postmenopausal women who reported having used estrogen (6). For all fractures, the relative risk was reduced by approximately 35% (22) to 50% (28) among current users.

Most observational studies have reported on the association between unopposed estrogen and fractures (29,30). However, addition of a progestin to

Table 6-1   Estrogen Doses That Preserve Bone Mineral Density (BMD) Based on Data from Placebo-Controlled Randomized Clinical Trials That Used Bone Densitometry Outcome Measurements

First Author	Participants and Treatments	Participant Characteristics	Spine or Arm BMD*	Hip BMD*
Writing Group for the PEPI Trial (10)	875 Total 174 Pbo 175 CEE 174 CEE-MPA (cyc) 174 CEE-MPA (con) 178 CEE-MP (cyc) 36 months duration Supplemental calcium used ad lib	• Mean age, 56 years (45–64) • Postmenopausal, 1 to 10 years, natural or surgical • 90% white • No BMD or fracture criteria	Spine, DEXA, 36 months • Pbo ↓ 1.8% • CEE, CEE-MPA (cyc), CEE-MP (cyc) ↑ 3.8%[†] • CEE-MPA (con) ↑ 5.0%[‡]	DEXA, 36 months • Pbo ↓ 1.7% • Each active Rx ↑ 1.7%[†]
Genant (11)	120 Total 28 Pbo 30 0.3 mg E_1S 32 0.625 mg E_1S 32 1.25 mg E_1S 12 months duration 1000 mg elemental calcium daily	• Mean age, 51 years • Postmenopausal, 6 months to 4 years • Excluded those with low BMD (<80 mg/cm³)	Spine, QCT, 12 months • Pbo ↓ 0.9% • E_1S, 0.3 ↓ 2.1% • E_1S, 0.625 ↑ 1.9%[†] • E_1S, 1.25 ↑ 2.5%[†]	Not done
Harris (12)	121 Total 28 Pbo 30 0.3 mg E_1S (0.375 mg EP) 32 0.625 mg E_1S (0.75 mg EP) 32 1.25 mg E_1S (1.5 mg EP) 24 months duration 1000 mg elemental calcium daily	• Mean age, 51 years • Postmenopausal, 2 months to no upper limit, natural or surgical • No BMD or fracture criteria	Spine, QCT, 24 months • Pbo ↓ 3.6% • E_1S, 0.3 ↓ 5.1% • E_1S, 0.625 ↓ 0.8% • E_1S, 1.25 ↑ 0.7%[†]	Not done

Study	Sample	Patient characteristics	Results	
Ettinger (13)	63 Total 16 Pbo 15 0.5 mg micronized E_2 16 1.0 mg micronized E_2 16 2.0 mg micronized E_2 12 months duration Calcium carbonate supplements calculated to raise daily intake to 1500 mg	• Mean age, 53 years (40–58) • Postmenopausal, 6 months to 5 years, natural or surgical • 75% white • No BMD or fracture criteria	Spine, DPA, 12 months • Pbo ↓ 0.9% • Active Rx ↑ between 1% and 3%	Not done
Adami (14)	34 Total 17 Pbo 17 50 mg transdermal E_2 for 3 of 4 weeks 18 months duration Diet containing 1200 mg calcium and 600–800 IU vitamin D recommended	• Mean age, 50 years (42–58) • Postmenopausal, 2–4 years previously, natural only	Forearm, DPA, 18 months • Pbo ↓ 3.5% • E_2 ↑ 4.3%†	Not done
Field (15)	123 Total 43 Pbo 25 0.025 mg transdermal E_2 28 0.05 mg transdermal E_2 27 0.10 mg transdermal E_2 24 months duration Daily minimum of 700 mg elemental calcium	• Mean age, 47 years (40 or greater) • Surgically postmenopausal, 6 weeks to 2 years • No BMD or fracture criteria	Mid-radius, SPA, 24 months • Pbo ↓ 4.9% • 0.025 mg E_2 ↓ 1.8%† • 0.05 mg E_2 ↓ 0.8%† • 0.10 mg E_2 ↓ 1.1%† Lumbar spine, DPA, 24 months • Pbo ↓ 6.4% • 0.025 mg E_2 ↓ 3.0%† • 0.05 mg E_2 ↑ 0.8%†§ • 0.10 mg E_2 ↑ 3.7%†§	Not done

(Cont'd.)

Table 6-1 Estrogen Doses That Preserve Bone Mineral Density (BMD) Based on Data from Placebo-Controlled Randomized Clinical Trials That Used Bone Densitometry Outcome Measurements (Cont'd)

First Author	Participants and Treatments	Participant Characteristics	Spine or Arm BMD*	Hip BMD*
Weiss (16)	175 Total 46 Pbo 32 0.025 mg transdermal E_2 31 0.05 mg transdermal E_2 31 0.06 mg transdermal E_2 35 0.10 mg transdermal E_2 Supplementation to achieve 1500 mg calcium daily	• Mean age, 51 years • Hysterectomy • If ovaries are intact, must have had hot flashes for between 1 and 5 years pre-enrollment • Serum $E_2 \leq 20$ pg/mL and FSH ≥ 50 µ/L • Spinal BMD (L2–L4) ≥ 0.09 g/cm^2 (Lunar) or 0.086 g/cm (Hologic)	Lumbar spine, DEXA, 24 months • Pbo ↓ 2.5% • 0.025 mg E_2 ↑ 2.4%† • 0.05 mg E_2 ↑ 3.4%† • 0.06 mg E_2 ↑ 4.0%† • 0.10 mg E_2 ↑ 4.7%†	Hip DEXA, 24 months • Pbo ↓ 2.0% • 0.025 mg E_2 ↑ 0.3%† • 0.05 mg E_2 ↑ 2.7%† • 0.06 mg E_2 ↑ 3.0%† • 0.10 mg E_2 ↑ 2.0%†
Genant (17)	406 Total 103 Pbo 101 0.3 mg EE daily 102 0.625 mg EE daily 100 1.25 mg EE daily 24 months duration 1000 mg elemental calcium daily	• Mean age, 51 years • Postmenopausal, 6 months to 4 years • Baseline BMD within 2.0 SD of young normals • Baseline endometrial biopsy showing atrophic, mildly proliferative, or moderately proliferative endometrium	Spine, DXA, 24 months • Pbo ↓ 2.5% • 0.3 EE ↑ 1.8%† • 0.6 EE ↑ 2.8%† • 1.25 EE ↑ 5.1%‡	Hip DEXA, 24 months • Pbo ↓ 0.8% • 0.3 EE ↑ 1.5%† • 0.6 EE ↑ 2.4%† • 1.25 EE ↑ 3.4%†

| Speroff (CHART) (18) | 1265 Total
137 Pbo
139 0.2 mg Neta/1.0 µg Ee
136 0.5 mg Neta/2.5 µg Ee
146 1.0 mg Neta/5 µg Ee
145 1.0 mg Neta/10 µg Ee
141 1.0 µg Ee
137 2.5 µg Ee
141 5.0 µg Ee
143 10.0 µg Ee

24 months duration

1000 mg elemental calcium daily | • Mean age, 52 years (40 or older)
• Naturally menopausal, intact uterus, less than 5 years postmenopausal
• Spinal trabecular BMD (QCT) between 90 and 150 mg/cm^3 | Spinal trabecular, QCT, 24 months
• Pbo ↓ 7.4%
Combination arms
• 0.2/1 ↓ 3.0%
• 0.5/2.5 ↓ 0.5%[†]
• 1.0/5 ↑ 2.2%[†]
• 1.0/10 ↑ 4.2%[†]

Ee-only arms
• 1.0 ↓ 2.0%[†]
• 2.5 ↓ 1.7%[†]
• 5.0 ↓ 1.5%[†]
• 10.0 ↑ 2.5%[†] | Not done |

* All BMD percent changes are relative to baseline. Values are not necessarily statistically significantly different from baseline. In some cases, when exact change figures were not cited in the reference, percents were calculated by the authors from raw BMD data or were extrapolated from graphs.
† Result statistically significantly different from placebo ($P < 0.05$).
‡ Result in this treatment arm statistically significant ($P < 0.05$) from all other active treatments.
§ Result in this treatment arm significantly different ($P < 0.05$) from the 0.025 mg E$_2$ treatment arm.

CEE, conjugated equine estrogens 0.625 mg daily; CEE + 5MPA (con), 0.625 mg conjugated equine estrogen and 5.0 mg medroxyprogesterone acetate daily; DEXA, dual-energy x-ray absorptiometry; DPA, dual-photon absorptiometry; E$_1$S, estrone sulfate; E$_2$, 17β estradiol; Ee, ethinyl estradiol; EE, esterified estrogens (75%–85% sodium estrone sulfate and 6%–15% sodium equilin sulfate); EP, estropipate; MP (cyc), micronized progesterone, 12 days per month; MPA (con), medroxyprogesterone acetate daily; MPA (cyc), medroxyprogesterone acetate, 12 days per month; Neta, norethindrone acetate; Pbo, placebo; QCT, quantitative computed tomography; Rx, treatment(s); SPA, single-photon absorptiometry.

Table 6-2   FDA-Approved Estrogens for Osteoporosis Prevention

Generic Names	Trade Names	Prevention Dose
Estrogens		
Conjugated equine estrogens	Premarin	0.625 mg
	Prempro*	0.625 mg
	Premphase†	0.625 mg
Estropipate‡	Ogen	0.625 mg
	Ortho-Est	0.625 mg
Estradiol (oral)	Estrace	0.5 mg
Estradiol (transdermal)	Estraderm	0.05 mg
	Climara	0.025 mg
Esterfied estrogens	Estratab	0.3 mg
Estrogen/Progestin Fixed Combinations§		
Ethinyl estradiol (Ee) and norethindrone acetate (Neta)	Femhrt	5 µg Ee and 1 mg Neta
Estradiol and norgestimate	Ortho-Prefest	1.0 mg E_2 and 0.09 mg norgestimate

* Prempro is a fixed combination product. In addition to conjugated estrogen, each pill contains 2.5 mg of medroxyprogesterone acetate. Each Prempro dose pack is a 28-day supply.

† Premphase is a fixed combination product. The first 14 pills contain conjugated equine estrogen only. The last 14 pills of each 28-day pill pack contains 5 mg of medroxyprogesterone acetate in addition to the estrogen.

‡ Estropipate was formerly known as estrone sulfate. References cited in support of its bone indication use the older terminology.

§ Indicated only for women who have not undergone hysterectomy.

estrogen had no additional effect on the risk of fracture: relative risk for wrist fracture among current unopposed estrogen users was 0.42 (CI, 0.25 to 0.70), and this risk among current users of estrogen plus progestin was 0.31 (CI, 0.11 to 0.84) (22).

The decrease in fracture risk associated with estrogen use is greatest among current or recent users, and the decreased risk tends to diminish with time after stopping estrogen (25,31,32). In the Study of Osteoporotic Fractures (SOF), a large prospective cohort study of almost 10,000 women, there was no association with fracture even among previous users who had used estrogen for 10 or more years (22).

In most studies, long-duration estrogen use was more beneficial in reducing fracture than was short duration of use (22). Case-control studies have suggested that at least 5 years of use may be needed to reduce fractures (25,30,31,33). Another study found that among women younger than age 75 years, at least 7 years of estrogen use was needed to reduce fracture risk (34). In SOF, 10 or more years of estrogen use was associated with a substantial reduction in the risk of wrist and hip fractures (22).

The association between estrogen therapy and reduction in risk of fracture is also more pronounced if estrogen is initiated close to menopause (22,30). Of importance, long-term users who had initiated therapy after 5 years of menopause had no significant reduction in the risk of nonspine fractures, despite an average duration of use of 16 years. This suggests that the time at which estrogen is initiated with respect to menopause may be more important than the total duration of use (22).

Observational studies may be biased because women who use HRT for long periods are healthier, have access to medical care, and maintain healthier lifestyles (35). Although these studies have been adjusted for these factors, there may be other confounders that could not be assessed. Only a randomized clinical trial comparing hormone use with placebo can provide conclusive evidence that treatment causes a reduction in fractures.

Randomized Controlled Trials

There have been few randomized trials of hormone replacement and fractures (Table 6-3); key findings of these studies are summarized here. Nachtigall et al (36) followed 84 pairs of institutionalized women who were treated daily with placebo or conjugated estrogen 2.5 mg/day and MPA, 10 mg per day, 7 days per month for 10 years. There were seven fractures in the control group and none in the treatment group. Lindsay et al (37) studied 100 women who were enrolled in a longitudinal study of bone loss after oophorectomy; about one half of the women were given mestranol (average dose, 23 µg/day), and the other half were given placebo. After a median follow-up of 9 years (range 6–12 years), estrogen treatment significantly reduced the incidence of vertebral compression. A 1-year trial in 75 postmenopausal women with established osteoporosis reported a 40% reduction in radiographic vertebral fracture rate in the group treated with 0.1 mg/day of transdermal estrogen compared with placebo (38). However, the reduction in risk was not statistically significant when analyzed by the number of women who developed vertebral fractures rather than the number of vertebrae that fractured (39). In a randomized trial of 464 non-osteoporotic Finnish women aged 47 to 56 years, HRT reduced the risk of non-vertebral fractures by about 60%, but the results were statistically significant only after they were adjusted for BMD and history of previous fractures (40). Furthermore, the hormone regimen used in this study (estradiol valerate and cyproterone acetate) is not approved in the United States.

In the Danish Osteoporosis Prevention Study, 1006 women were randomized to receive estradiol only (if hysterectomized), estradiol and norethisterone (if uterus intact), or no estrogen and followed for about 5 years (41). Forearm fracture risk was reduced by about 60% in the hormone group, but

Table 6-3　Randomized Controlled Trials of Estrogen Therapy with Fracture Outcomes

First Author	Intervention	Subject Characteristics	Fracture Outcomes	Results
Nachtigall (36)	• CEE 2.5 mg daily and MPA 10 mg daily for 7 days ($n = 67$) • Placebo ($n = 62$) • 10 years	• Age matched • 76.7% completed study • 40%, < 3 years since menopause • 10 years	Self-report of fracture	No. of fractures: CEE and MPA: 0 Placebo: 7
Lindsay (37)	• Mestranol, average dose 23.3 μg/day (range, 10 to 38 μg) ($n = 58$) • Placebo ($n = 42$) • 9 years (range, 6 to 12)	• Oophorectomized • Subset of original trial: women who attended clinic visits consistently and for longest period of time • Mean age about 48 years	Vertebral morphometry • Thoracic vertebrae (9) and lumbar vertebrae (2) • Subjective assessment of wedging and collapse • Compression of vertebral heights measured by calipers • Total spine score based on wedging or collapse	• Mestranol: 4%–7% greater anterior height ($P < 0.10$) • Mestranol: 34%–56% smaller wedge angle ($P < 0.05$) • Mestranol: 9%–13% greater ratio of central height to anterior height ($P < 0.06$)
Lufkin (38) & Windeler (39)	• Estraderm 0.1 mg E$_2$ plus MPA 10 mg/day for 10 days ($n = 36$) • Placebo ($n = 39$) • 1 year	• Osteoporotic women: prevalent vertebral fracture or BMD < 10th percentile of normal premenopausal women • All white • Mean age, 65 years (55 to 72)	• Vertebral morphometry • Anterior (ha), posterior (hp) and central biconcave heights (hm) • Decrease of >15% of ha/hp, hm/hp or hp < 85% hp adjacent vertebral • Fracture rate (total number of new fractures per 100 PY) • Number with ≥ 1 new fracture	No. of new fractures: • Pbo: 20 new fractures in 12 women • E$_2$ + MPA: 8 new fractures in 7 women Fracture rate per 100 PY • Pbo: 58 • E$_2$ + MPA: 23 ($P = 0.04$) No. of women with ≥ 1 new fracture • Pbo: 12 • E$_2$ + MPA: 7 ($P = 0.28$)

Komulainen (40)	• E$_2$ valerate 2 mg (days 1–21) and CPA 1 mg (days 12–21) (n = 116) • Vitamin D 300 IU and 93 mg calcium (n = 116) • E$_2$ valerate plus vitamin D (n = 116) • Placebo (n = 116) • 4.3 years	• Subset of Kuopio Osteoporosis Study • 6–24 months since last menstruation • T-score > −2.5 • Mean age, 53 years (47 to 56)	• All symptomatic nonvertebral fractures • Validated by medical reports	ITT (RR (95% CI*)) • E$_2$ valerate + CPA: 0.38; (0.15 − 0.99) • Vitamin D: 0.64 (0.29 − 1.42) • E$_2$ valerate + CPA + vitamin D: 0.48 (0.19 − 1.18) • Placebo: 1.0

Cauley (44)	• 0.625 mg CEE in combination with 2.5 MPA daily (n = 1380)
	• Placebo (n = 1383)
	• 4.1 years
		• Documented coronary heart disease
		• 89% Caucasian
		• Postmenopausal
		• Intact uterus
		• Mean age, 67 years (44 to 79)
			• Secondary outcome
			• Documented by radiographic report
			• All clinical fractures
			  —Hip
			  —Wrist
			  —Vertebral
			  —Other
			• Height loss ≥ 2 cm
				ITT (RR (95% CI))
				• All clinical fractures: 0.94 (0.75–1.19)
				  —Hip: 1.09 (0.51–2.31)
				  —Wrist: 0.97 (0.58–1.62)
				  —Spine: 0.69 (0.34–1.40)
				  —Other: 0.92 (0.69–1.23)
				≥ 2 cm height loss: 0.86 (0.67–1.10)

Mosekilde (41)	• 2 mg estradiol (12 days) and 2 mg estradiol and 1 mg norethisterone acetate (10 days) and 1 mg estradiol (6 days) in women with an intact uterus
	• Hysterectomized: 2 mg estradiol
	• No HRT
	• Not blinded
	• 5 years
		• Age 45–58 years
		• 3–24 months since menopause
			• Documented by radiographic report
			• All fractures
			  —Forearm
			  —Vertebral
			  —Other
				RR (95% CI) (randomized results)
				All fractures: 0.82 (0.53–1.29)
				Forearm: 0.42 (0.16–1.01)
				Vertebral: 2.00 (0.62–6.49)
				Other: 0.96 (0.57–1.64)

CEE, conjugated equine estrogen; CPA, cyproterone acetate; E2, estradiol; ITT, intention to treat; MPA, medroxyprogesterone acetate; Pbo, placebo.

this relationship was of borderline significance, and there was no effect on other fractures. Thirty-one percent of the women stopped taking HRT by the end of the trial.

The Heart and Estrogen/Progestin Replacement Study (HERS) was a randomized, double blind, placebo-controlled secondary prevention trial of daily use of conjugated equine estrogen (CEE) plus MPA on the occurrence of non-fatal myocardial infarction or CHD death among women with documented heart disease (42). Fractures were a secondary endpoint to the HERS trial. There was no evidence that 4 years of treatment with CEE (0.625 mg) and MPA (2.5 mg) daily substantially reduced the incidence of fractures or height loss among these older, non-osteoporotic women with established CHD (43,44).

Interpreting the Results of Randomized Trials and Observational Studies

How do we interpret the differences between the results of randomized trials of HRT with fracture outcomes and observational studies of HRT use and fracture occurrence? First, HERS is the largest randomized trial of HRT, but the women were selected because of heart disease, and only about 15% had osteoporosis by BMD criteria. Additionally, HERS did not include spine radiographs to assess the effect of HRT on vertebral fractures. Finally, the duration of three of the five intervention trials (Table 6-3) was relatively short, 4 years or less, and observational studies, noted earlier, suggest that more that 10 years of HRT may be needed before treatment substantially reduces the risk of non-spine fractures (22).

The lack of randomized trials of HRT with fracture outcomes emphasizes the need to clarify the effect of HRT on fractures in women, in those with and without low bone density at baseline. The overall benefits and risks of estrogen, including its effects on fracture risk, may be clarified by ongoing trials, particularly the Womens' Health Initiative. In the meantime, given the proven benefit of HRT on bone density, the biological plausibility of an effect of HRT on bone, and the consistent finding that HRT reduces fracture risk in observational studies, it is reasonable to consider using HRT for prevention of osteoporotic fractures.

Duration of Estrogen Treatment for the Prevention of Fracture

Bone loss resumes after estrogen is stopped (45). Observational data indicate that the lower risk of fractures associated with long-term use of estrogen also disappears when a woman stops taking estrogen, even if she has taken it for a decade (22). These results suggest that for estrogen to be effective for prevention of fractures lifelong, it must be continued lifelong. Thus, patients and physicians should consider the potential long-term risks and benefits of HRT when considering use of estrogen for prevention of fractures.

Hormone Replacement Therapy in Elderly Women

Women who begin estrogen treatment in later life appear to enjoy the same degree of BMD responsiveness as do younger women. For example, in PEPI, BMD gains did not vary by postmenopausal age (from 1 to 10 years since the last menstrual period) or by chronological age (45 to 64 years) (10). In a randomized, placebo-controlled trial that enrolled only women with established osteoporosis (defined as one or more vertebral fractures present), treatment with 0.1 mg of estradiol by patch produced statistically significant increases in spinal, radial, and trochanteric BMD (38). As noted earlier, however, the long-term benefits of estrogen appear to be greater for women who start treatment within 5 years of the onset of menopause.

Lower Doses of Estrogen in Older Women

Low doses of estrogen also seem to improve BMD in elderly women. For example, Recker and colleagues tested a 0.3 mg dose of CEE, 0.3 mg combined with 2.5 mg of MPA daily, supplemental calcium, and vitamin D (the latter two treatments titrated to each participant's dietary intake) in women 65 years of age and older (45). At 3 years, spinal BMD increased by about 4% and 5% and hip BMD by about 2% in adherent women. Does this allow us to recommend a lower dose (0.3 mg) of CEE (along with patient-specific amounts of calcium and vitamin D) to prevent osteoporosis in older women? The evidence about low-dose estrogen is limited to small trials of bone density, whereas virtually all observational studies (on which the anti-fracture efficacy of estrogen is based) included women who used higher doses of estrogen. Therefore, women should take standard doses if they are able to tolerate them; if side-effects limit treatment, then other agents to prevent fractures should be considered.

Other Outcomes of Postmenopausal Hormone Therapy

Postmenopausal hormone therapy is a complex intervention that may produce many outcomes in addition to the skeletal ones that are the primary focus of this book. Physicians and patients must consider many other effects: menopausal symptom amelioration, unwanted side effects, and effects on several chronic diseases. Individual patient preferences and goals must also be factored in when deliberating about whether to use estrogens or estrogens and progestins for osteoporosis prevention. Therefore, we consider the non-bone effects of estrogen and estrogen in combination with specific progestins. In keeping with our emphasis on data from randomized, placebo-controlled studies, we concentrate on information derived from this level of evidence.

Hormone Replacement Therapy and Symptom Relief

Vasomotor symptoms and vaginal atrophy generally improve with estrogen therapy. Clinical trials consistently demonstrate that estrogen substantially reduces the frequency and severity of hot flashes (46). For example, in PEPI, 3 years of treatment with CEE, CEE/micronized progesterone, or CEE/MPA reduced the frequency of hot flashes by 72% to 83% compared with results in placebo-treated women (47). Combination estrogen/progestin treatment was not more effective for hot flashes than was CEE alone. Estrogen also helps relieve symptoms and signs of vaginal atrophy by restoring a thicker, more mature vaginal epithelium (48).

Effect of Hormone Replacement Therapy on Other Conditions Potentially Related to Menopause

The following symptoms and conditions are *possibly* related to menopause: skin thinning and wrinkling, difficulty with memory, dysphoric mood, sexual dysfunction, stress and urge urinary incontinence, and recurrent urinary tract infection. To date, there is no strong evidence that these conditions respond to the oral or transdermal doses of estrogens or estrogen/progestins that are approved for osteoporosis prevention (49). However, it should be noted that vaginal estrogen, which would not be adequate for osteoporosis prevention, is effective for prevention of recurrent urinary tract infection (50,51).

Observational studies suggest associations between hormone therapy and numerous chronic diseases (49,52); an extensive review cannot be done here. Major examples of *possible* benefits include tooth retention (53), diminished risk of colon cancer (54), preservation of cognitive function, and prevention of Alzheimer dementia (55). The relations between heart disease, breast cancer, and HRT are discussed in more detail below.

Heart Disease

Estrogen increases high-density lipoprotein (HDL) and decreases low-density lipoprotein (LDL) cholesterol, and the addition of progestins blunts these effects (56,57). The impact of estrogens and estrogens plus progestins on many other proposed mediators of cardiac risk, including insulin resistance, fibrinogen, clotting factors, vascular reactivity, anti-oxidant function, and blood pressure, are reviewed in detail elsewhere (58). Large observational studies report an approximate 50% risk reduction in CHD events and mortality among current users of estrogen (7,59). Smaller observational studies also suggest that estrogen users with established CHD have improved survival (60). Combined estrogen and progestin use has been associated with a similar reduction in risk of CHD as that seen with unopposed estrogen (61).

In the HERS trial, older women (mean age of 67) with established CHD who were randomized to daily continuous combined HRT (0.625 mg CEE and 2.5 mg MPA) had a 50% increased risk of CHD events and CHD mortality during the first year of treatment. Subsequently, decreased risk during the third and fourth years of treatment resulted in an overall neutral effect of combined estrogen/progestin on CHD events (Table 6-4) (43).

Table 6-4   Adverse Events Related to 0.625 mg Conjugated Equine Estrogen and 2.5 mg Medroxyprogesterone Acetate (CEE + MPA) in the Heart and Estrogen/Progestin Replacement Study (HERS)

Outcome and Time On-study	Event Rate per 1000 Woman-Years and Relative Hazard (RH) (95% CI)			P-value for Trend in Log-Relative Hazard
	CEE + MPA	Placebo	Relative Hazard	
Primary CHD event				
Year 1	42.5	28.0	1.52 (1.01,2.29)	
Year 2	37.0	37.1	1.00 (0.67,1.49)	0.009
Year 3	28.8	33.1	0.87 (0.55,1.37)	
Year 4+5	23.0	34.4	0.67 (0.43,1.04)	
Nonfatal myocardial infarction				
Year 1	31.1	21.4	1.47 (0.91,2.36)	
Year 2	26.8	28.6	0.94 (0.59,1.49)	0.01
Year 3	16.5	23.4	0.70 (0.40,1.24)	
Year 4+5	13.9	23.9	0.58 (0.34,1.02)	
Venous thromboembolic event				
Year 1	9.6	2.9	3.29 (1.07,10.08)	
Year 2	6.1	1.5	4.09 (0.87,19.27)	0.28
Year 3	5.5	2.3	2.40 (0.62,9.28)	
Year 4+5	4.0	2.0	2.05 (0.15,8.18)	

Outcome During Entire Study	Cumulative Number of Events and Relative Hazard (95% CI)			P-value
	CEE + MPA	Placebo	Relative Hazard	
Deep vein thrombosis	25	8	3.18 (1.43,7.04)	0.004
Pulmonary embolism	12	4	2.79 (0.89,8.75)	0.080
Any thromboembolic event	34	12	2.89 (1.50,5.58)	0.002
Gallbladder disease	84	62	1.38 (1.00,1.92)	0.050

Based on the finding of no overall CHD benefit of the HRT regimen tested in HERS, as well as the temporal pattern of an *initial increase* in CHD risk when HRT was begun, it is prudent to avoid *starting* HRT for osteoporosis prevention in women with established CHD.

Breast Cancer

No randomized trials have been large enough or long enough to evaluate whether postmenopausal estrogen causes breast cancer. To understand the effects of postmenopausal estrogen use on breast cancer risk, we must first consider the effect of menopause on breast cancer risk. Among thinner postmenopausal women (body mass index [BMI] < 25), the age-adjusted relative risk (RR) of breast cancer declines with menopause. This protective effect of menopause is absent in women with a BMI greater than 25. In both a large meta-analysis of observational studies (62) and a large cohort study (63), only current and recent long-term users of estrogen with lower BMI (less than 24.4 or 25) had an increased breast cancer risk related to taking estrogen. In the meta-analysis, thinner postmenopausal women who took estrogen for 5 or more years had a 10% increase in breast cancer risk (62). In addition, a cohort study found that current/recent combination estrogen and progestin use for 4 years or more was associated with a 2-fold increase in risk only in the thinner women (63).

In general, the results of observational studies of HRT and breast cancer risk indicate that: 1) Ever-use and former use (used longer ago than 4 to 5 years) of postmenopausal estrogen is not associated with an increased risk of breast cancer (62,64); 2) More than 5 years of current/recent estrogen use has been associated with 10% to 35% increase in breast cancer risk (62,63,65); 3) Breast cancer risk is greater with estrogen/progestin use compared with use of estrogen only, but precise estimates of this risk differential are limited by smaller numbers of long-term estrogen/progestin users; and 4) The increased postmenopausal breast cancer risk associated with estrogen replacement therapy (ERT) and HRT appears to only affect thinner women (BMI < about 24).

Endometrial Cancer

In the 1970s, landmark observational studies reported an association between unopposed postmenopausal estrogen use and endometrial carcinoma (66,67). Endometrial hyperplasia (particularly atypical and complex hyperplasia) is a precursor to endometrial cancer; therefore, trials use hyperplasia as a surrogate endpoint for endometrial safety. In PEPI, 62% of women treated with CEE only developed any grade of hyperplasia during 3 years of follow-up (68).

In contrast, when estrogen is combined with adequate doses of an approved progestin (Table 6-5), endometrial hyperplasia occurs uncommonly (<3% over 2 to 3 years) and at a similar rate as found in placebo-treated women (18,68,69). Importantly, prevention of hyperplasia is well documented only for the exact doses and durations of the progestins tested in studies; deviation from them is not recommended. Specifically, there are no long-term tests of daily treatment using low-dose (100 mg) daily MPA (70); this is not an approved method of hyperplasia prevention. Although less-than-monthly progestin dosing initially looked promising, a recent study using quarterly administration of progestin was halted because of unacceptable rates of endometrial cancer development (71).

Low-dose (0.3 mg) esterified estrogen (EE), which recently gained approval for osteoporosis prevention (Table 6-2), unexpectedly had the same 2-year hyperplasia rate as placebo treatment (17). Although this encouraging finding warrants additional investigation, use of low-dose EE without a progestin is not approved or recommended for women with a uterus.

Table 6-5   FDA-Approved Progestogens* for Prevention of Endometrial Hyperplasia in Postmenopausal Women Who Are Using Estrogen Therapy

Progestogens	Trade Names	Dose and Duration	Expected Vaginal Bleeding Pattern
Medroxyprogesterone acetate (MPA)	Provera[†]	2.5[‡] mg daily (continuous combined HRT)	• Light spotting or bleeding for up to 1 year • No bleeding after 1 year • Absence of bleeding
		5[§] or 10[‡] mg daily for 12 to 14 consecutive days/month (cyclical HRT)	• Cyclical bleeding commencing on or after day 9 of progestogen use • Absence of bleeding
Micronised progesterone (MP)	Prometrium[†]	200[‡] mg daily for 13 to 14 consecutive days/month (cyclical HRT)	• Cyclical bleeding commencing on or after day 9 of progestogen use • Absence of bleeding

* Norethindrone acetate and norgestimate are also approved in fixed combination products (see Table 6-2). Expected bleeding pattern for the fixed combinations shown in Table 6-2 is the same as that for continuous, combined HRT.

[†] Cycrin is another brand of MPA but it does not have a formal FDA approval for this indication.

[‡] Data from The PEPI Trial Investigators (10). Effects of hormone replacement therapy on endometrial histology in postmenopausal women. The Postmenopausal Estrogen/Progestin Interventions (PEPI) Trial. JAMA 1996;275:370-5.

[§] Data from Woodruff JD, Pickar JH. Incidence of endometrial hyperplasia in postmenopausal women taking conjugated estrogens (Premarin) with medroxyprogesterone acetate or conjugated estrogens alone. Am J Obstet Gynecol. 1994;170:1213–23.

Side Effects

Estrogen therapy increases the risk of venous thrombosis and pulmonary embolism (Table 6-4). It should not be prescribed for women with previous thrombotic or embolic disease or for those who are at high risk of deep vein thrombosis. Oral estrogens increase the lithogenicity of bile, and women assigned to CEE/MPA treatment in HERS experienced about a 40% increase in risk of clinical gallbladder disease (Table 6-4).

Although it is widely believed that estrogen causes breast discomfort, the PEPI trial found that breast sensitivity and pain were confined to combination estrogen/progestin treatments; women taking CEE only did not report any increase in mastalgia compared with women taking placebo (47). Micronized progesterone and MPA treatments produced equivalent risks of breast pain. Many women express concern that HRT causes weight gain. However, the converse was observed in PEPI (57). On average, during 3 years placebo-assigned women gained 1.3 kilograms, while those assigned to active treatments gained between 0.4 and 0.8 kilograms. The weight gain that is often attributed to HRT in the clinical setting probably reflects the natural history of weight gain with menopause (72).

Table 6-5 outlines the expected patterns of vaginal bleeding produced by continuous and cyclical progestin administration. Continuous combined HRT is often referred to as the method that avoids vaginal bleeding; however, it may take up to 1 full year for endometrial atrophy to occur and for bleeding to cease. All cyclical regimens have the same normal bleeding pattern: if bleeding occurs, it should commence on or after day 9 of the progestin component.

Contraindications to and Precautions with Hormone Replacement Therapy

Absolute contraindications to estrogen or estrogen/progestin therapy are undiagnosed vaginal bleeding, breast cancer, endometrial cancer, and a history of deep vein thrombosis or pulmonary embolism. Gynecological opinion holds that estrogen is permissible after cured, stage I, endometrial cancer (73). Uterine fibroids are not a contraindication, but vaginal bleeding may be heavier. Because oral estrogens raise triglycerides and increase the rate of gallbladder disease, transdermal therapy should be considered for women with high baseline triglycerides (>300 mg/dL) or with gallbladder disease (74). Use of estrogen by women who have had melanoma remains debated (75). Use of HRT after breast cancer is also controversial (76), and non-HRT therapies should be considered.

Patient Education

Meticulous patient education is central to promoting optimal adherence to and safe use of estrogen or estrogen/progestin treatment. The first step is a complete discussion of benefits and risks of treatment and a mutual determination of the suitability of HRT. Patients must next be counseled about how to take their hormones, what bleeding patterns to expect, symptoms of possible complications, and what actions to take if potential problems develop. Tables 6-6 and 6-7 summarize key points related to bleeding patterns and possibly urgent side effects. These can be given as patient handouts. Women should have mammograms and clinical breast examinations annually while taking HRT.

When cyclical estrogen and progestin are prescribed as separate pills, we recommend giving the estrogen every day of the month (irrespective of the length of the month) and the progestin on calendar days 1 to 12. If a transdermal estrogen patch is used, it should be changed once or twice per week, depending on the patch. This schedule makes it easy to remember when progestin pills are to be taken. It also simplifies patient reporting of bleeding patterns: if bleeding starts before calendar day 9 of the month, it may signal a problem and should be reported (Table 6-6) (77). The same principles apply

Table 6-6   Patient Education Points When Prescribing Estrogen or Estrogen-Progestin: Vaginal Bleeding

Hormone Prescription	Expected Bleeding	Patient Action if Unexpected Bleeding Occurs
Estrogen daily and progestogen for 12 days per month (cyclical HRT)	• Bleeding is expected to start on or after day 9 of progestogen use; bleeding before that time is unexpected • Some women do not bleed when taking cyclical HRT; this is not problematic	• Notify provider if bleeding begins *before day 9* of the progestogen part of the treatment • Notify provider if bleeding is uncharacteristically *heavy or prolonged*
Estrogen daily and progestogen daily (continuous combined HRT)	• Light and unpredictable spotting and bleeding is expected for the first 12 months of continuous combined HRT; after 12 months, bleeding should cease	• During first year of continuous combined HRT use, notify provider if bleeding is unusual or prolonged compared to typical bleeding. • After the first year, report any bleeding.
Estrogen only* (unopposed estrogen)	• None	• Notify provider if any bleeding occurs

* When unopposed estrogen is used in a woman with an intact uterus, annual endometrial check-ups must be done. In addition, any vaginal bleeding requires evaluation.

Table 6-7   Patient Education Points When Prescribing Estrogen or Estrogen/Progestins: Possible Complications, Symptoms, and Patient Actions

Symptom	Possible Complication	Patient Action
Right upper quadrant pain or dyspepsia syndrome	Gallbladder stones	• Non-urgent report, if mild • If severe, urgent report and stop hormones until consultation with physician
One-sided leg swelling and/or pain	Blood clot in leg	Urgent report: Stop hormones until consultation with physician
Sudden shortness of breath, pain in chest, bloody sputum	Blood clot in lung	Urgent report: Stop hormones until consultation with physician

when patients use Premphase, but the provider must realize that the combination pills are at the end of the pack. The dose pack consists of 0.625 mg CEE and 5 mg MPA (as one pill) for the last 14 doses and CEE only for the first 14 doses. Patients should report bleeding that commences before the ninth combination pill of each pack, which would correspond to "pack-day" 23. Lack of bleeding when using cyclical HRT is not cause for concern.

Instructions for using continuous combined HRT, whether prescribed as two separate estrogen and progestin pills, patch and progestin, or single combination, are identical. Both hormones are used continuously. The vaginal bleeding patterns experienced with continuous combined HRT can be quite annoying (or even alarming) to the patient, especially if she is not forewarned. During the first 12 months, patterns are unpredictable and range from spotting to bleeding (78). A departure from the patient's norm (e.g., prolonged or heavy bleeding compared with her usual) or bleeding after 1 year of continuous combination therapy should be reported (Table 6-6). Rarely, women who have not undergone hysterectomy will opt to take unopposed estrogen; this should be done only with guidance by a physician experienced in the endometrial monitoring that is required. In such cases, any bleeding is abnormal and merits evaluation. Because HRT can lead to gallbladder problems or to thromboembolic complications, women should be advised about symptoms that might signal the presence of these conditions (Table 6-7).

REFERENCES

1. **Eriksen B.** A randomized, open, parallel-group study on the preventive effect of an estradiol-releasing vaginal ring (Estring) on recurrent urinary tract infections in postmenopausal women. Am J Obstet Gynecol. 1999;180:1072–1079.

2. **Oursler MJ, Osdoby P, Pyfferoen J, et al.** Avian osteoclasts as estrogen target cells. Proc Natl Acad Sci U S A. 1991;88:6613–6617.

3. **Garnero P, Sornay-Rendu E, Chapuy MC, Delmas PD.** Increased bone turnover in late postmenopausal women is a major determinant of osteoporosis. J Bone Miner Res. 1996;11:337–349.

4. **Pacifici R.** Cytokines estrogen and postmenopausal osteoporosis: the second decade [editorial, comment]. Endocrinology. 1998;139:2659–2661.

5. **Riggs BL, Khosla S, Melton LJ 3rd.** A unitary model for involutional osteoporosis: estrogen deficiency causes both type I and type II osteoporosis in postmenopausal women and contributes to bone loss in aging men. J Bone Miner Res. 1998;13:763–773.

6. **Grady D, Rubin SM, Petitti DB, et al.** Hormone therapy to prevent disease and prolong life in postmenopausal women. Ann Intern Med. 1992;116:1016–1037.

7. **Grodstein F, Stampfer M.** The epidemiology of coronary heart disease and estrogen replacement in postmenopausal women. Prog Cardiovasc Dis. 1995;38:199–210.

8. **Cauley JA, Seeley DG, Browner WS, et al.** Estrogen replacement therapy and mortality among older women. The Study of Osteoporotic Fractures. Arch Intern Med. 1997;157:2181–2187.

9. **Grodstein F, Stampfer MJ, Colditz GA, et al.** Postmenopausal hormone therapy and mortality. N Engl J Med. 1997;336:1769–1775.

10. **The Postmenopausal Estrogen/Progestin Interventions (PEPI) Trial Writing Group.** Effects of hormone therapy on bone mineral density: results from the Postmenopausal Estrogen/Progestin Interventions (PEPI) trial. JAMA. 1996;276:1389–1396.

11. **Genant HK, Baylink DJ, Gallagher JC, et al.** Effect of estrone sulfate on postmenopausal bone loss. Obstet Gynecol. 1990;76:579–584.

12. **Harris ST, Genant HK, Baylink DJ, et al.** The effects of estrone (Ogen) on spinal bone density of postmenopausal women. Arch Intern Med. 1991;151:1980–1984.

13. **Ettinger B, Genant HK, Steiger P, Madvig P.** Low-dosage micronized 17β-estradiol prevents bone loss in postmenopausal women. Am J Obstet Gynecol. 1992;6:479–488.

14. **Adami S, Suppi R, Bertoldo F, et al.** Transdermal estradiol in the treatment of postmenopausal bone loss. Bone Miner. 1989;7:79–86.

15. **Field CS, Ory SJ, Wahner HW, et al.** Preventive effects of transdermal 17-beta-estradiol on osteoporotic changes after surgical menopause. A two-year placebo-controlled trial. Am J Obstet Gynecol. 1993;168:114–121.

16. **Weiss SR, Ellman H, Dolker M, for the Transdermal Estradiol Investigator Group.** A randomized controlled trial of four doses of transdermal estradiol for preventing postmenopausal bone loss. Obstet Gynecol. 1999;94:330–336.

17. **Genant HK, Lucas J, Weiss S, et al.** Low-dose estrified estrogen therapy: effects on bone, plasma estradiol concentrations, endometrium and lipid levels. Arch Intern Med. 1997;157:2609–2615.

18. **Speroff L, Rowan J, Symons J, et al.** The comparative effect on bone density, endometrium, and lipids of continuous hormones as replacement therapy (CHART Study). JAMA. 1996;276:1397–1403.

19. **Ribot C, Tremollieres F, Pouilles JM.** Effect of 17-beta-oestradiol and norethisterone acetate on vertebral bone mass and lipid metabolism in early postmenopausal women. Maturitas. 1992;15:217–223.

20. **Christiansen C, Riss BJ.** 17-Beta-estradiol and continuous norethistrone: a unique treatment for established osteoporosis in elderly women. J Clin Endocrinol Metab. 1990;71:835–841.

21. **National Osteoporosis Foundation.** Osteoporosis: review of the evidence for prevention, diagnosis, and treatment and cost-effectiveness analysis. Osteoporos Int. 1998; Suppl 4:S1–S86.

22. **Cauley JA, Seeley DG, Ensrud K, et al.** Estrogen replacement therapy and fractures in older women. Ann Intern Med. 1995;122:9–16.

23. **Naessen T, Persson I, Adami HO, et al.** Hormone replacement therapy and the risk for the first hip fracture. A prospective, population-based cohort study. Ann Intern Med. 1990;133:95–103.

24. **Maxim P, Ettinger B, Spitalny GM.** Fracture protection provided by long-term estrogen treatment. Osteoporos Int. 1995;5:23–29.

25. **Weiss NS, Ure CL, Ballard JH, et al.** Decreased risk of fractures of hip and lower forearm with postmenopausal use of estrogen. N Engl J Med. 1980;303:1195–1198.

26. **Ettinger B, Grady D.** Maximizing the benefit of estrogen therapy for prevention of osteoporosis. Menopause. 1994;1:19–36.

27. **Kiel DP, Baron A, Anderson JJ, et al.** Smoking eliminates the protective effect of oral estrogens on the risk for hip fracture among women. Ann Intern Med. 1992;117:716–721.

28. **Hammond CB, Jelovsek FR, Lee KL, et al.** Effects of long-term estrogen replacement therapy. Am J Obstet Gynecol. 1979;122:525–536.

29. **Ettinger B, Genant HK, Camnn CE.** Long-term estrogen replacement therapy prevents bone loss and fractures. Ann Intern Med. 1985;102:319–324.

30. **Kiel DP, Felson DT, Anderson JJ, et al.** Hip fracture and the use of estrogens in postmenopausal women. The Framingham Study. N Engl J Med. 1987;317:1169–1174.

31. **Paganini-Hill A, Chao A, Ross RK, Henderson BE.** Exercise and other factors in the prevention of hip fracture. The Leisure World Study. Epidemiology. 1991;2:16–25.

32. **Krieger N, Kelsey JL, Holford TR, O'Connor T.** An epidemiologic study of hip fracture in postmenopausal women. Am J Epidemiol. 1982;116:141–148.

33. **Paganini-Hill A, Ross RK, Gerkins VR, et al.** Menopausal estrogen therapy and hip fractures. Ann Intern Med. 1981;95:28–31.

34. **Felson DT, Zhang Y, Hannon MT, et al.** The effect of postmenopausal estrogen therapy on bone density in elderly women. N Engl J Med. 1993;329:1141–1146.

35. **Cauley JA, Cummings SR, Black DM, et al.** Prevalence and determinants of estrogen replacement therapy in elderly women. Am J Obstet Gynecol. 1990;163:1438–1444.

36. **Nachtigall LE, Nachtigall RH, Nachtigall RD, Beckman EM.** Estrogen replacement therapy I. A 10-year prospective study in the relationship to osteoporosis. Obstet Gynecol. 1979;53:277–281.

37. **Lindsay R, Hart DM, Forrest C, Baird C.** Prevention of spinal osteoporosis in ooporectomized women. Lancet. 1980;2:1151–1153.

38. **Lufkin EG, Wahner HW, O'Fallon WM, et al.** Treatment of postmenopausal osteoporosis with transdermal estrogen. Ann Intern Med. 1992;117:1–9.

39. **Windeler J, Lange S.** Events per person year: a dubious concept. BMJ. 1995;310:454–456.

40. **Komulainen MH, Kroger H, Tuppurainen MT, et al.** HRT and Vitamin D in prevention of non-vertebral fractures in postmenopausal women. A 5 year randomized trial. Maturitas. 1998;31:45–54.

41. **Mosekilde L, Beck-Nielsen H, Sorensen OH, et al.** Hormonal replacement therapy reduces forearm fracture incidence in recent postmenopausal women. Results of the Danish Osteoporosis Prevention Study. Maturitas. 2000;36:181–193.

42. **Grady D, Applegate W, Bush T, et al.** Heart and Estrogen Replacement Study (HERS): design, methods and baseline characteristics. Control Clin Trials. 1998;19:314–335.

43. **Hulley S, Grady D, Bush T, et al.** Randomized trial of estrogen plus progestin for secondary prevention of coronary heart disease in postmenopausal women. Heart and Estrogen/Progestin Replacement Study (HERS) Research Group. JAMA. 1998;380: 605–613.

44. **Cauley JA, Black DM, Barrett-Connor E, et al.** Effects of hormone replacement therapy on clinical fractures and height loss. The Heart and Estrogen/Progestin Replacement Study (HERS). Am J Med. 2001;110:442–450.

45. **Greendale GA, Espeland ME, Slone S, et al.** Bone mass response to discontinuation or long-term use of hormone replacement therapy: Results from the PEPI Safety Follow-up Study. Arch Intern Med; in press.

46. **Recker RR, Davies M, Dowd RM, Heaney RP.** The effect of low-dose continuous estrogen and progesterone therapy with calcium and vitamin D on bone in elderly women. A randomized controlled trial. Ann Intern Med. 1999;130:897–904.

47. **Greendale GA, Reboussin BA, Hogan P, et al.** Symptom relief and side effects of postmenopausal hormones. Results from the Postmenopausal Estrogen/Progestin Interventions Trial. Obstet Gynecol. 1998;92:982–988.

48. **Nilsson K, Risberg B, Heimer G.** The vaginal epithelium in the postmenopause: cytology, histology and pH as methods of assessment. Maturitis. 1995;21:51–56.

49. **Greendale GA, Lee NP, Arriola ER.** The menopause. Lancet. 1999;353:571–580.

50. **Raz R, Stamm WE.** A controlled trial of intravaginal estriol in postmenopausal women with recurrent urinary tract infections. N Engl J Med. 1993;329:753–760.

51. **Eriksen B.** A randomized, open, parallel-group study on the preventive effect of an estradiol-releasing vaginal ring (Estring) on recurrent urinary tract infections in postmenopausal women. Am J Obstet Gynecol. 1999;180:1072–1079.

52. **Sowers MFR, La Pietra MT.** Menopause: its epidemiology and association with chronic diseases. Epidemiologic Rev. 1995;17:287–302.

52. **Grodstein F, Colditz GA, Stampfer MJ.** Postmenopausal hormone use and tooth loss. A prospective study. J Am Dent Assoc. 1996;127:370–377.

53. **Krall EA, Dawson-Hughes B, Hannan MT, et al.** Postmenopausal estrogen replacement and tooth retention. Am J Med. 1997;102:536–542.

54. **Crandall CJ.** Estrogen replacement therapy and colon cancer: a clinical review. J Womens Health Gender-Based Med. 1999;8:1155–1166.

55. **Yaffee K, Sawaya G, Lieberburg I, Grady D.** Estrogen therapy in postmenopausal women: effects on cognitive function and dementia. JAMA. 1998;279:688–695.

56. **Jensen J.** Effects of sex steroids on serum lipids and lipoproteins. Baillères Clin Obstet Gynaecol. 1991;5:867–887.

57. **The Postmenopausal Estrogen/Progestin Interventions (PEPI) Trial Writing Group.** Effects of estrogen or estrogen/progestin regimens on heart disease risk factors in postmenopausal women. The Postmenopausal Estrogen/Progestin Interventions (PEPI) trial. JAMA. 1995;273:199–208.

58. **Chai CU, Redker PM, Manson JE.** Postmenopausal hormone replacement and cardiovascular disease. Thromb Haemost. 1997;78:70–80.

59. **Manson JE.** Postmenopausal hormone therapy and atherosclerotic disease. Am Heart J. 1994;128:1337–1343.

60. **Sullivan JM, El-Zeky E, Vander Zwaag R, Ramanathan KB.** Effect on survival of estrogen replacement therapy after coronary artery bypass grafting. Am J Cardiol. 1997;79:847–850.

61. **Grodstein F, Stampfer MJ, Manson JE, et al.** Postmenopausal estrogen and progestin use and the risk of cardiovascular disease. N Engl J Med. 1996;335:453–461.

62. **Collaborative Group on Hormonal Factors in Breast Cancer.** Breast cancer and hormone replacement therapy. Lancet. 1997;350:1047–1059.

63. **Schairer C, Lubin J, Troisi R, et al.** Menopausal estrogen and estrogen-progestin replacement therapy and breast cancer risk. JAMA. 2000;283:485–491.

64. **Brinton LA.** Hormone replacement therapy and risk for breast cancer. Endocrinol Metab Clin North Am. 1997;26:361–378.

65. **Colditz GA, Hankinson SE, Hunter DJ, et al.** The use of estrogens and progestins and the risk of breast cancer in postmenopausal women. N Engl J Med. 1995;332: 1589–1593.

66. **Smith DC, Prentice R, Thompson DJ, Herrmann WL.** Association of exogenous estrogen and endometrial carcinoma. N Engl J Med. 1975;293:1164–1167.

67. **Ziel HK, Finkle WD.** Increased risk of endometrial carcinoma among users of conjugated estrogens. N Engl J Med. 1975;293:1167–1170.

68. **The Postmenopausal Estrogen/Progestin Interventions (PEPI) Trial Writing Group.** Effects of hormone replacement therapy on endometrial histology in postmenopausal women. The Postmenopausal Estrogen/Progestin Interventions (PEPI) trial. JAMA. 1996;275:370–375.

69. **Woodruff JD, Pickar JH.** Incidence of endometrial hyperplasia in postmenopausal women taking conjugated estrogens (Premarin) with medroxyprogesterone acetate or conjugated estrogens alone. Am J Obstet Gynecol. 1994;170:1213–1223.

70. **Gillet JY, Andre G, Faguer B, et al.** Induction of amenorrhea during hormone replacement therapy: optimal micronized progesterone dose. A multicenter study. Maturitas. 1994;19:103–115.

71. **Cerin A, Heldaas K, Moeller B.** Adverse endometrial effects of long-cycle estrogen and progestin replacement therapy. N Engl J Med. 1996;334:668–689.

72. **Matthews KA, Meilahn E, Kuller LH, et al.** Menopause and risk factors for coronary heart disease. N Engl J Med. 1989;321:641–646.

73. **Committee Opinion. Committee on Gynecologic Practice.** Estrogen replacement therapy and endometrial cancer. J Gynecol Obstet. 1993;43:89.

74. **Crook D.** The metabolic consequences of treating postmenopausal women with nonoral hormone replacement therapy. Br J Obstet Gynaecol. 1997;104:S4–S13.

75. **Smith MA, Fine JA, Barnhill RL, Berwick M.** Hormonal and reproductive influences and risk of melanoma in women. Int J Epidemiol. 1998;37:751–757.

76. **Cobleigh MA, Berris RF, Bush T, et al.** Estrogen replacement in breast cancer survivors: a time for change. JAMA. 1995;273:378.

77. **ACOG Technical Bulletin.** Washington, DC: American College of Obstetricians and Gynecologists, April 1992;166.

78. **Archer DF, Pickar JH, Bottoglioni F, for the Menopause Study Group.** Bleeding patterns in postmenopausal women taking continuous combined or sequential regimens of medroxyprogesterone acetate. Obstet Gynecol. 1997;83:686–692.

CHAPTER 7

Selective Estrogen-Receptor Modulators

FELICIA COSMAN, MD

Key Points

- Raloxifene and tamoxifen are selective estrogen-receptor modulators (SERMs).

- Raloxifene is approved by the FDA for treatment and prevention of osteoporosis. Tamoxifen is approved by the FDA for treatment and prevention of breast cancer in women at high risk.

- Both increase the risk of venous thromboembolism to the same degree as estrogen, and both can cause or worsen hot flashes.

- Randomized trials have shown that raloxifene improves bone mineral density by a small amount throughout the skeleton and that it decreases bone turnover.

- Four years of raloxifene reduces the risk of vertebral fracture but not other types of fractures in postmenopausal women with osteoporosis.

- Raloxifene is most useful in women of middle menopausal age (55 to 65 years); in these women, hot flashes and hip fractures are uncommon.

- Raloxifene appears to substantially reduce the risk of breast cancer but has not been approved by the FDA for this indication.

Cont'd

Table 7-1   Effect of Tamoxifen on Bone Mass and Bone Turnover: Randomized Clinical Trials

Author	No. of Subjects	Age	Characteristics	Intervention	Bone Mineral Density Results	Bone Turnover Results
Love et al, 1992 (3)	140 postmenopausal women	Mean = 57.7 yr	• Axillary node negative breast cancer within 10 years • Spine and radius BMD > 80% of age-matched women • No active breast disease	Tamox 10 mg bid vs Pbo for 2 years	*Spine:* Pbo: −1.0%/year ($P \le 0.01$); Tamox: 0.6%/year ($P \le 0.01$); *Radius:* Pbo: −1.3%/year ($P \le 0.01$); Tamox: −0.7%/year ($P \le 0.01$)	OC: NSC Pbo; 50% Tamox ($P < 0.001$); AP: NSC Pbo; 21% Tamox ($P < 0.001$)
Love et al, 1994 (7)	62 women enrolled in above trial	Mean = 57.6 yr	As above	As above for 5 years	*Spine:* Pbo: −0.7% ($P = 0.06$); Tamox: 0.8% at 5 years ($P = 0.06$)	OC: Tamox 50% vs Pbo at 5 years ($P < 0.001$)
Kristensen et al, 1994 (2)	50 postmenopausal women; randomized but open trial	Median = 57.3 yr	• Low-risk breast cancer diagnosis • Axillary node negative • Age ≤ 65	Tamox 30 mg/day vs Con group; no Pbo for 2 years	*Spine:* Con: 2%/year; Tamox: 1.5%/year; *Forearm:* Con: 3%/year ($P < 0.02$); Tamox: 1%/year (NS)	AP: NSC Con; 20% Tamox

Study	Subjects	Age	Population	Treatment	Results	Markers
Grey et al, 1995 (4)	57 postmenopausal women	Mean = 59 yr	• Healthy • Mean years from menopause = 11 (all at least 3 years from LMP)	Tamox 20 mg/day one dose vs Pbo for 2 years	*TBBM:* *Spine:* Tamox vs Pbo: 0.5% *Hip:* Tamox vs Pbo: 2.9% Tamox vs Pbo: NSD	AP: 29% Tamox ($P < 0.001$ vs Pbo) OHP: 26% Tamox ($P < 0.05$ vs Pbo) NTX: 55% Tamox ($P < 0.05$ vs Pbo)
Powles et al, 1996 (9)	54 postmenopausal women	Mean = 57.8 yr	Healthy women in European Breast Cancer Prevention Trial	Tamox 20mg/day one dose vs Pbo for 3 years	**Postmenopausal** *Spine:* Tamox: 1.2%/year ($P < 0.01$) *Hip:* Tamox: 1.7%/year ($P < 0.01$) *Spine & Hip:* Pbo: NS loss	
	125 premenopausal women	Mean = 43.7 yr			**Premenopausal** *Spine:* Tamox: 1.4%/year Pbo: 0.3%/year *Hip:* Tamox & Pbo: NS change	
Gotfredsen et al, 1984 (10)	31 postmenopausal women	Mean = 45.5 yr Range = 30–56 yr	Recent mastectomy for breast cancer	Tamox 10 mg 3×/day vs Pbo for 1 year	*Forearm:* Pbo: 2.5% Tamox: 3.2%	

LMP = last menstrual period; NSD = not significantly different; NS = not significant; Pbo = placebo; Tamox = tamoxifen; AP = alkaline phosphatase; OC = osteocalcin.

Table 7-2   Randomized Clinical Trials of Tamoxifen: Fracture Outcomes

Author	No. of Subjects	Age	Characteristics	Intervention	Follow-up	Results		
							Controls	**Tamoxifen**
Kristensen et al, 1996 (Danish Cooperative Group) (11)	1716 postmenopausal women	Median = 66.64 yr	High-risk breast cancer (node positive, large tumor, deep invasion); all s/p radiotherapy	1 year tamoxifen 30 mg/d or no additional Rx	Median follow-up, 6.3 yr	Total # femoral fractures	51	64
						% women with femoral fracture	6%	7.4%
						NSD between tamoxifen and Pbo		
							Placebo	**Tamoxifen**
Fisher et al, 1998 (BCPT) (12)	13,388 premenopausal and postmenopausal women	• 39% ≤ 49 yr • 31% 50–59 yr • 24% 60–69 yr • 6% ≥ 70 yr	All women at risk of breast cancer (5-year risk ≥ 1.66%) but no previous cancer diagnosis	Tamoxifen 20 mg/day vs placebo	Mean follow-up, 47.7 mo; median follow-up, 54.6 mo	% women with any fracture	7.3%	7.2%
						Hip #	22	12
						Clinical spine #	31	23
						Colles' #	23	14
						Other radius #	63	66
						Total #	**137**	**111**
						NSD between tamoxifen and placebo groups for any fracture		

NSD = no significant difference.

compared to placebo-treated women. This suggests that in women with high endogenous concentrations of estrogen, tamoxifen may inhibit estrogen's effects on bone.

Only two randomized trials have reported the effect of tamoxifen on fracture risk (Table 7-2; 11,12), one in which tamoxifen was used as adjuvant therapy in breast cancer patients and one in a large breast cancer prevention trial. Neither study was primarily designed to evaluate the effect of tamoxifen on osteoporosis, and methodological problems limit applicability of the results, particularly regarding the study in breast cancer patients. Furthermore, neither study was comprehensive in investigating fracture occurrence. In the first, 1716 postmenopausal women with high-risk breast cancer were randomized (after mastectomy and radiotherapy) to tamoxifen 30 mg/day (or no additional treatment) for only 1 year (11). Hip fracture occurrence, but no other fracture incidence, was investigated through the Danish Breast Cancer Cooperative Group for up to 8 years. This study was flawed by inclusion of fractures caused by bone metastases, lack of complete registration of hip fracture cases, and misclassification of fracture cases, as well as increased survival in the tamoxifen group. This study provided no evidence, however, that 1 year of tamoxifen protects against hip fracture occurrence in patients with high-risk breast cancer. This is not at all unexpected because 1 year of treatment with a SERM is very unlikely to be sufficient to provide long-term skeletal protection.

The better fracture data come from the Breast Cancer Prevention Trial (BCPT), performed in 13,388 healthy premenopausal and postmenopausal women who were at increased risk of future breast cancer (12). This study found a trend toward a reduction in the risk of selected fractures (hip, symptomatic spine, and Colles' fractures) in those women 50 years of age or older but no reduction at other skeletal sites and no protection against fractures in younger women. Although fracture recording in this study was more comprehensive than it was in the breast cancer trial discussed earlier, there were no spine radiographs done routinely to evaluate asymptomatic vertebral compression deformity. This study was flawed by lack of data about occurrence of other specific types of fracture in the 955 women who had fractures over the course of the study. In fact, the overall incidence of all fractures was the same in tamoxifen-treated and placebo-treated women. Furthermore, there were so few bone density tests done that the prevalence of osteoporosis in this group is totally unknown. This group of women was theoretically at lower risk of osteoporosis, because they were at increased risk of breast cancer. When evaluating other medications for osteoporosis, a greater effect is usually seen against fracture in women with osteoporosis than in women with normal bone mass. Thus, there is still uncertainty about the effects of tamoxifen on fracture occurrence and how these effects might differ in women with a greater prevalence of osteoporosis.

Effects on Other Organ Systems

Breast
Women with ER-positive breast cancer should be treated with tamoxifen for 5 years because it reduces the risk of mortality, recurrent tumors, and contralateral new primary tumors, and it increases disease-free survival (13–16). In addition, in the BCPT trial (12), tamoxifen administration during a 4- to 5-year period reduced the incidence of new breast cancers (invasive and noninvasive) by approximately 50% in both premenopausal and postmenopausal women who were at elevated risk (more than 1.7% risk per year) for breast cancer (Table 7-3). The incidence of ER-positive breast cancers was reduced by 69%, without any effect on the risk of ER-negative cancer. Two smaller, ongoing European studies on tamoxifen for breast cancer prevention have so far found no reduction in breast cancer risk (17,18). Differences between the BCPT and the European studies could be caused by inadequate study power, differences in study populations (with inclusion of women at greater risk of ER-negative cancer), or poor compliance with therapy in the latter studies.

Vascular Disease
Tamoxifen reduces serum total and LDL cholesterol, lipoprotein(a), LDL oxidation, and fibrinogen, with no effect on HDL (1). Two European randomized trials of adjuvant tamoxifen treatment in breast cancer survivors (19-21)

Table 7-3   Effects of Tamoxifen on Nonskeletal Outcomes: 4-Year Cumulative Incidence*

Event	Incidence over 4 Years (%)		Tamoxifen vs Placebo	
	Placebo	Tamoxifen	Relative Risk	95% CI
Invasive breast cancer	2.7	1.4	0.5	0.4–0.7
Noninvasive breast cancer	1.0	0.5	0.5	0.3–0.8
All ischemic CVD	0.9	1.1	1.2	0.8–1.6
Stroke	0.4	0.6	1.6	0.9–2.8
Transient ischemic attack	0.4	0.3	0.8	0.4–1.4
Pulmonary embolism	0.1	0.3	3.0	1.2–9.3
Deep vein thrombosis	0.3	0.5	1.6	0.9–2.9
Endometrial cancer	0.4	0.9	2.5[†]	1.4–5.0

* Data from Fisher B, Costantino JP, Wickerham DL, et al. Tamoxifen for prevention of breast cancer. Report of the National Surgical Adjuvant Breast and Bowel Project P-1 Study. J Natl Cancer Inst. 1998;90: 1371–1388.
[†] Relative risk of endometrial cancer is particulary high in women 50 years of age or older (RR, 4.0; CI, 1.7–10.9).

found that tamoxifen significantly reduced the incidence of cardiovascular events by approximately 30% to 60%. These results were similar to one U.S. trial in which a modest but insignificant reduction in cardiovascular mortality was seen (22). No reduction in the risk of stroke has been described (19-22). The larger BCPT trial (12), however, found no trend toward protection against cardiovascular disease (Table 7-3) but in contrast suggested that tamoxifen could possibly increase the risk of cerebrovascular disease.

The potential thrombotic risk of tamoxifen has been documented. Tamoxifen decreases serum levels of antithrombin III (1) and increases the risk of venous thromboembolic disease approximately 3-fold in breast cancer patients (20,23-27) and in premenopausal and postmenopausal healthy women (12; Table 7-3). Approximately 1 in every 100 postmenopausal women who is taking tamoxifen for 5 years will have a venous thromboembolic event (either deep vein thrombosis or pulmonary embolism).

Reproductive Organs

Tamoxifen increases the occurrence of uterine cancer as well as that of benign uterine disease, including fibroid tumors, adenomyosis, and hyperplasia (1,12,23,28-32). The relative risk of invasive uterine cancer in women who are older than 50 years and without hysterectomy was 4 (Table 7-3), but all cancers in the women carefully followed in the BCPT were localized stage 1 tumors. Although tamoxifen might increase occurrence of ovarian cysts, there are no data suggesting an increased risk of ovarian cancer (12,23,28). Increased vaginal discharge has been described (22).

Central Nervous System

Tamoxifen increases hot flashes (22,33-35) but does not appear to affect mood, anxiety, or overall quality of life (12,35). There is an increase in cataract development with tamoxifen use and an increase in rate of cataract surgery (12).

Clinical Recommendations

The most important use of tamoxifen is for adjuvant treatment of breast cancer at multiple stages of the disease. Tamoxifen can also be recommended to some women who are at increased risk of breast cancer. The risk-benefit ratio in regard to the skeleton and perhaps other organ systems may very well be different for postmenopausal versus premenopausal women. In the skeleton, tamoxifen (20 mg/day) increases BMD in the spine and perhaps hip in postmenopausal women; however, the effect on fracture risk is unclear. Therefore, for postmenopausal women who are at the highest risk of osteoporotic fracture (those with established disease and/or with T scores below –2.5), consideration

Table 7-4   Effects of Raloxifene on Bone Mass and Bone Turnover in Randomized Controlled Trials

Author	No. of Subjects	Age	Characteristics	Intervention	Bone Mineral Density Results for 60-mg Dose		Bone Turnover Results for 60-mg Dose	
Johnston et al, 2000 (41)	1145 healthy postmenopausal women 2–8 yr from LMP from European (n = 601) and North American (n = 544) studies combined	Mean = 59.6 yr Range = 45–60 yr	Normal lumbar spine T score above –2.5 and below +2.0	• 30, 60, or 150 mg Rlx or Pbo • All received 400–600 mg elemental supplemental calcium • No vitamin D • 3-yr interim analysis	*Spine:* *Hip:* *TBBM:* *Ultradistal radius:*	Rlx 2.7% vs Pbo Rlx 2.2% vs Pbo Rlx 1.7% vs Pbo Rlx 1.8% vs Pbo but losses in both	*OC:* *BSAP:* *UCTX:* *UNTX:*	Rlx 14% vs Pbo Rlx 7% vs Pbo Rlx 19% vs Pbo Rlx 12% vs Pbo
Eli Lilly Product Circular (37)	619 women s/p hysterectomy	Median = 54 yr	Normal, as above	• 60 mg Rlx, Pbo, or CEE 0.625 mg/d • 400–600 mg Ca • 2 yr	*Spine:* *Total hip:*	Rlx 1.8% vs Pbo Rlx 1.3% vs Pbo		—
Lufkin et al, 1998 (43)	143 postmenopausal women with osteoporosis	Mean = 68.4 yr	Lumbar spine or hip ≤10th percentile vs. normal premenopausal and at least 1 prevalent vertebral fracture	• Rlx 60, Rlx 120, or no drug (control) • All received Ca 750 mg/d and vitamin D to total 800 IU/d • 1 yr	*Spine:* *Total hip:*	Rlx 2.8% vs Con Rlx 2.7% vs Con	*BSAP:* *OC:* *UCTX:*	Rlx 15% vs Con Rlx 21% vs Con Rlx 12% vs Con
Ettinger et al, 1999 (MORE) (42)	7705 postmenopausal women with osteoporosis	Mean = 67 yr Range = 31–80 yr	• Group 1: BMD <–2.5 T score • Group 2: Prevalent vertebral fracture ± <–2.5 T score	• Rlx 60, Rlx 120, or Pbo • All received 500 mg Ca and 400–600 IU vitamin D/d • 3 year interim analysis	*Spine:* *FN:*	Rlx 2.6% vs Pbo Rlx 2.1% vs Pbo	*OC:* *UCTX:*	Rlx 18% vs Pbo Rlx 26% vs Pbo

LMP = last menstrual period; BSAP = bone serum alkaline phosphatase; FN = femoral neck; Pbo = placebo; OC = osteocalcin; Rlx = raloxifene; Con = control.

should be given to the addition of an agent that is shown to have efficacy against fractures (such as bisphosphonates), even while these women are on tamoxifen. For women at only modest or moderate risk, with bone density above the osteoporosis range (T score above –2.5), tamoxifen is probably adequate for 5 years of use. Potentially serious adverse effects include venous thromboembolism, uterine cancer, benign uterine disease, and cataracts.

Raloxifene

Skeletal Effects

High-dose raloxifene (200 mg) reduces bone turnover to a similar degree that conjugated equine estrogen does (36), with estrogenic effects on bone remodeling (37) and calcium metabolism (38). Bone biopsy data in 65 normal postmenopausal women indicated that raloxifene doses of 60 to 120 mg/day reduce bone formation rate and remodeling activation frequency, confirming that raloxifene is an antiresorptive drug (39).

In osteoporosis prevention studies in healthy postmenopausal women with bone density above the osteoporosis range, raloxifene's effects are similar at multiple skeletal sites. Raloxifene increases spine, hip, and total body bone mass by 1.4% to 2.8% versus placebo, and reduces bone formation 7% to 21% and bone resorption 12% to 26% versus placebo (37,40–43; Table 7-4). Overall, raloxifene's effects on bone mass are similar to those of tamoxifen.

Three years of treatment with raloxifene 60 mg/day in women with osteoporosis (MORE study) reduced risk of vertebral fracture (but no other fractures) by approximately 40% (42; Table 7-5). Vertebral fracture was defined as radiographic deformity and therefore included both symptomatic and asymptomatic compressions. As expected, women in the placebo group who had prevalent vertebral fractures at baseline had a higher incident fracture rate (21.2%) over 3 years compared with women in the placebo group with osteoporosis who did not have prevalent fractures at entry (4.5%). In the former group, there appeared to be a slightly greater reduction in incident vertebral fractures in women in the 120-mg subgroup compared with women in the 60-mg raloxifene group. The trial indicated that 46 women with osteoporosis, without previous vertebral fracture, would need to be treated for 3 years to prevent one vertebral fracture. The corresponding number for women with a previous vertebral fracture would be only 16 (because the baseline incidence is so much higher in this latter group). Raloxifene did not reduce the risk of wrist, hip, or all nonvertebral fractures during 3 or 4 years of use in this study. Four-year data confirm continued protection against vertebral fracture of similar magnitude to that seen after 3 years (43a).

Table 7-5   Effects of Raloxifene on Multiple Outcomes Over 3 to 3.5 Years (Cumulative Incidence) in MORE Randomized Trial*

Event	Placebo (%)	Raloxifene (%)	RR (95% CI)
Incident vertebral fracture (subgroup—no prevalent fracture)	4.5	2.3	0.5 (0.4–0.8)
Incident vertebral fracture (subgroup—prevalent fracture)	21.2	14.7	0.7 (0.6–0.9)
Incident vertebral fracture (study group—combined)	10.1	6.6	0.6 (0.5–0.8)
All nonvertebral fractures	9.3	8.5	0.9 (0.8–1.1)
Wrist fracture	3.3	2.9	0.9 (0.6–1.1)
Ankle fracture	1.1	0.7	0.6 (0.4–1.0)
Hip fracture	0.7	0.8	1.1 (0.6–1.9)
Invasive breast cancer	1.0	0.3	0.2 (0.1–0.4)
Noninvasive or uncertain invasiveness breast cancer	0.2	0.2	—
Venous thromboembolism[†]	0.3	1.0	3.1 (1.5–6.2)
Endometrial cancer	0.2	0.2	0.8 (0.2–2.7)

* Data from Ettinger B, Black DM, Mitlak BH, et al. Reduction of vertebral fracture risk in post-menopausal women with osteoporosis treated with raloxifene. Results from a 3-year randomized clinical trial. JAMA. 1999;282:637–645; and Cummings SR, Eckert S, Krueger KA, et al. The effect of raloxifene on risk of breast cancer in postmenopausal women. Results from the MORE randomized trial. JAMA. 1999;281:2189–2197.

† Including both deep vein thrombophlebitis and pulmonary embolism. For incident vertebral fracture, data are presented for 60 mg raloxifene dose. For all other outcomes, data are from pooled raloxifene groups (60 and 120 mg).

Effects on Other Organ Systems

Breast

The occurrence of invasive breast cancer was 76% lower in women taking raloxifene for over 3 years, owing entirely to a reduction in ER-positive disease (Table 7-5; 44). A similar reduction was seen in women taking raloxifene for 4 years (44a). Approximately 93 women would need to be treated with raloxifene for 4 years to prevent one case of invasive breast cancer. Women in the raloxifene trial were recruited because of osteoporosis, not elevated breast cancer risk. Nevertheless, the average age in MORE was older than that in the BCPT, and therefore these women were probably at increased risk of breast cancer by age. The potency of effects of raloxifene versus tamoxifen on breast cancer prevention, however, cannot be directly compared from the available data. A study comparing the two drugs regarding effects on breast cancer occurrence and other outcomes, called STAR (Study of Tamoxifen and Raloxifene), is underway.

Vascular Disease

Raloxifene reduces serum total cholesterol, LDL cholesterol, lipoprotein a, and plasma fibrinogen, while increasing the HDL subclass HDL-2 (36,40–41,45). No end-organ effects of cardiovascular or cerebrovascular disease have been published. Venous thromboembolic disease is increased to a 3-fold degree, as is seen with tamoxifen and estrogen (42). Of approximately 155 women treated with raloxifene for 3 years, one case of venous thromboembolism would be diagnosed. In the MORE study after 4 years cardiovascular and cerebrovascular disease occurrences were not increased in the overall population and were decreased by 40% in patients with established disease or those at high risk (45a). An ongoing study, Raloxifene Use for the Heart (RUTH), will assess the effect of raloxifene on cardiovascular disease in postmenopausal women who have heart disease or who are at high risk.

Reproductive Organs

In contrast to tamoxifen, raloxifene is not associated with an increased risk of uterine cancer (Table 7-5) or any benign disease. Serial transvaginal ultrasounds reveal no increase in endometrial proliferation or other benign uterine disease, including polyps, although clinically insignificant increases in fluid have been documented within the endometrial cavity (44). Raloxifene does not increase pelvic organ prolapse and might actually reduce the need for pelvic floor surgery (45b).

Central Nervous System

Raloxifene increases hot flashes similarly to tamoxifen (44). A systematic study of cognitive function in 143 women with osteoporosis revealed no differences in performance between raloxifene and placebo groups on tests of memory and mood (46). Cognitive function was not significantly affected in postmenopausal women from the MORE study (47).

Other

Raloxifene can be associated with leg cramps, leg swelling, and an influenza-like syndrome.

Clinical Recommendations

Raloxifene (60 mg/day) protects against vertebral fractures in women with osteoporosis, produces small increases in bone mass of the spine, hip, and total body, and reduces bone turnover in postmenopausal women with or without osteoporosis. No significant effect on nonvertebral fracture is seen after 3 years of treatment. Raloxifene has the additional benefit of substantially reducing the risk of ER-positive invasive breast cancer without increasing the risk of uterine disease, as seen with tamoxifen. Raloxifene increases the risk of venous thromboembolic disease to the same degree as do tamoxifen and estrogen. Therefore, both SERMS and estrogens are generally contraindicated in women with a previous history of venous thromboembolism or those at significantly increased risk of same.

Raloxifene is probably most useful in those women who have osteoporosis (T score ≤ -2.5) or who are at risk (T score < -1.5 with clinical risk factors) in the middle menopausal period (age 55–65) or in the early menopausal period (for women who have no significant hot flashes). At this stage in life, vertebral fractures are common, but hip fractures are not. Therefore, women who take raloxifene can expect a reduction in the likelihood of having a vertebral fracture, and possibly breast cancer, but the lack of proven efficacy against hip fracture is not a major deterrent to use of this agent in this age group.

Summary

Raloxifene (60 mg/day) improves BMD, albeit by only a small amount, and decreases bone turnover. In postmenopausal women with osteoporosis, it has been shown to reduce the risk of vertebral fracture but not other types of fractures. Raloxifene has been approved by the FDA for the treatment and prevention of osteoporosis. This agent also appears to reduce substantially the risk of breast cancer, although it has not been approved by the FDA for this indication. Raloxifene might be most useful in women with osteoporosis who also have a high risk of breast cancer or in women who are at high risk of vertebral fracture. There are no data yet that confirm that raloxifene reduces the risk of hip fracture, so it may be less useful in elderly women who are at particularly high risk of hip fracture.

Tamoxifen, which is used for the treatment and prevention of breast cancer, has similar effects on bone density and bone turnover as raloxifene. Like raloxifene, there are no data confirming that tamoxifen reduces the risk of non-spine fractures. Its effects on the risk of vertebral fracture have not been as well studied as those of raloxifene, and it has not been approved by the FDA for the prevention or treatment of postmenopausal osteoporosis.

REFERENCES

1. **Cosman F, Lindsay R.** Selective estrogen receptor modulators: clinical spectrum. Endocr Rev. 1999;20:418–434.

2. **Kristensen B, Ejlertsen B, Dlagaard P, et al.** Tamoxifen and bone metabolism in postmenopausal low-risk breast cancer patients. A randomized study. J Clin Oncol. 1994;12:992–997.

3. **Love RR, Mazess RB, Barden HS, et al.** Effects of tamoxifen on bone mineral density in postmenopausal women with breast cancer. N Engl J Med. 1992;326:852–856.

4. **Grey AB, Stapleton JP, Evans MC, et al.** The effect of the antiestrogen tamoxifen on bone mineral density in normal late postmenopausal women. Am J Med. 1995;99: 636–641.

5. **Wright CDP, Garrahan NJ, Stanton M, et al.** Effect of long-term tamoxifen therapy on cancellous bone remodeling and structure in women with breast cancer. J Bone Miner Res. 1994;9:153–159.

6. **Kenny AM, Prestwood KM, Pilbeam CC, Raisz LG.** The short-term effects of tamoxifen on bone turnover in older women. J Clin Endocrinol Metab. 1995;80:3287–3291.

7. **Love RR, Barden HS, Mazess RB, et al.** Effect of tamoxifen on lumbar spine bone mineral density in postmenopausal women after 5 years. Arch Intern Med. 1994;154: 2585–2588.

8. **Wright CDP, Mansell RE, Gazet JC, Compston JE.** Effect of long term tamoxifen treatment on bone turnover in women with breast cancer. BMJ. 1993;306:429–430.

9. **Powles TJ, Hickish T, Kanis JA, et al.** Effect of tamoxifen on bone mineral density measured by dual energy x-ray absorptiometry in healthy premenopausal and postmenopausal women. J Clin Oncol. 1996;14:78–84.

10. **Gotfredsen A, Christiansen C, Palshof T.** The effect of tamoxifen on bone mineral content in premenopausal women with breast cancer. Cancer. 1984;53:853–857.

11. **Kristensen B, Ejlertsen B, Mouridsen HT, et al.** Femoral fractures in postmenopausal breast cancer patients treated with adjuvant tamoxifen. Breast Cancer Res Treat. 1996;39:321–326.

12. **Fisher B, Costantino JP, Wickerham DL, et al.** Tamoxifen for prevention of breast cancer. Report of the National Surgical Adjuvant Breast and Bowel Project P-1 Study. J Natl Cancer Inst. 1998;90:1371–1388.

13. **Early Breast Cancer Trialists' Collaborative Group.** Systemic treatment of early breast cancer by hormonal, cytotoxic, or immune therapy. 133 randomised trials involving 31,000 recurrences and 24,000 deaths among 75,000 women. Lancet. 1992;339:1–15, 71–85.

14. **Early Breast Cancer Trialists' Collaborative Group.** Tamoxifen for early breast cancer. An overview of the randomised trials. Lancet. 1998;351:1451–1467.

15. **Osborne CK.** Drug Therapy: tamoxifen in the treatment of breast cancer. N Engl J Med. 1998;339:1609–1618.

16. **Hortobagyi GN.** Treatment of breast cancer. N Engl J Med. 1998;339:974–984.

17. **Powles T, Eeles R, Ashley S, et al.** Interim analysis of the incidence of breast cancer in the Royal Marsden Hospital tamoxifen randomised chemoprevention trial. Lancet. 1998;352:98–101.

18. **Veronesi U, Maisonneuve P, Costa A, et al.** Prevention of breast cancer with tamoxifen: preliminary findings from the Italian randomised trial among hysterectomised women. Lancet. 1998;352:93–97.

19. **McDonald CC, Stewart HJ.** Fatal myocardial infarction in the Scottish adjuvant tamoxifen trial. The Scottish Breast Cancer Committee. BMJ. 1991;303:435–437.

20. **McDonald CC, Alexander FE, Whyte BW, et al.** Cardiac and vascular morbidity in women receiving adjuvant tamoxifen for breast cancer in a randomised trial. The Scottish Cancer Trials Breast Group. BMJ. 1995;311:977–980.

21. **Rutqvist LE, Mattsson A.** Cardiac and thromboembolic morbidity among postmenopausal women with early stage breast cancer in a randomized trial of adjuvant tamoxifen. The Stockholm Breast Cancer Study Group. J Natl Cancer Inst. 1993;85:1398–1406.

22. **Costantino JP, Kuller LH, Ives DG, et al.** Coronary heart disease mortality and adjuvant tamoxifen therapy. J Natl Cancer Inst. 1997;89:776–782.

23. **Fisher B, Costantino JP, Redmond CK, et al.** Endometrial cancer in tamoxifen-treated breast cancer patients. Findings from the National Surgical Adjuvant Breast and Bowel Project (NSABP) B-14. J Natl Cancer Inst. 1994;86:527–537.

24. **Fisher B, Costantino, JP, Redmond C, et al.** A randomized clinical trial evaluating tamoxifen in the treatment of patients with node-negative breast cancer who have estrogen-receptor-positive tumors. N Engl J Med. 1989;320:479–484.

25. **Fisher B, Redmond C.** Systemic therapy in node-negative patients. Updated findings from NSABP clinical trials. National Surgical Adjuvant Breast and Bowel Project. J Natl Cancer Inst Monogr. 1992;11:105–116.

26. **Saphner T, Tormey DC, Gray R.** Venous and arterial thrombosis in patients who received adjuvant therapy for breast cancer. J Clin Oncol. 1991;9:286–294.

27. **"Nolvadex" Adjuvant Trial Organisation.** Controlled trial of tamoxifen as a single adjuvant agent in the management of early breast cancer. Br J Cancer. 1998;57:608–611.

28. **Cook LS, Weiss NS, Schwartz SM, et al.** Population-based study of tamoxifen therapy and subsequent ovarian, endometrial, and breast cancers. J Natl Cancer Inst. 1995;87:1359–1364.

29. **Rutqvist LE, Johansson H, Signomklao T, et al.** Adjuvant tamoxifen therapy for early stage breast cancer and second primary malignancies. Stockholm Breast Cancer Study Group. J Natl Cancer Inst. 1995;87:645–651.

30. **Neven P, DeMulder X, van Belle Y, et al.** Tamoxifen and the uterus. BMJ. 1994;309:1313–1314.

31. **Jaiyesimi IA, Buzdar AU, Decker DA, Hortobagyi GN.** Use of tamoxifen for breast cancer: twenty-eight years later. J Clin Oncol. 1995;113:513–529.

32. **Kedar RP, Bourne TH, Powles TJ, et al.** Effects of tamoxifen on uterus and ovaries of postmenopausal women in a randomized breast cancer prevention trial. Lancet. 1994;343:1318–1321.

33. **Fisher B, Dignam J, Bryant J, et al.** Five versus more than five years for tamoxifen therapy for breast cancer patients with negative lymph nodes and estrogen receptor-positive tumors. J Nat Cancer Inst. 1996;88:1529–1542.

34. **Love RR, Cameron L, Connell BL, Leventhal H.** Symptoms associated with tamoxifen treatment in postmenopausal women. Arch Intern Med. 1991;151:1842–1947.

35. **Love RR, Cameron L, Connell BL, Leventhal H.** Symptoms associated with tamoxifen treatment in postmenopausal women. Arch Intern Med. 1991;151:1842–1847.

36. **Draper MW, Flowers DE, Huster WJ, et al.** A controlled trial of raloxifene (LY139481) HC1: impact on bone turnover and serum lipid profile in healthy postmenopausal women. J Bone Miner Res. 1996;11:835–842.

37. Product Circular 1997: Evista (Raloxifene Hydrochloride). Eli Lilly and Company, Indianapolis, IN.

38. **Heaney RP, Draper MW.** Raloxifene and estrogen: comparative bone remodeling kinetics. J Clin Endocrinol Metab. 1997;82:3425–3429.

39. **Ott SM, Oleksik A, Lu Y, et al.** Bone histomorphometric results of a 2-year randomized, placebo controlled trial of raloxifene in postmenopausal women. Bone. 1998;23(S1):TS295.

40. **Delmas PD, Bjarnason NH, Mitlak BH, et al.** Effects of raloxifene on bone mineral density, serum cholesterol concentrations, and uterine endometrium in postmenopausal women. N Engl J Med. 1997;337:1641–1647.

41. **Johnston CC, Bjarnason NH, Cohen FJ, et al.** Long-term effects of raloxifene on bone mineral density, bone turnover, and serum lipid levels in early postmenopausal women: three-year data from 2 double-blind, randomized, placebo-controlled trials. Arch Intern Med. 2000;160:3444–3450.

42. **Ettinger B, Black DM, Mitlak BH, et al.** Reduction of vertebral fracture risk in postmenopausal women with osteoporosis treated with raloxifene. Results from a 3-year randomized clinical trial. JAMA. 1999;282:637–645.

43. **Lufkin EG, Whitaker MD, Nickelsen T, et al.** Treatment of established postmenopausal osteoporosis with raloxifene. A randomized trial. J Bone Miner Res. 1998;13:11.

43a. **Pols H, Eastell R, Delmas P, et al.** Early onset and sustained efficacy of raloxifene on incident vertebral fractures in postmenopausal women with osteoporosis: 4 year results from the MORE trial. Bone. 2001;28(suppl 5):585–586.

44. **Cummings SR, Eckert S, Krueger KA, et al.** The effect of raloxifene on risk of breast cancer in postmenopausal women. Results from the MORE randomized trial. JAMA. 1999;281:2189–2197.

44a. **Cauley JA, Norton L, Lippman ME, et al.** Continued breast cancer risk reduction in postmenopausal women treated with raloxifene: 4-year results from the MORE trial. Breast Cancer Res Treat. 2001;65:125–134.

45. **Nickelsen T, Lifkin EG, Riggs BL, et al.** Raloxifene hydrochloride, a selective estrogen receptor modulator: safety assessment of effects on cognitive function and mood in postmenopausal women. Psychoneuroendocrinology. 1999;24:115–128.

45a. **Barrett-Connor E, Grady P, Sashegyi A, et al.** Raloxifene and cardiovascular events in osteoporotic postmenopausal women. Four-year results from the MORE (Multiple Outcomes of Raloxifene Evaluation) randomized trial. JAMA. 2002;287:847–857.

45b. **Goldstein SR, Neven P, Zhou L, et al.** Raloxifene effect on frequency of surgery for pelvic floor relaxation. Obstet Gynecol. 2001;98:91–96.

46. **Walsh BW, Kuller LH, Wild RA, et al.** Effects of raloxifene on serum lipids and coagulation factors in healthy postmenopausal women. JAMA. 1998;279:1445–1455.

47. **Yaffe K, Krueger K, Sarkar S, et al.** Cognitive function in postmenopausal women treated with raloxifene. N Engl J Med. 2001;344:1207–1213.

CHAPTER 8

Phytoestrogens and DHEA

SUNDEEP KHOSLA, MD

Key Points

- Early evidence suggests that dietary and low-dose pharmacologic phytoestrogens may have tissue-specific effects, with beneficial effects on bone and the vascular system. Recent trials have failed to establish a beneficial effect of phytoestrogens on bone density.

- Phytoestrogens appear to have neutral or inhibitory effects on breast and uterine tissue.

- The safety of pharmacologic doses of phytoestrogens is unknown.

Although traditional hormone replacement therapy (HRT) is effective in the prevention of hot flashes, osteoporosis, and, possibly, vascular disease, there are significant concerns about its effects on the risk of breast cancer and of unopposed estrogen on the risk of uterine cancer. The availability of synthetic selective estrogen-receptor modulators (SERMs), such as tamoxifen and raloxifene (see Chapter 7), has supplied new options for postmenopausal women, providing many of the benefits of HRT without some of the risks. Nonetheless, there is tremendous interest among postmenopausal women in potentially "natural" alternatives to estrogen or the SERMs. The principal compounds generating this interest are the phytoestrogens and related compounds such as natural progesterone. Indeed, there is widespread belief in the scientific and lay press that phytoestrogens are "natural" SERMs. In addition, there is considerable interest among aging women and men in dehydroepiandrosterone (DHEA) as an "anti-aging" hormone, with putative benefits for the skeleton and an improved sense of well-being, increased muscle mass, and enhanced immune function. This has led to an abundance of phyto-estrogen, natural progesterone, and DHEA preparations at health food stores and at Internet sites. However, because these are considered "dietary supplements," there is no significant, authoritative supervision of the manufacture of these compounds or of the claims placed on their use by manufacturers. In this chapter, our current understanding of the biology of these compounds and the available data on their efficacy, particularly on the skeleton, are reviewed.

Dietary and Synthetic Phytoestrogens

Classification of Phytoestrogens

There are three main classes of phytoestrogens: isoflavones, lignans, and coumestans (Fig. 8-1). They are found principally in plants or their seeds, and a single dietary source often contains more than one class of phytoestrogens. Isoflavones (genistein, daidzein, glycitein, equol) are found principally in legumes (soybeans, lentils, beans, and chickpeas) and soybean products (1). Lignans (enterolactone, enterodiol) are found principally in fruits and vegetables and in alcoholic sources (beer, bourbon), and coumestans (coumestrol) are found in bean sprouts and fodder crops (1). Among the "other" phytoestrogens, perhaps the ones of greatest interest are resveratrol and black

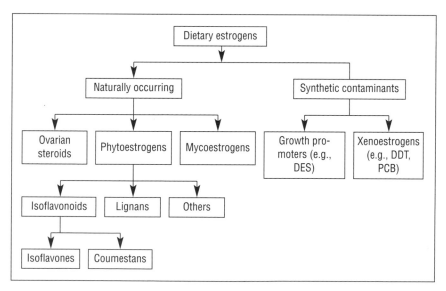

Figure 8-1   Classification of dietary estrogens, including phytoestrogens.

cohosh. Resveratrol is found in dark-skinned grapes and, hence, in red wine (2). Black cohosh is an herbal preparation that is very popular at health food stores. It contains an estrogenic compound, 27-deoxytriterpene glycoside, with putative benefits on menopausal symptoms. In addition, there is a synthetic isoflavone, ipriflavone, which has been the most extensively studied.

Mechanism of Action

The discovery of a second estrogen receptor (ER), called ER-β (3,4) (distinct from the first ER found, ER-α) has added a new level of complexity to our understanding of tissue-specific actions of estrogen and SERMs as well as of phytoestrogens.

Human osteoblasts express significant amounts of ER-β and lower levels of ER-α (5). Note that although phytoestrogens are structurally similar to estrogen (Fig. 8-2) and bind the ER, the binding affinity of the phytoestrogens for either ER-α or ER-β is lower than that for estrogen. In addition, although estrogen binds equally to ER-α and ER-β, phytoestrogens have a higher binding affinity for ER-β (6). Furthermore, although the overall potency of phytoestrogens is substantially lower than that of estradiol, circulating phytoestrogen levels on traditional Chinese or Japanese diets may be 1000-fold or higher than those of estradiol (7). Collectively, these data indicate that phytoestrogens have the potential to have significant biological effects, although

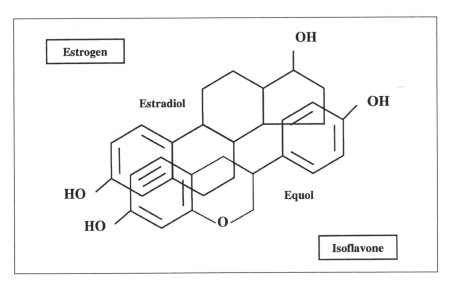

Figure 8-2 Structural similarity of the major isoflavone metabolite, equol, to estradiol. (Adapted from Setchell KDR, Cassidy A. Dietary isoflavones: biological effects and relevance to human health. J Nutr. 1999;129:748S–767S.)

clearly the spectrum of these effects may be quite different from that of estrogen or SERMs.

Phytoestrogen Effects on Bone Metabolism

The most convincing evidence for phytoestrogen effects on bone comes from animal studies. In most rat and mice models, dietary soybean protein (8), soy isoflavones (9), genistein (10-14), daidzein (11), and coumestrol and zearalanol (15) have all prevented or ameliorated bone loss immediately after ovariectomy, although soy isoflavones did not reverse established bone loss (16), and resveratrol did not affect radial bone growth in normal growing rats (17).

Observational studies in humans indicate considerable variation worldwide in the rates of hip fractures in different populations, with generally lower rates in Asian populations (18). This has led to speculation that the ethnic differences in hip fracture rates could be related to dietary factors, such as the high phytoestrogen intake in most Asian populations. For example, gender-specific hip fracture rates in people 85 years of age or older in Hong Kong are 30% of those in the United States (19). Similarly, the incidence rates of hip fracture in mainland China (20) and in Japan (21) are consistently lower than those in Caucasian populations. However, vertebral fracture rates are, in fact, higher in Japanese women compared with Caucasian women (21), and bone mineral density (BMD) (at both the spine and hip) of Asian women is similar to that of Caucasian women, after adjusting for weight and height (22). Thus, other factors such as differences in hip axis length, lower incidence of falls, or other lifestyle factors are perhaps more likely explanations for the lower hip fracture rates in Asian populations than the high phytoestrogen intake, although a potential role for the latter certainly cannot be excluded. In support of this, a recent study of Southern Chinese women (23) found that postmenopausal women with a habitually high intake of dietary isoflavones had higher BMD values at both the spine and hip.

Direct evidence for a protective effect of phytoestrogens on BMD in humans is extremely sparse at present. In a preliminary study, 6 months of treatment with 90 mg/d of isoflavones from soy protein increased spine BMD by 2.2%, compared with a 0.6% decrease in the control group ($P < 0.05$; 24). In another short-term study, isoflavone treatment from 40 g/day of soy protein each day prevented bone loss at the lumbar spine in perimenopausal women compared with placebo (25). Clearly, more studies in humans to assess the possible effects of phytoestrogens on bone are needed.

In contrast to the natural phytoestrogens, there are considerably more human data on the synthetic isoflavone, ipriflavone. Data from some small, randomized, clinical trials suggest that ipriflavone might be efficacious in preventing bone loss at the radius and spine in postmenopausal women (Table 8-1)

Table 8-1   Randomized Clinical Trials on Skeletal Effects of Ipriflavone

Author	Number of Subjects	Age (yr)	Characteristics	Change in BMD in Treatment Group Compared with Placebo
Gambacciani et al. (26)	40 women 10–30 days following ovariectomy	Mean = 48.1	• Ipf 600 mg/day vs control • All: Ca 500 mg/day • 12-month study	• Radius: 5.7%, $P < 0.01$
Gambacciani et al. (27)	100 premeno-pausal women treated with a GnRH agonist	Mean = 39.1	• Ipf 200 mg tid vs placebo • All: Ca 500 mg/day • 12-month study	• Lumbar spine: 4.7%, $P < 0.01$ • Total body: 6.9%, $P < 0.01$
Valente et al. (28)	40 postmeno-pausal women	Range = 47–65	• Ipf 300 mg bid vs placebo • All: Ca 1000 mg/day • 12-month study	• Radius: 4.2%, no significant difference • Lumbar spine: 3.4%, $P < 0.05$
Agnusdei et al. (29)	83 early post-menopausal women	Mean = 50.3	• CEE 0.3 mg/day vs CEE 0.3 mg/day + Ipf 200 mg tid vs placebo • All: Ca 1000 mg/day + MPA 10 mg for 15 days q 3 months • 12-month study	• Forearm: CEE + Ipf: 7.3%, $P < 0.05$
Adami et al. (30)	255 post-menopausal women	Range = 50–65	• Ipf 200 mg tid vs placebo • All: Ca 1000 mg/day • 24-month study	• Radius: 3.5%, $P < 0.05$
Gambacciani et al. (31)	80 early post-menopausal women	Range = 40–48	• Ipf 200 mg tid vs CEE 0.3 mg/day vs Ipf 200 mg bid + CEE vs control • All: Ca 500 mg/day • 24-month study	• Lumbar spine: Ipf 4.9%, $P < 0.05$ • CEE + Ipf: 4.9%, $P < 0.05$
Agnusdei et al. (32)	198 postmeno-pausal women	Range = 50–65	• Ipf 200 mg tid vs placebo • All: Ca 1000 mg/day • 24-month study	• Lumbar spine: 1.7%, $P < 0.05$
Gennari et al. (33)	255 postmeno-pausal women	Mean = 57.4	• Ipf 200 mg tid vs placebo • All: Ca 1000 mg/day • 24-month study	• Radius: 3.5%, $P < 0.05$
Alexandersen et al. (34)	474 postmeno-pausal women; vertebral T score < −2	Mean = 63	• Ipf 200 mg tid vs placebo • All: Ca 500 mg/day	• Lumbar spine: no significant difference • Total hip: no significant difference • Forearm: no significant difference • Incident vertebral fractures: no significant difference

Ipf = ipriflavone; Ca = calcium; CEE = conjugated equine estrogens; MPA = medroxyprogesterone acetate.

(26-34). In addition, a trial in premenopausal women treated with a gonadotropin-releasing hormone (GnRH) agonist for heavy menstrual bleeding indicated that ipriflavone could prevent the bone loss associated with estrogen deficiency in this setting (30). In these studies, ipriflavone was generally associated with decreases in bone turnover, although these effects were relatively modest when compared with those seen with HRT. In contrast to these small, relatively positive studies, however, are the recently reported findings of the largest study of the longest duration (3 years) (34), which found no effect of ipriflavone over placebo on lumbar spine, hip, or forearm BMD, bone resorption markers, or incident vertebral fractures. Moreover, ipriflavone was associated with significant lymphopenia in 29 of the 234 treated women (33). The findings of this study indicate that ipriflavone is unlikely to be a useful agent for the treatment of women with established low bone mass.

Tissue-Specific Effects of Phytoestrogens

In the animal studies reviewed earlier, genistein (11-14) and soy protein (8) did not increase uterine weights, consistent with a neutral or antagonistic effect of these phytoestrogens on the uterus. In contrast, daidzein increased uterine weight in a manner similar to estrogen (11). Human data on the effects of phytoestrogens come from one study in premenopausal women treated with GnRH agonist therapy; there was no effect of ipriflavone on uterine weight decline (27), consistent with a lack of uterine stimulation with this agent. Thus, it seems likely that different phytoestrogens may have different actions, not only on bone but also in terms of possible tissue specificity.

Animal studies suggest that phytoestrogens may retard the development of breast cancer (35-39). However, cell data suggest that phytoestrogens can stimulate or inhibit the proliferation of breast cancer cells, depending on the particular phytoestrogen, the dose of phytoestrogen, and the cancer cell line (35). Thus, certain phytoestrogens at certain doses may behave as estrogen agonists on breast tissue, raising obvious concerns about their widespread use.

Animal studies in both rats and primates demonstrate that some phytoestrogens (soy and genistein) have a protective effect on the vascular system (40-43). Consistent with the animal data, observational studies in humans have found that Asian populations with a high phytoestrogen intake have lower rates of cardiovascular disease (44), as well as lower rates of breast and uterine cancer (45,46). However, it is unclear how much of this is related to phytoestrogen intake rather than a number of other genetic or environmental factors. Soy protein consumption benefits blood lipids (reductions in total and low-density lipoprotein [LDL] cholesterol and triglycerides) (47), and 40 mg of phytoestrogen in pill form increases serum high-density lipoprotein (HDL) cholesterol (48). In addition, soy phytoestrogens may also have other beneficial vascular effects via inhibition of platelet aggregation and antioxidant effects (49). Additionally, some studies have found beneficial effects of phytoestrogens in reducing hot flashes in postmenopausal women (1).

In summary, there is some preliminary evidence (from animal and observational human studies) that indicates that dietary and low-dose pill phytoestrogens may have tissue-specific effects, with beneficial effects on bone and the vascular system. However, the effects on the breast and uterus are antagonistic or neutral, and the largest clinical trial using a synthetic phytoestrogen did not demonstrate any benefit on bone. Furthermore, the safety of pharmacologic doses of phytoestrogens is completely unknown.

Natural Progesterone

Many postmenopausal women are also turning to "natural" progesterone in the form of yam extracts for a number of putative benefits. Currently, however, there are no rigorous clinical trial data to support the use of these agents.

DHEA

DHEA and its sulfate ester (DHEAS) are the major circulating adrenal androgens (50). Serum DHEA levels peak by the second decade of life and then steadily decline by an average of 10% per decade (50); the decline is even more rapid after the age of 80. Indeed, no other hormone declines as profoundly with aging as DHEA. Some (51,52) but not all (53,54) cross-sectional studies have noted associations between serum DHEAS levels and BMD. In addition, postmenopausal women with primary adrenal failure were noted to have decreased serum DHEA levels and decreased distal forearm bone density compared to control postmenopausal women (55), further suggesting a role for adrenal androgens in the maintenance of bone mass, particularly in postmenopausal women.

The potential regulatory role of adrenal androgens in bone metabolism has also been assessed in several animal studies. In rats, adrenalectomy resulted in loss of metaphyseal trabecular bone to an extent similar to that produced by oophorectomy (56). In addition, treatment with DHEA reduced loss of cancellous bone after oophorectomy, indicating that adrenal androgens may prevent the bone loss induced by estrogen deficiency (57).

Although these studies suggest that adrenal androgens may have important effects on the skeleton, there are few data on the potential effects of therapy with adrenal androgens on bone and calcium metabolism in humans. A few small clinical trials indicate that administration of synthetic anabolic steroids to women with postmenopausal osteoporosis may be associated with a modest increase in BMD. Several investigators have used either pharmacologic (58) or physiologic (59) doses of DHEA and have found variable effects on blood lipids or body composition, although none of these studies examined the effects of adrenal androgen replacement on the skeleton. Of interest, a preliminary report of DHEA therapy in six patients with systemic lupus erythematosus who were on corticosteroids suggested that DHEA might have some utility in preventing steroid-induced bone loss (60). In addition, in an uncontrolled study, daily application of 10% DHEA cream in 14 postmenopausal women produced a significant (2.0%) increase in hip BMD associated with a decrease in bone turnover markers (61). Despite the absence of any clear data indicating beneficial effects of DHEA replacement on any age-related changes, this agent has stimulated a great deal of attention among the media and the public, and a significant number of individuals use DHEA to prevent or reverse these age-related changes.

Summary and Recommendations

It is clear that, despite the availability of HRT and SERMs for menopausal symptoms and osteoporosis, there is tremendous interest among postmenopausal women in potential "natural" alternatives such as phytoestrogens. In addition, DHEA has also generated considerable interest as an anti-aging hormone to prevent or reverse a number of age-related changes, including osteoporosis. Although some small studies suggest possible beneficial effects of phytoestrogens on the skeleton, this has not been confirmed in larger studies. Therefore, it is premature to advocate the widespread use of these compounds. More studies are needed to assess possible skeletal benefits and to assess potential benefits or adverse effects on the breast, uterus, and cardiovascular system.

This leads, then, to the issue of what practical advice the physician can offer the patient who presents with interest in the use of these agents. First, it is important to point out to the patient that our knowledge about the benefits and risks of these compounds is, at present, quite incomplete. Therefore, it is probably beneficial for most individuals to institute modest dietary changes, such as reducing the intake of animal protein and substituting soy protein, with its potential beneficial lipid and antioxidant effects. Traditional Japanese or Chinese diets contain up to approximately 50 mg/day of total isoflavones, and, in the absence of direct data, this is probably a reasonable guideline as an upper limit for patients. In terms of dietary sources, most soy products contain about 2 mg/g of isoflavones, and tofu contains about 0.3 mg/g isoflavones (62). Table 8-2 lists the isoflavone content of common foods and supplements. Although it is probably better to institute dietary changes, if the patient chooses to use isoflavone products from health food stores, they should aim

Table 8-2   Isoflavone Content of Common Foods and Supplements*

Limited Information About Effectiveness

Common foods

Soybeans	2 mg/g
Tofu	0.3 mg/g
Soy flour	2 mg/g
Soy hot dog	0.2 mg/g
Tofu yogurt	0.3 mg/g

Common supplements

Soy powders	13–103 mg/oz
Soy drinks	3-40 mg/oz

No Evidence About Effectiveness or Safety

Black cohosh

* Isoflavone content is approximate and given per ounce or gram. If an individual chooses to use supplemental phytoestrogens, the upper limit for isoflavone intake, until additional data are available, should be approximately 50 mg/day from all sources (diet and supplements).

to limit the isoflavone supplementation to the guidelines noted earlier. There is at present little efficacy or safety data on black cohosh, and DHEA supplementation should be deferred until the results of ongoing studies with this agent become available.

REFERENCES

1. **Murkies AL, Wilcox G, Davis SR.** Phytoestrogens. J Clin Endocrinol Metab. 1998; 83:297–303.

2. **Kopp P.** Resveratrol, a phytoestrogen found in red wine: a possible explanation for the conundrum of the 'French paradox'? Eur J Endocrinol. 1998;138:619–620.

3. **Kuiper GG, Enmark E, Pelto-Huikko M, et al.** Cloning of a novel estrogen receptor expressed in rat prostate and ovary. Proc Natl Acad Sci U S A. 1996;93:5925–5930.

4. **Kuiper GG, Carlsson B, Grandien K, et al.** Comparison of the ligand binding specificity and transcript tissue distribution of estrogen receptor α and β. Endocrinology. 1997;138:863–870.

5. **Arts J, Kuiper GG, Janssen JM, et al.** Differential expression of estrogen receptors alpha and beta mRNA during differentiation of human osteoblast SV-HFO cells. Endocrinology. 1997;138:5067–5070.

6. **Kuiper GG, Jansen JM, Lemmen JG, Carlsson B, et al.** Interaction of estrogenic chemicals and phytoestrogens with estrogen receptor β. Endocrinology. 1998;139: 4252–4263.

7. **Setchell KDR, Cassidy A.** Dietary isoflavones: biological effects and relevance to human health. J Nutr. 1999;129:758S–767S.

8. **Arjmandi BH, Alekel L, Hollis BW, et al.** Dietary soybean protein prevents bone loss in an ovariectomized rat model of osteoporosis. J Nutr. 1995;126:161–167.

9. **Arjmandi BH, Birnbaum R, Goyal NV, et al.** Bone-sparing effect of soy protein in ovarian hormone-deficient rats is related to its isoflavone content. Am J Clin Nutr. 1998;68(Suppl):1364S–1368S.

10. **Blair HC, Jordan SE, Peterson TG, Barnes S.** Variable effects of tyrosine kinase inhibitors on avian osteoclastic activity and reduction of bone loss in ovariectomized rats. J Cell Biochem. 1996;61:629–637.

11. **Ishida H, Uesugi T, Hirai K, et al.** Preventive effects of the plant isoflavones, daidzin and genistin, on bone loss in ovariectomized rats fed a calcium-deficient diet. Biol Pharm Bull. 1998;21:62–66.

12. **Fanti P, Monier-Faugere MC, Geng Z, et al.** The phytoestrogen genistein reduces bone loss in short-term ovariectomized rats. Osteoporos Int. 1998;8:274–281.

13. **Anderson JJB, Ambrose WW, Garner SC.** Biphasic effects of genistein on bone tissue in the ovariectomized, lactating rat model. Proc Soc Exp Biol Med. 1998;217: 345–350.

14. **Ishimi Y, Miyaura C, Ohmura M, et al.** Selective effects of genistein, a soybean isoflavone, on B-lymphopoiesis and bone loss caused by estrogen deficiency. Endocrinology. 1999;140:1893–1900.

15. **Draper CR, Edel MJ, Dick IM, et al.** Phytoestrogens reduce bone loss and bone resorption in oophorectomized rats. J Nutr. 1997;127:1795–1799.

16. **Arjmandi BH, Getlinger MJ, Goyal NV, et al.** Role of soy protein with normal or reduced isoflavone content in reversing bone loss induced by ovarian hormone deficiency in rats. Am J Clin Nutr. 1998;68(Suppl):1358S–1363S.

17. **Turner RT, Evans GL, Zhang M, et al.** Is resveratrol an estrogen agonist in growing rats? Endocrinology. 1999;140:50–54.

18. **Lau EMC.** The epidemiology of osteoporosis in Asia. In: Lau EMC (ed). Osteoporosis in Asia. Singapore: World Scientific Press; 1997;1–20.

19. **Ho SC, Bacon WE, Harris T, et al.** Hip fracture rates in Hong Kong and the United States, 1988 through 1989. Am J Public Health. 1993;83:694–697.

20. **Lu AM, Xu S, Cumming R, et al.** Very low rates of hip fractures in Beijing. A validated population-based study of rates and causes of hip fractures in China (Abstr). J Bone Miner Res. 1995;S467.

21. **Fujiwara S, Ross PD.** Epidemiological studies of osteoporosis in Japan. In: Lau EMC (ed). Osteoporosis in Asia. Singapore: World Scientific Press; 1997;21–29.

22. **Russell-Aulet M, Wang J, Thornton JC, et al.** Bone mineral density and mass in a cross-sectional study of white and Asian women. J Bone Miner Res. 1993;8:575–582.

23. **Mei J, Yeung SSC, Kung AWC.** High dietary phytoestrogen intake is associated with higher bone mineral density in postmenopausal but not premenopausal women. J Clin Endocrinol Metab. 2001;86:5217–5221.

24. **Potter SM, Baum JA, Teng H, et al.** Soy protein and isoflavones: their effects on blood lipids and bone density in postmenopausal women. Am J Clin Nutr. 1998; 68(Suppl):1375S–1379S.

25. **Alekel DL, Peterson C, St Germain A, Hanson K.** Isoflavone-rich soy isolate exerts significant bone-sparing in the lumbar spine of perimenopausal women. J Bone Miner Res. 1999;14(Suppl 1):S208.

26. **Gambacciani M, Spinetti A, Cappagli B, et al.** Effects of ipriflavone administration on bone mass and metabolism in ovariectomized women. J Endocrinol Invest. 1993;16:333–337.

27. **Gambacciani M, Cappagli B, Piaggesi L, et al.** Ipriflavone prevents the loss of bone mass in pharmacological menopause induced by GnRH-agonists. Calcif Tissue Int. 1997;61(Suppl 1):S15–S18.

28. **Valente M, Bufalino L, Castiglione GN, et al.** Effects of 1-year treatment with ipriflavone on bone in postmenopausal women with low bone mass. Calcif Tissue Int. 1994;54:377–380.

29. **Agnusdei D, Gennari C, Bufalino L.** Prevention of early postmenopausal bone loss using low doses of conjugated estrogens and the non-hormonal, bone-active drug ipriflavone. Osteoporosis Int. 1995;5:462–466.

30. **Adami S, Bufalino L, Cervetti R, et al.** Ipriflavone prevents radial bone loss in postmenopausal women with low bone mass over 2 years. Osteoporos Int. 1997;7:119–125.

31. **Gambacciani M, Ciaponi M, Cappagli B, et al.** Effects of combined low dose of the isoflavone derivative ipriflavone and estrogen replacement on bone mineral density and metabolism in postmenopausal women. Maturitas. 1997;28:75–81.

32. **Agnusdei D, Crepaldi G, Isaia G, et al.** A double blind, placebo-controlled trial of ipriflavone for prevention of postmenopausal spinal bone loss. Calcif Tissue Int. 1997;61:142–147.

33. **Gennari C, Adami S, Agnusdei D, et al.** Effect of chronic treatment with ipriflavone in postmenopausal women with low bone mass. Calcif Tissue Int. 1997;61:S19–S22.

34. **Alexandersen P, Toussaint A, Reginster J, et al.** Ipriflavone in the treatment of postmenopausal osteoporosis. A randomized controlled trial. JAMA. 2000;285:1482–1488.

35. **Barnes S.** Effect of genistein on in vitro and in vivo models of cancer. J Nutr. 1995;125:777S–783S.

36. **Lamartiniere CA, Murrill WB, Manzolillo PA, et al.** Genistein alters the ontogeny of mammary gland development and protects against chemically induced mammary cancer in rats. Proc Soc Exper Biol Med. 1998;217:358–364.

37. **Li Y, Upadhyay S, Bhuiyan M, Sarkar FH.** Induction of apoptosis in breast cancer cells MDA-MB-231 by genistein. Oncogene. 1999;18:3166–3172.

38. **Constantinou AI, Kamath N, Murley JS.** Genistein inactivates bcl-2, delays the G2/M phase of the cell cycle, and induces apoptosis of human breast adenocarcinoma MCF-7 cells. Eur J Cancer. 1998;34:1927–1934.

39. **Shao Z-M, Alpaugh ML, Fontana JA, Barsky SH.** Genistein inhibits proliferation similarly in estrogen receptor-positive and negative human breast carcinoma cell lines characterized by P21$^{WAF1/CIP1}$ induction, G_2/M arrest, and apoptosis. J Cell Biochem. 1998;69:44–54.

40. **Anthony MS, Clarkson TB, Bullock BC, Wagner JD.** Soy protein versus soy phytoestrogens in the prevention of diet-induced coronary artery atherosclerosis of male cynomolgus monkeys. Arterioscler Thromb Vasc Biol. 1997;17:2524–2531.

41. **Clarkson TB, Anthony MS, Williams JK, et al.** The potential of soybean phytoestrogens for postmenopausal hormone replacement therapy. Proc Soc Exp Biol Med. 1998;217:365-368.

42. **Honore EK, Williams JK, Anthony MS, Clarkson TB.** Soy isoflavones enhance coronary vascular reactivity in atherosclerotic female macaques. Fertil Steril. 1997;67:148–154.

43. **Makela S, Savolainen H, Aavik E, et al.** Differentiation between vasculoprotective and uterotrophic effects of ligands with different binding affinities to estrogen receptors α and β. Proc Natl Acad Sci U S A. 1999;96:7077–7082.

44. **Keys A, Menotti A, Aravanis C, et al.** The seven countries study: 2,289 deaths in 15 years. Prev Med. 1984;13:141–154.

45. **Parkin DM.** Cancers of the breast, endometrium, and ovary: geographic correlations. Eur J Cancer Clin Oncol. 1989;25:1917–1925.

46. **Rose DP, Boyar AP, Wynder EL.** International comparisons of mortality rates for cancer of the breast, ovary, prostate and colon, and per capita food consumption. Cancer. 1986;58:2363–2371.

47. **Anderson JW, Johnstone BM, Cook-Newell ME.** Meta-analysis of the effects of soy protein intake on serum lipids. N Engl J Med. 1995;333:276–282.

48. **Eden JA, Knight DC, Howes JB.** A controlled trial of isoflavones for menopausal symptoms (Abstr). Eighth International Congress on the Menopause, Sydney, Australia, 1996.

49. **Wilcox JN, Blumenthal BF.** Thrombotic mechanisms in atherosclerosis: potential impact of soy proteins. J Nutr. 1995;125:631S–638S.

50. **Meikle AW, Daynes RA, Araneo BA.** Adrenal androgen secretion and biologic effects. Endocrinol Metab Clin North Am. 1991;20:381–400.

51. **Szathmari M, Szucs J, Feher T, Hollo I.** Dehydroepiandrosterone sulphate and bone mineral density. Osteoporos Int. 1994;4:84–88.

52. **Rozenberg S, Ham H, Bosson D, et al.** Age, steroids and bone mineral content. Maturitas. 1990;12:137–143.

53. **Davidson BJ, Riggs BL, Wahner HW, Judd HL.** Endogenous cortisol and sex steroids in patients with osteoporotic spinal fractures. Obstet Gynecol. 1983;61: 275–278.

54. **Barrett-Connor E, Kritz-Silverstein D, Edelstein SL.** A prospective study of dehydroepiandrosterone sulfate (DHEAS) and bone mineral density in older men and women. Am J Epidemiol. 1993;137:201–206.

55. **Devogelaer JP, Crabbe J, De Deuxchaisnes CN.** Bone mineral density in Addison's disease: evidence for an effect of adrenal androgens on bone mass. BMJ. 1987;294: 798–800.

56. **Durbridge TC, Morris HA, Parsons AM, et al.** Progressive cancellous bone loss in rats after adrenalectomy and oophorectomy. Calcif Tissue Int. 1990;47:383–387.

57. **Turner RT, Lifrak ET, Beckner M, et al.** Dehydroepiandrosterone reduces cancellous bone osteopenia in ovariectomized rats. Am J Physiol. 1990;258:E673–E677.

58. **Nestler JE, Barlascini CD, Clore JN, Blackard WG.** Dehydroepiandrosterone reduces serum low density lipoprotein levels and body fat but does not alter insulin sensitivity in normal men. J Clin Endocrinol Metab. 1994;78:1360–1367.

59. **Morales AJ, Nolan JJ, Nelson JC, Yen SSC.** Effects of replacement dose of dehydroepiandrosterone in men and women of advancing age. J Clin Endocrinol Metab. 1994;78:1360–1367.

60. **Van Vollenhoven RF.** Increased bone mineral density in patients with SLE treated with DHEA. Arth Rheum. 1996;39:S292.

61. **Labrie F, Diamond P, Cusan L, et al.** Effect of 12-month dehydroepiandrosterone replacement therapy on bone, vagina, and endometrium in postmenopausal women. J Clin Endocrinol Metab. 1997;82:3498–3505.

62. **Tham DM, Gardner CD, Haskell WL.** Potential health benefits of dietary phytoestrogens: a review of the clinical, epidemiological, and mechanistic evidence. J Clin Endocrinol Metab. 1998;83:2223–2235.

CHAPTER 9

Bisphosphonates

MARC C. HOCHBERG, MD, MPH

Key Points

- Alendronate and risedronate are FDA approved for the prevention and treatment of osteoporosis in postmenopausal women and patients taking glucocorticoids. Alendronate is also approved for the treatment of osteoporosis in men.

- Randomized controlled trials demonstrate that patients with vertebral fractures or osteoporosis, as determined by bone mineral density testing, who take these drugs decreased their risk of vertebral fractures by 50% and nonvertebral fractures by about 30% to 49%. Both drugs appear to reduce the risk of hip fracture.

- In women without osteoporosis, bisphosphonates improve bone mass, but their value for the prevention of fractures is unclear.

- Patients should be instructed to take bisphosphonates on an empty stomach with a full glass of water and to have nothing to eat for at least 30 minutes afterwards. Failure to do so may interfere with absorption and increase side effects.

- The ideal duration of treatment with bisphosphonates is not known.

Bisphosphonates bind to hydroxyapatite crystals in bone and inhibit bone resorption. This results in an increase in the density and mineral content of bone, with a resultant increase in bone strength (1). More importantly, these agents have also been documented to decrease fracture rate.

Bisphosphonates are commonly used for the prevention and treatment of osteoporosis among postmenopausal women. They are also the first choice of treatment for men with osteoporosis and for most patients with glucocorticoid-induced osteoporosis (see Chapter 12). Bisphosphonates are also used to treat Paget's disease of the bone and hypercalcemia of malignancy, and in some cases may decrease the risk of bone metastases caused by breast cancer (2,3).

Bisphosphonates are divided into two major groups: the nitrogen-free agents etidronate and clodronate and the more potent nitrogen-containing agents alendronate, pamidronate, and risedronate. In the United States, three bisphosphonates are available for oral use: etidronate, alendronate, and risedronate. The year each agent was introduced for general use in the United States and the Food and Drug Administration indications for its use are listed in Table 9-1.

In this chapter, we review the evidence for the use of etidronate, alendronate, and risedronate in the prevention and treatment of osteoporosis in women and men. The use of bisphosphonates for patients receiving glucocorticoids is reviewed in Chapter 12.

Treatment and Prevention of Osteoporosis

Etidronate

Etidronate has not been approved by the FDA for the prevention and treatment of osteoporosis. However, etidronate is used, particularly in Canada and

Table 9-1   Oral Bisphosphonates Approved for Use in the United States

Agent	Type	Year Introduced for General Use	FDA Indications
Etidronate	Nonnitrogen	1977	1. Paget's disease of the bone 2. Prevention and treatment of heterotopic ossification following total hip replacement or spinal cord injury
Alendronate	Nitrogen	1995	1. Paget's disease of the bone 2. Prevention and treatment of osteoporosis in postmenopausal women 3. Treatment and prevention of glucocorticoid-induced osteoporosis 4. Treatment of osteoporosis in men
Risedronate	Nitrogen	2000	1. Paget's disease of the bone 2. Prevention and treatment of osteoporosis in postmenopausal women 3. Prevention and treatment of glucocorticoid-induced osteoporosis

in Europe, for this purpose. Etidronate is given cyclically: patients are instructed to take 400 mg for 2 weeks every 3 months. Patients should also be instructed to take nothing by mouth but plain water for 2 hours before and 2 hours after the etidronate is taken. Because of these dosing instructions, patients are typically advised to take the drug before bed.

Four randomized controlled studies have examined the efficacy of intermittent cyclical etidronate in women with established osteoporosis (4–7). These studies have all been small (66 to 423 patients) and ranged in duration from 1 to 4 years. All of these studies demonstrate an increase in lumbar spine bone mineral density (BMD) among patients taking etidronate compared with placebo (the increase ranges from 4% to 8%). Two of the three studies that measured femoral neck BMD also reported an increase (2% to 4%) at this site (4,5).

In the four trials designed to evaluate the effect of etidronate on BMD, radiographs of the spine at baseline and at completion of the study were obtained. Two of the four studies demonstrated an approximately 50% reduction in the rate of new vertebral fractures (6,7). Larger studies and studies on the effects of etidronate on hip and other fractures are lacking.

There have been five small (36 to 152 patients), short (average 2 years), randomized placebo-controlled trials that have examined the effects of cyclic etidronate on the prevention of osteoporosis (8–11). These studies demonstrate that women taking cyclical etidronate have higher lumbar spine BMD compared with women taking placebo. Only one study (8) demonstrated a higher femoral neck BMD among women taking cyclical etidronate.

Alendronate

Alendronate is one of the most commonly used agents for the treatment of osteoporosis. Randomized placebo-controlled clinical trials demonstrate that alendronate, at daily doses of 5 mg and 10 mg, increases BMD at the lumbar spine, femoral neck, and total body in postmenopausal women with osteoporosis (Table 9-2) (12–15). The increases in BMD are dose related, with greatest increases at the treatment dose of 10 mg a day (average lumbar spine increase: 6% to 9%; average femoral neck increase: 2.5% to 6%).

Alendronate does not have to be taken every day. Recent data from a large 1-year randomized trial in women with postmenopausal osteoporosis demonstrate that alendronate given either as 10 mg once daily, 35 mg twice weekly, or 70 mg once weekly results in similar increases in lumbar spine and hip BMD, although no fracture data is available for weekly treatment (16).

Alendronate also decreases the incidence of radiographic vertebral fractures by about 50% and is even more effective in decreasing the incidence of multiple vertebral fractures (Table 9-3) (12–14). Based on data from the Fracture Intervention Trial, about 40 women would need to be treated with alendronate

Table 9-2   Effect of Alendronate on BMD in Postmenopausal Women

Author	N	Age (yr)	Characteristics	Intervention	Follow-up (yr)	Mean Increase (%) in BMD in Treatment Group vs Placebo	
Liberman et al, 1995 (12)	994	45–80	L-spine T score ≤ –2.5	1. 5 mg aln × 3 yr 2. 10 mg aln × 3 yr 3. 20 mg × 2 yr and 5 mg × 1 yr 4. Placebo All: 500 mg calcium	3	10 mg: L-spine Femoral neck	8.8 5.9
Black et al, 1996 (13)	2047	55–81	≥ 1 vertebral fracture	1. 5 mg × 2 yr, then 10 mg 2. Placebo If calcium < 1000 mg, then 500 mg calcium and 250 IU vitamin D	2.9	L-spine Femoral neck	6.1 4.1
Cummings et al, 1998 (14)	4432	55–81	Femoral neck BMD ≤ 0.68 g/cm	Same as above	4.2	L-spine Femoral neck	6.6 4.6
Pols et al, 1999 (15)	1908	Mean = 62.8	< 85 yr; L-spine T score ≤ –2.0	1. 10 mg aln 2. Placebo All: 500 mg calcium	1	L-spine Femoral neck	4.9 2.5
Hosking et al, 1998 (27)	1609	45–59	Postmenopausal; in good health	1. 2.5 mg aln 2. 5 mg aln 3. HRT 4. Placebo	2	L-spine: 2.5 mg 5.0 mg HRT > 5.1 Total hip: 2.5 mg 5.0 mg HRT > 2.8	 3.1 4.6 2.2 2.7

Study	N	Age	Inclusion criteria	Treatment groups		Outcome
McClung et al, (1998) (28)	447	40–59	T score at lumbar spine > –2; no previous hip or spine fx	1. 1 mg aln × 3 yr 2. 5 mg aln × 3 yr 3. 10 mg aln × 3 yr 4. 20 mg × 2 yr and 1 yr Pbo 5. Placebo If calcium < 1000 mg/day, then 500 mg calcium	3	L-spine: 5 mg — 6.39 10 mg — 7.45 Total hip: 5 mg — 4.09 10 mg — 5.41
Ravn et al, 1999 (29)	1609	45–59	Same as in Ref 27 (Hosking et al)	1. 2.5 mg aln × 2 yrs, then Pbo × 2 yr 2. 5 mg × 2 yr, then Pbo × 2 yrs 3. 5 mg × 4 yr 4. HRT 5. Placebo	4	Femoral neck: 5 mg + pbo — 1.6 5 mg — 4.3

aln = alendronate; BMD = bone mineral density; fx = fracture; Pbo = placebo.

Table 9-3   Effect of Alendronate on Fracture in Postmenopausal Women

Author	N	Age (yr)	Characteristics	Intervention	Follow-up (yr)	Fracture Type	No. of Fractures (%) in Treatment and Placebo Groups			
							Placebo	Alendronate	Relative Hazard (95% CI)	P
Liberman et al, 1995 (12)	994	45–80	• T score at L-spine ≤ −2.5 SD	1. 5 mg aln × 3 yr 2. 10 mg aln × 3 yr 3. 20 mg aln × 2 yr and 5 mg aln × 1 yr 4. Placebo All: Calcium 500 mg	3	Vertebral 1 ≥ 2 Nonvertebral	22 (6.2%) 15 (4.2%) 38 (9.6%)	17 (3.2%) 3 (0.6%) 45 (7.5%)	0.52 (0.28–0.95) Not reported 0.79 (0.52–1.22)	0.03 ···
Black et al, 1996 (13)	2047	55–81	• At least one vertebral fx	1. 5 mg aln × 2 yr, then 10 mg aln 2. Placebo If calcium intake < 1000 mg/day, then 500 mg calcium and 250 IU vitamin D	2.9	Vertebral Hip Wrist Other*	50 (5%) 22 (2.2%) 41 (4.1%) 99 (9.9%)	23 (2.3%) 11 (1.1%) 22 (2.2%) 100 (9.8%)	0.45 (0.27–0.72) 0.49 (0.23–0.99) 0.52 (0.31–0.87) 0.99 (0.75–1.31)	<0.001 0.047 0.013 0.95
Cummings et al, 1998 (14)	4432 in FIT Clinical Fracture Arm	55–81	• Femoral neck BMD of 0.68 g/cm², no vertebral fx	Same as above	4.2	Vertebral 1 ≥ 2 Hip Wrist Other*	78 (3.8%) 10 (0.5%) 24 (1.1%) 70 (3.2%) 227 (10.2%)	42 (2.1%) 4 (0.2%) 19 (0.9%) 83 (3.7%) 182 (8.2%)	0.56 (0.39–0.80) 0.40 (0.13–1.24) 0.79 (0.43–1.44) 1.19 (0.87–1.64) 0.79 (0.65–0.96)	0.002 0.11 0.44 0.28 0.02
Pols et al, 1999 (15)	1908	62.8	• < 85 yr • T score at L-spine ≤ −2 SD	1. 10 mg aln 2. Placebo All: Calcium 500 mg	1	Nonvertebral	37 (4.4%)	19 (2.4%)	0.53 (0.30–0.90)	0.021

* Other than hip, wrist, spine.
aln = alendronate; fx, fracture.

for 3 years in order to prevent one vertebral fracture (13). The reduction in fracture risk appears to be independent of age at study entry, baseline femoral neck BMD, number of previous vertebral fractures, and history of previous osteoporotic fracture (17). Among women with vertebral fractures, 3 years of treatment with alendronate also reduced the number of the days of bed rest or limited activity because of back pain during an average of 2.9 years of follow-up (18).

Alendronate also decreases the occurrence of nonvertebral fractures in women with osteoporosis (defined as low BMD with a T score of less than –2.5, or previous osteoporotic fracture) (Table 9-3). In the Vertebral Fracture Arm of FIT, there was a 27% reduction in the risk of occurrence of all clinical fractures; this included about a 50% reduction in the risk of symptomatic vertebral fractures, hip fractures, and wrist fractures (13). Approximately 30 women would need to be treated for 3 years to prevent one nonvertebral fracture. Similarly, women in the Clinical Fracture Arm of FIT with a femoral neck T score of less than –2.5 had a significant 36% reduction in the risk of all clinical fractures and a 56% reduction in the risk of hip fractures (19). In contrast, there was not a significant decrease in nonspine fractures in women in this trial who did not have osteoporosis (14). In a multinational, 1-year study, alendronate-treated women (all of whom had a T score at the lumbar spine of ≤ –2.0) had a significant 47% reduction in the incidence of nonvertebral fractures (15).

Alendronate has recently been approved for the treatment of men with osteoporosis. Compared with placebo, 2 years of alendronate treatment at 10 mg/day was associated with a 5% higher bone mass at the lumbar spine and a 2.5% higher bone mass at the femoral neck ($P < 0.001$). The effect of alendronate of fracture rate is not clear. Using morphometric methods, men treated with alendronate had a lower incidence of vertebral fractures (0.8%), compared with men receiving placebo (7.1%; $P = 0.02$). However, the difference using semiquantitative methods (8.1% vs. 3.1%) was not statistically significant (20).

Risedronate

Randomized placebo-controlled clinical trials demonstrate that risedronate, at daily doses of 2.5 mg and 5 mg, increases BMD at the lumbar spine, femoral neck, radius, and total body in postmenopausal women with osteoporosis (Table 9-4) (21–25). The increases in BMD are greatest at the approved dose for treatment, 5 mg per day. The average increase in lumbar spine BMD was 4% to 7%, and average increase in femoral neck BMD was 3%. Recent data from a large 1-year randomized trial in women with postmenopausal osteoporosis demonstrate that risedronate given either as 5 mg once daily or 35 mg once weekly results in comparable increases in lumbar spine and hip BMD, although no fracture data is available as yet for weekly treatment (25a).

Table 9-4   Effect of Risedronate on Bone Mineral Density

Author	N	Age (yr)	Characteristics	Intervention	Follow-up (yr)	Mean Increase (%) in BMD in Treatment Group vs Placebo
Harris et al, 1999 (21)	2458	<85; mean = 69	• ≥ 1 vertebral fx and L-spine T score ≤ −2.0, or 2 vertebral fxs	1. 2.5 mg rsn, discontinued after 1 yr 2. 5 mg rsn 3. Placebo. All received 1000 mg calcium; those with low serum 25 (OH) vitamin D received 500 IU	3	L-spine: 4.4 / Femoral neck: 2.8
Reginster, et al, 2000 (22)	1226	<85; mean = 71	• At least 2 vertebral fxs, T4–L4	Same as above	3	L-spine: 5.9 / Femoral neck: 3.1
Geusens et al, 1999 (abstract) (23)	9497	>70; mean = 78	• Women 70–79 yr had fem neck T score <−3 and ≥1 risk factor for hip fx • Women >80 yr had ≥1 risk factor for hip fx	1. 2.5 mg rsn 2. 5 mg rsn 3. Placebo. All received 1000 mg calcium; those with low serum 25 (OH) vitamin D received vitamin D	3	L-spine: 2.5 mg: 5.37 / 5 mg: 7.02 / Femoral neck: 2.5 mg: 2.11 / 5 mg: 3.24
Fogelman et al, 2000 (24)	543	<80	• Lumbar spine T score ≤ −2.0	1. 2.5 mg rsn 2. 5.0 mg rsn 3. Placebo. All received 1000 mg calcium	2	L-spine: 2.5 mg: 1.4 / 5.0 mg: 4 / Femoral neck: 2.5 mg: 1.9 / 5.0 mg: 2.3
Mortensen et al, 1998 (25)	111	Range = 40–60	• Women with normal BMD	1. 5 mg rsn for 2 wk alt with Pbo for 2 wk × 2 yr, then Pbo × 1 yr 2. 5 mg rsn × 2 yr, then Pbo × 1 yr 3. Placebo	3	L-spine: 5 mg cyclic: 2.7 / 5 mg daily: 5.7

rsn = risedronate; fx = fracture; fem = femoral; Pbo = placebo.

Two randomized, placebo-controlled trials have examined the antifracture efficacy of risedronate (Table 9-5) (21,22) in postmenopausal women up to age 85 years with two or more vertebral fractures or one vertebral fracture and a lumbar spine BMD T score of –2 or less at baseline. Risedronate at 5 mg/day decreased new vertebral fractures by 41% at 36 months (21). There was also a 39% reduction in the cumulative incidence of pre-specified, non-vertebral fractures. Based on this data, approximately 20 women would need to be treated for 3 years to prevent one vertebral deformity, detectable by radiograph, and approximately 30 women would need to be treated for 3 years to prevent one nonvertebral fracture. A trial in Europe with an identical design involving 1226 women found that 3 years of risedronate decreased vertebral fractures by 49% and nonvertebral fractures by 33% (22).

A large trial involving women aged 70 years and older specifically studied the ability of risedronate to reduce the incidence of hip fractures (26). Among women aged 70 to 79 years with a femoral neck T score of –3.0 or less, rise-dronate at 2.5 or 5 mg/day reduced the risk of hip fracture by 40%. Among women with a vertebral fracture, risedronate reduced the risk of hip fracture by 60%. Risedronate had no significant effect on hip fracture incidence in women aged 80 and older who were enrolled on the basis of risk factors for hip fracture in whom BMD measurement had not been performed. Only 16% of these women had BMD T scores of less than –2.5 at the femoral neck.

Prevention of Bone Loss

Both alendronate and risedronate can be used for the prevention of osteo-porosis in postmenopausal women. In double-blind placebo-controlled trials of postmenopausal women 60 years old or younger, alendronate, at a dose of 5 mg/day, prevented bone loss in most women and induced a 1% to 7% increase in mean BMD at the lumbar spine, femoral neck, ultradistal radius, and total body, relative to placebo (Table 9-2) (27–29). In postmenopausal women, 24 months of risedronate also increased BMD by 6% in the spine and 3% in the hip (Table 9-4) (25). Twelve months after treatment stopped, lumbar-spine bone mass declined to levels below those at study entry in all groups. This may indicate that the effects of risedronate on bone mass are only maintained while taking the drug. The effects on fracture are not known.

Adverse Events

Although patients taking bisphosphonates often complain of gastrointestinal side effects, data from the FIT suggest that the incidence of adverse events

Table 9-5   Effect of Risedronate on Fracture in Postmenopausal Women

Author	N	Age (yr)	Characteristics	Intervention	Follow-up (yr)	Fracture Type	Placebo	Risedronate	Relative Hazard (95% CI)	P
Harris et al, 1999 (21)	2458	<85; mean = 69	• ≥ 1 vertebral fx and L-spine T score ≤ –2.0, or 2 vertebral fxs	1. 2.5 mg rsn, discontinued after 1 yr 2. 5 mg rsn 3. Placebo All received 1000 mg calcium; those with low serum 25 (OH) vitamin D received 500 IU	3	Vertebral Nonvertebral (6 sites)	93 (16.3%) 52 (8.4%)	61 (11.3%) 33 (5.2%)	0.59 (0.43–0.82) 0.61 (0.39–0.94)	0.003 0.02
Reginster, et al 2000 (22)	1226	<85; mean = 71	• At least 2 vertebral fxs, T4–L4	Same as above	3	Vertebral Nonvertebral (6 sites)	89 (29.0%) 51 (16.0%)	53 (18.1%) 36 (10.9%)	0.51 (0.36–0.73) 0.67 (0.44 –1.04)	<0.001 0.063
McClung et al, 2000 (26)	9331	>70	• Women 70–79 yr had fem neck T score < –3 and ≥ 1 risk factor for hip fx • Women >80 yr had ≥ 1 risk factor for hip fx	Same as above	3	In women aged 70–79 (Group 1) incidence of hip fx was reduced by 39% (P = 0.02); no effect on incidence of hip fx was observed in women aged 80+ (Group 2)				

fx = fracture; rsn = risedronate; fem = femoral.

was similar among placebo- and alendronate-treated women. This was true even for women aged 75 years and older, those with a history of previous upper gastrointestinal tract disease, and those who were concomitantly using nonsteroidal anti-inflammatory drugs (30). Severe esophagitis with alendronate therapy has been reported to occur at a rate of approximately one case per 1000 patient years of therapy (31). The risk of this complication may be reduced by taking the medication properly. Proper instructions for patients are outlined in detail elsewhere (32). The risk of irritating or eroding gastrointestinal mucosa appears to depend more on the frequency and duration of exposure than on the dose of alendronate. Therefore, high doses given less frequently might lower the risk of gastrointestinal side effects. No significant differences were found in the rate of gastrointestinal side effects between women receiving 10 mg of alendronate daily and those receiving greater than 70 mg weekly (16).

Other adverse effects of bisphosphonates are theoretical and are related to the long half-life (10 years) of these agents. With only 7 years of follow-up data, it is not known if bone remodeling in the future can occur normally in bone containing bisphosphonate that was incorporated earlier. If remodeling cannot occur normally, weakness in bone strength may result. If remodeling can proceed normally, when bone is reabsorbed the bisphosphonate will be released into the circulation. This may be beneficial, decreasing bone resorption, or it may suppress bone turnover to such a degree that old or damaged bone might not be replaced, thus increasing the risk of fracture (33). Because there are no head-to-head clinical trials of alendronate versus risedronate, it is difficult to know whether there are any differences with regard to efficacy or tolerability.

Clinical Recommendations

Bisphosphonates have several pharmacokinetic properties that influence how and in whom these drugs are prescribed. These compounds are poorly absorbed from the upper gastrointestinal tract; therefore, patients should be instructed to take them on an empty stomach. Bisphosphonates are excreted by the kidneys and should not be prescribed for patients with renal failure (creatinine clearance of less than 35 mL/min). Finally, as mentioned previously, these drugs are slowly released from bone during skeletal remodeling, and the terminal half-life is estimated at 10 years. Therefore, they have the potential to exert effects long after the treatment has been discontinued. Because newer agents have been in general use less than decades, not all long-term effects can be assessed.

Patients who are prescribed alendronate or risedronate should be instructed to take the medication properly (Table 9-6). This decreases adverse

Table 9-6   How to Prescribe a Bisphosphonate to Maximize Efficacy and Minimize GI Side Effects

Indication	Agent	Dose	Instructions to Patient
Prevention of osteoporosis	Alendronate	5 mg daily or 35 mg weekly	Take the pill first thing in the morning on an empty stomach with a full glass (6–8 ounces) of water. Stay upright (sitting or standing) for at least half an hour after taking the medication and wait at least 30 minutes before eating or drinking.
	Risedronate	5 mg daily or 35 mg weekly	
Treatment of osteoporosis	Alendronate	10 mg daily or 35 mg twice weekly, or 70 mg weekly	
	Risedronate	5 mg daily 35 mg weekly	

events and enhances absorption. Waiting less than 30 minutes after eating or taking the drug with food, beverages other than plain water, or other medications, particularly calcium supplements, will lessen the effect of the bisphosphonate by decreasing absorption.

Currently, the optimum duration of treatment is not known, and only expert opinion is available on this issue (33). We suggest that it may be reasonable to limit treatment to 4 years because there are very few data about the effects of bisphosphonates beyond 4 years. At that time, a bone density measurement could be repeated, and, for patients with a T score of less than –2.5 or ongoing fractures, it may be reasonable to treat for an additional 3 years because biochemical and BMD data do not demonstrate any adverse effects with 7 years of treatment. For those whose bone mass has increased to a T score of more than –2.5, it may be reasonable to discontinue treatment. Then, bone density testing could be repeated at 2-year intervals, and, if substantial bone loss ensues (e.g., greater than 4% at the spine or 6% at the hip), the physician and patient could consider restarting the bisphosphonate. Note that among patients taking these medications for the prevention of osteoporosis, a shorter duration of treatment may be reasonable with a similar follow-up.

Summary

Alendronate, risedronate, and etidronate increase bone density and substantially decrease bone resorption. Three- or 4-year treatment with alendronate and risedronate have been shown to decrease the risk of vertebral fractures by about half in women who have osteoporosis indicated by the presence of a vertebral fracture or low hip-bone density. These drugs have also been shown to reduce the risk of non-spine and hip fractures in women with osteoporosis defined as a femoral neck T score of less than –2.5 (alendronate) or less than –3.0 (risedronate). Both alendronate and risedronate have been approved by the FDA for the prevention and treatment of osteoporosis in postmenopausal women, treatment of osteoporosis in men, and treatment of osteoporosis in patients taking glucocorticoids. The value of these agents for prevention of fractures in women without osteoporosis is not clear.

REFERENCES

1. **Rodan GA, Fleisch HA.** Bisphosphonates: mechanisms of action. J Clin Invest. 1996; 97:2692–2696.

2. **Delmas PD, Meunier PJ.** The management of Paget's disease of bone. N Engl J Med. 1997;336:558–566.

3. **Mundy GR, Yoneda T.** Bisphosphonates as anticancer drugs. N Engl J Med. 1998; 339:398–400.

4. **Montessori MLM, Scheele WH, Netelenbos JC, et al.** The use of etidronate and calcium versus calcium alone in the treatment of postmenopausal osteopenia: results of three years of treatment. Osteoporos Int. 1997;7:52–58.

5. **Harris ST, Watts NB, Jackson RD, et al.** Four-year study of intermittent cyclic etidronate treatment of postmenopausal osteoporosis: three years of blinded therapy followed by one year of open therapy. Am J Med. 1993;95:557–567.

6. **Storm T, Thamsborg G, Steiniche T, et al.** Effect of intermittent cyclical etidronate therapy on bone mass and fracture rate in women with postmenopausal osteoporosis. N Engl J Med. 1990;322:1265–1271.

7. **Watts NB, Harris ST, Genant HK, et al.** Intermittent cyclical etidronate treatment of postmenopausal osteoporosis. N Engl J Med. 1990;323:73–79.

8. **Meunier PJ, Confavreux E, Tupinon I, et al.** Prevention of early postmenopausal bone loss with cyclical etidronate therapy (a double-blind, placebo-controlled study and 1-year follow-up). J Clin Endocrinol Metab. 1997;82:2784–2791.

9. **Herd RJM, Dalena R, Blake GM, et al.** The prevention of early postmenopausal bone loss by cyclical etidronate therapy: a 2-year, double-blind, placebo-controlled study. Am J Med. 1997;103:92–99.

10. **Tobias JH, Dalzell N, Pazianas M, Chambers TJ.** Cyclical etidronate prevents spinal bone loss in early postmenopausal women. Br J Rheumatol. 1997;36:612–613.

11. **Pouilles JM, Tremollieres F, Roux C, et al.** Effects of cyclical etidronate therapy on bone loss in early postmenopausal women who are not undergoing hormonal replacement therapy. Osteoporos Int. 1997;7:213–218.

12. **Liberman UA, Weiss SR, Broll J, et al.** Effect of oral alendronate on BMD and the incidence of fractures in postmenopausal osteoporosis. N Engl J Med. 1995;333:1437–1443.

13. **Black DM, Cummings SR, Karpf DB, et al.** Effect of alendronate on risk of fracture in women with existing vertebral fractures. Results of the Fracture Intervention Trial. Lancet. 1996;348:1535–1541.

14. **Cummings ST, Black DM, Thompson DE, et al.** Effect of alendronate on risk of fracture in women with low bone density but without vertebral fractures. JAMA. 1998; 280:2077–2082.

15. **Pols HAP, Felsenberg D, Hanley DA, et al.** Multinational, placebo-controlled, randomized trial of the effects of alendronate on bone density and fracture risk in postmenopausal women with low bone mass. Results of the FOSIT Study. Osteoporos Int. 1999;9:461–468.

16. **Schnitzer T, Bone HG, Crepaldi G, et al.** Therapeutic equivalence of alendronate 70 mg once-weekly and alendronate 10 mg daily in the treatment of osteoporosis. Alendronate Once-Weekly Study Group. Aging (Milano). 2000;12:1–12.

17. **Ensrud KE, Black DM, Palermo L, et al.** Treatment with alendronate prevents fractures in women at highest risk. Results from the Fracture Intervention Trial. Arch Intern Med. 1997;157:2617–2624.

18. **Nevitt MC, Thompson DE, Black DM, et al.** Effect of alendronate on limited-activity days and bed-disability days caused by back pain in postmenopausal women with existing vertebral fractures. Fracture Intervention Trial Research Group. Arch Intern Med. 2000;160:77–85.

19. **Black D, Thompson DE, Bauer D, et al.** Fracture risk reduction with alendronate in women with osteoporosis. The Fracture Intervention Trial. J Clin Endocrinol Metab. 2000;85:4118–4124.

20. **Orwoll E, Ettinger M, Weiss S, et al.** Alendronate for the treatment of osteoporosis in men. N Engl J Med. 2000;343:604–610.

21. **Harris ST, Watts NB, Genant HK, et al.** Effects of risedronate treatment on vertebral and nonvertebral fractures in women with postmenopausal osteoporosis. A randomized controlled trial. JAMA. 1999;282:1344–1352.

22. **Reginster JY, Minne H, Sorensen O, et al.** Randomized trial of the effects of risedronate on vertebral fractures in women with established postmenopausal osteoporosis. Osteoporos Int. 2000;11:83–91.

23. **Geusens P, Burge D, Zippel H, et al.** Risedronate increases BMD at the hip and spine in elderly, osteoporotic women (Abstr). Arthritis Rheum. 1999;42(Suppl 9): S287.

24. **Fogelman I, Ribot C, Smith R, et al.** Risedronate reverses bone loss in postmenopausal women with low bone mass. Results from a multinational, double-blind, placebo-controlled trial. JCEM. 2000;85:1895–1900.

25. **Mortensen L, Charles P, Bekker PJ, et al.** Risedronate increases bone mass in an early postmenopausal population: two years of treatment plus one year of follow-up. J Clin Endocrinol Metab. 1998;83:396–402.

25a. **Lindsay R, Kendler D, McClung MR, et al.** Risedronate 35 mg once a week is as effective as 5 mg daily in postmenopausal women. Arthritis Rheum. 2001;44:S153 (Abstr 604).

26. **McClung M, Eastell R, Bensen W, et al.** Risedronate reduces hip fracture risk in elderly women with osteoporosis (Abstr). Osteoporos Int. 2000;11(Suppl 2):S207.

27. **Hosking D, Chilvers CE, Christiansen C, et al.** Prevention of bone loss with alendronate in postmenopausal women under 60 years of age. Early Postmenopausal Intervention Cohort Study Group. N Engl J Med. 1998;338:485–492.

28. **McClung M, Clemmesen B, Daifotis A, et al.** Alendronate prevents postmenopausal bone loss in women without osteoporosis. A double-blind, randomized, controlled trial. Alendronate Osteoporosis Prevention Study Group. Ann Intern Med. 1998;128:253–261.

29. **Ravn P, Bidstrup M, Wasnich RD, et al.** Alendronate and estrogen-progestin in the long-term prevention of bone loss. Four-year results from the early postmenopausal intervention cohort study. A randomized, controlled trial. Ann Intern Med. 1999;131: 935–942.

30. **Bauer DC, Black D, Ensrud K, et al.** Upper gastrointestinal tract safety profile of alendronate. The Fracture Intervention Trial. Arch Intern Med. 2000;160:517–525.

31. **de Groen PC, Lubbe DF, Hirsch LF, et al.** Esophagitis associated with the use of alendronate. N Engl J Med. 1996;335:1016–1021.

32. **Yates AJ, Rodan GA.** Alendronate and osteoporosis. Drug Discovery Today. 1998;3: 69–78.

33. **Cosman F, Cummings SR, Lindsay R.** How long should patients with osteoporosis be treated with bisphosphonates? J Womens Health. 2000;9:81–84.

CHAPTER 10

Calcitonin

STUART L. SILVERMAN, MD

Key Points

- Calcitonin is FDA approved for the treatment of osteoporosis in late postmenopausal women.

- Randomized controlled trials have shown that calcitonin reduces the rate of bone loss in late postmenopausal women but not in early postmenopausal women.

- Intranasal calcitonin can reduce the risk of vertebral fractures but not other types of fractures among women with osteoporosis and previous vertebral fracture.

- Calcitonin may have some analgesic benefit, especially in patients with acute, painful vertebral fractures.

- Treatment with calcitonin should be considered for older women with osteoporosis who fail to respond to, or cannot take, other treatments.

Calcitonin is a small polypeptide hormone that is produced predominantly by the parafollicular "C" cells of the thyroid (1). Calcitonin may play a major role in the protection of the maternal skeleton, with large increases seen during pregnancy and lactation. Parathyroid hormone (PTH) and 1,25-dihydroxyvitamin D are the major regulators of calcium homeostasis in the nonpregnant or lactating woman, but calcitonin may play a minor role. Calcitonin levels increase in response to increases in serum calcium (2). Calcitonin binds to receptors on osteoclasts, inhibiting bone resorption (3).

In this chapter, we review the evidence for use of injectable and nasal calcitonin for the prevention and treatment of osteoporosis.

Injectable Calcitonin

Injectable salmon-derived calcitonin is approved by the FDA for the treatment of hypercalcemia, Paget's disease of bone, and postmenopausal osteoporosis. For many years, this agent was the only option available for Paget's disease and the only alternative to hormone therapy for osteoporosis management. Now that several other options are available, patient acceptance of this medication is limited by common side effects and need to inject daily.

Effect on Bone Mineral Density

There are three small, randomized, controlled trials of injectable calcitonin for the treatment of postmenopausal osteoporosis (4–6) and two studies on prevention (7,8) (Table 10-1). Injectable calcitonin, given daily or every other day at 50 IU to 100 IU intramuscularly or subcutaneously, improved distal radius bone mass or metacarpal radiogammetry by 6% to 23% and lumbar spine dual photon absorptiometry by 79% compared with placebo in postmenopausal women (4–8). The effects of injectable calcitonin on hip bone mineral density (BMD) are unknown.

Effect on Fracture

Data on the efficacy of injectable calcitonin for the prevention of osteoporotic fractures are limited. In a nonrandomized, observational study, the Mediterranean Osteoporosis Study (MEDOS), the rate of hip fracture in patients taking injectable calcitonin was modestly but not significantly reduced compared with the rate in patients not taking calcitonin (9).

Injectable calcitonin significantly reduced the risk of vertebral fracture by 84% over 2 years in a small randomized single-center study of postmenopausal women with prevalent vertebral fractures (6) (Table 10-2). There have been no randomized trials with injectable calcitonin using vertebral fracture as an endpoint. There are no data on the efficacy of injectable calcitonin on nonvertebral fracture.

Side Effects

The use of injectable calcitonin is limited by the inconvenience of injection, side effects of nausea with or without vomiting (20%), local reactions at the injection site (3%), and flushing of the face and hands (20%) (12).

Table 10-1   Effect of Injectable Calcitonin on Bone Mineral Density (BMD) in Postmenopausal Women

Authors	N	Age (yr)	Characteristics	Intervention	Follow-up (yr)	BMD Compared with Placebo When Available
Mazzuoli et al, 1986 (4)	60	65	At least one vert comp fx	1. 100 IU IM qod 2. Placebo injection qod All received 500 mg calcium bid	1	• 23% mean change in BMD distal radius DPA compared with placebo
Agnusdei et al, 1989 (5)	40	65	At least one vert comp fx	1. 100 IU IM qod 2. 100 IU nasal qd 3. Calcium only All received 1 g calcium	1	• BMD distal radius DPA increased in both calcitonin groups (P < 0.01) compared with baseline and decreased in control group (P < 0.05) compared with baseline
Mazzuoli et al, 1990 (7)	28	39–51	S/p ovariectomy for uterine fibromatosis	1. 100 IU IM qod for 12 mos 2. Placebo inj qod for 6 mos, then 100 IU IM qod for 6 mos All received 500 mg calcium bid	1	• 6% increase in BMD ultradistal radius by DPA compared with placebo • P < 0.01 at 6 mos between groups • NS at 12 mos
Meschia et al, 1992 (8)	104	NA	1–10 yr post-menopause	1. 40 IU calcitonin IM biw 2. 40 IU calcitonin IM biw+ HRT (1.25 mg oral conjugated estrogen + 10 mg MPA 10 d/mo) 3. HRT 4. No treatment	1	Compared to baseline: • Calcitonin increased 2.4% • HRT + calcitonin increased 10% (P < 0.001) • HRT increased 3.2% (P < 0.05) • Control decreased 5% (P < 0.001)
Rico et al, 1995 (6)	72	69	> 1 vert fx	1. 100 IU IM calcitonin 10 d/mo 2. Calcium only All received 500 mg calcium 10 d/mo	2	• Calcitonin group had 12% increase by metacarpal radiogrammetry compared with baseline (all patients) and 3.5% by total body BMD using DXA (only 10 patients) with a 5% loss on calcium alone compared with baseline

DPA = dual photon absorptiometry; DXA = dual energy x-ray absorptiometry; HRT = hormone replacement therapy; NS = not significant.

Table 10-2   Effect of Calcitonin on Fracture in Postmenopausal Women

Authors	N	Age (yr)	Characteristics	Intervention	Follow-up (yr)	No. of Fractures in Treatment and Placebo Groups
Rico et al, 1995 (6)	72	69	>1 vert fx	1. 100 IU IM 10 d/mo 2. Calcium only All received 500 mg calcium for 10 d/mo	2	Vert fx: Calcitonin: 5/36 Placebo: 32/36 P < 0.001
Overgaard et al, 1992 (10)	124	70	BMC distal forearm ≤ 2 SD	1. Nasal calcitonin 50 IU qd 2. Nasal calcitonin 100 IU qd 3. Nasal calcitonin 200 IU qd 4. Placebo nasal spray All received 500 mg calcium qd	2	Vert fx: 50 IU CT: 2/40 100 IU CT: 0/43 200 IU CT: 2/41 Placebo: 6/40 P = 0.017 using pooled data (50+100+200) vs placebo
Chesnut et al, 2000 (PROOF Study) (11)	1255	68	817 with 1–5 prevalent fx; BMD < 2.0 in all	1. Nasal calcitonin 100 IU qd 2. Nasal calcitonin 200 IU qd 3. Nasal calcitonin 400 IU qd 4. Placebo nasal spray All received 1000 mg calcium and 400 IU vitamin D daily	5	*see sub-table below*

Fx Type	Treatment	Incidence	RR (95% CI)	P
Entire study cohort				
Vert	Placebo	70 (26%)		
	100 IU	59 (22%)	0.85 (0.6–1.21)	
	200 IU	51 (18%)	0.67 (0.47–0.97)	<0.05
	400 IU	61 (22%)	0.84 (0.59–1.18)	
Participants with 1–5 prevalent fx				
Vert	Placebo	60 (30%)		
	200 IU	40 (19%)	0.64 (0.43–0.96)	<0.05
Entire study cohort				
Nonvert	Placebo	48 (16%)		
	100 IU	32 (10%)	0.64 (0.41–0.99)	<0.05
	200 IU	46 (15%)	0.88 (0.59–1.32)	
	400 IU	41 (13%)	0.81 (0.53–1.23)	

Nasal Spray Calcitonin

Nasal spray calcitonin has been available since 1995 in the United States. The bioavailability of nasal calcitonin is less than that of the intramuscular or subcutaneous preparation. For this reason, nasal calcitonin is given in higher dosages (13). Nasal spray calcitonin is FDA approved for treatment of osteoporosis in late postmenopausal women.

Effect on Bone Mineral Density and Bone Turnover

There are 12 published randomized clinical trials on the efficacy of nasal salmon calcitonin on BMD for the prevention and treatment of postmenopausal osteoporosis (Table 10-3). Most of these studies are small, single-center trials.

The efficacy of nasal spray calcitonin in postmenopausal women appears to be dependent on the number of years since menopause. In early postmenopausal women (less than or equal to 5 years since the last menstrual period), nasal calcitonin prevented bone loss, compared with placebo, in the lumbar spine (14–19) in some studies but did not slow radial bone loss (15). No published data on hip-bone mass are available. However, two unpublished large multicenter studies indicated that calcitonin did not prevent bone loss from the hip or spine (23) in early postmenopausal women. FDA approval and labelling reflect these negative results (24).

In late postmenopausal women (greater than 5 years since the last menstrual period), daily nasal calcitonin was found to increase lumbar spine BMD by an average of 1% to 2%, which was significant over 2 years in most (10,11,16,20,21) but not all studies (21). Intermittent calcitonin did not have an effect on BMD (19). There was no significant increase at cortical bone sites (forearm or hip) (11,22). In most cases, nasal spray calcitonin modestly reduces both urine and serum markers of bone turnover (11,22). Compared to other antiresorptive agents, the increase in bone mass and reduction in bone turnover is more modest with nasal calcitonin.

Effect on Fracture

There are three published trials on the effect of nasal spray calcitonin on fracture (Table 10-2). All show efficacy against risk of vertebral fracture but not hip fracture. In a 2-year study in 208 postmenopausal women with low bone mass, nasal spray calcitonin significantly reduced the rate of new vertebral fractures to about one third of the rate seen in patients taking calcium alone (10).

In the PROOF study (11), which used an intent-to-treat analysis of patients enrolled with a prevalent vertebral fracture ($N = 910$), there was a significant (36%) reduction in the number of patients with new single vertebral fractures

Table 10-3　Effect of Nasal Calcitonin on Bone Mineral Density (BMD) in Postmenopausal Women

Authors	N	Age (yr)	Characteristics	Intervention	Follow-up (yr)	BMD Compared with Placebo When Available
Reginster et al, 1987 (14)	30	NA	< 36 mos post-menopause	1. 50 IU 5 d/wk 2. Placebo All received 500 mg calcium 5 d/wk	1	• 4.54% difference in BMD lumbar spine between calcitonin and placebo (P < 0.01)
Overgaard et al, 1989 (15)	52	55?	2.5–5.0 yrs post-menopause	1. 100 IU q day 2. Nasal placebo q day All received 500 mg calcium	2	• 8.2% difference in BMD lumbar spine between calcitonin and placebo (P < 0.001)
Overgaard et al, 1989 (17)	40	65	Postmenopause with wrist fx	1. 100 IU bid 2. Placebo nasal bid All received 500 mg calcium	1	• Using valid completers (N = 37), 2.1% difference BMD spine • DPA vs placebo: 2.1% difference in prox radius BMD 2.3% difference in distal radius
Agnusdei et al, 1989 (5)	40	NA?	Established PMO	1. 100 IU nasal q day 2. 100 IU IM qod 3. Calcium only All received 1000 mg calcium q day	1	• BMD increased in treatment groups (P < 0.01), decreased in control group (P < 0.05)
Overgaard et al, 1992 (10)	208	70	BMD distal forearm < −2	1. 50 IU q day 2. 100 IU q day 3. 200 IU q day 4. Placebo nasal q day All received 500 mg calcium q day	2	• 0.7% increase in BMD lumbar spine at 2 yr with 50 IU and 100 IU compared with placebo at 2 yr • 2.0% increase in BMD lumbar spine at 2 yr with 200 IU compared with placebo
Gennari et al, 1992 (16)	21		< 5 yrs post-menopause	1. 200 IU qod 2. Placebo nasal q day	1	• 6.8% difference in BMD lumbar spine between calcitonin and placebo using DPA (P < 0.05)
Reginster et al, 1994 (18)	287	NA	6–36 mos post-menopause	1. 50 IU 5 d/wk 2. Placebo All received 500 mg calcium 5 d/wk	3	• 7.6% difference in BMD lumbar spine DPA with calcitonin compared with placebo (P < 0.01)

Study	N	Age	Entry criteria	Treatment groups	Duration (yr)	Results
Reginster et al, 1994 (19)	100	NA	2-yr extension of above trial	1. 50 IU 5 d/wk 2. Calcium only All received 500 mg calcium 5 d/wk	5	• 7.8% difference in BMD lumbar spine DPA calcitonin compared with placebo at 5 yr ($P < 0.001$)
Ellerington et al, 1996 (20)	117	55	T score of <1.2 at spine or hip	1. 200 IU calcitonin q day 2. 200 IU calcitonin tiw 3. Placebo nasal spray q day 4. Placebo nasal spray tiw No additional calcium	2	• BMD lumbar spine DPA mean change compared with placebo: • 200 IU q day 2% ($P < 0.025$) • 200 IU tiw 1.2% NS • 200 IU q day late postmenopausal 3.1% ($P < 0.01$) • 200 IU q day early postmenopausal 0.5% NS
Flicker et al, 1997 (21)	123	70	At least one fx of spine, forearm, or FN or BMD lumbar spine T score ≤ 1	1. Placebo nasal spray 2. 400 IU daily 3. 20 injections of nandrolone decanoate plus placebo nasal spray 4. Nandrolone + calcitonin	2	• Significant difference from baseline in DXA BMD lumbar spine in calcitonin group 5.0%: • 1.1% in placebo group • 4.7% with nandrolone • 0.7% with nandrolone and calcitonin
Chesnut et al, 2000 (11)	1255	68	817 with 1–5 prevalent vert fx, all with BMD T score of <2.0	1. 100 IU daily 2. 200 IU daily 3. 400 IU daily 4. Placebo All received 1000 mg calcium and 400 IU vitamin D	5	• All doses significantly different from baseline to 5 yrs • 0.8–1.0% difference at 5 yrs between calcitonin and placebo at lumbar spine using DXA • All doses significantly different from placebo at years 1 and 2 ($P < 0.05$) • At year 3 only 400 IU significantly different from placebo ($P = 0.01$) • No treatment effect at femoral neck using DXA
Downs et al, 2000 (22)	299	64	T score ≤ –2 at spine or FN and T score ≤ 1 at other site	1. 200 IU daily 2. Placebo	1	• No significant differences between calcitonin and placebo at lumbar spine and trochanter using DXA • Difference between calcitonin and placebo at femoral neck using DXA • Significant change from baseline at lumbar spine (1.18%) but not at femoral neck (0.6%)

DPA = dual photon absorptiometry; DXA = dual energy x-ray absorptiometry; FN = femoral neck; NA = not applicable; PMO = postmenopausal osteoporosis.

and a 45% reduction in the number of patients with multiple new vertebral fractures. These reductions were seen only in the 200 IU group and surprisingly not seen in the 400 IU group (11). If patients who did not have prevalent vertebral fractures were included in the analysis, vertebral fracture risk was significantly reduced by 33%, and multiple vertebral fracture occurrence was reduced by 35%. Vertebral fracture reduction in PROOF was independent of some variables known to influence fracture risk, such as baseline BMD and bone markers (11). Although there was a very high discontinuation rate (59%), withdrawal was seen equally across groups, and analyses limited to women who adhered to treatment did not alter the results. A post hoc analysis of women with prevalent vertebral fracture indicated that 12.5 women would need to be treated with 200 IU each day for 3 years to prevent a vertebral fracture. No significant reduction in the risk of nonvertebral fracture was observed in the PROOF study (11).

The PROOF study suggests that the FDA-approved dose of 200 IU nasal spray salmon calcitonin daily safely reduces the risk of new vertebral compression fractures over 5 years in postmenopausal women with established osteoporosis. The lack of significant vertebral fracture efficacy at the higher (400 IU) dose and the very high discontinuation rate limit the conclusions that can be drawn from this study.

Glucocorticoid-Induced Osteoporosis

Data on the use of calcitonin for glucocorticoid-induced osteoporosis are limited but discussed in Chapter 12. A few small studies demonstrate that injectable calcitonin may reduce the rate of bone loss in lumbar spine and radius in patients both initiating and receiving corticosteroid therapy (25,26). Data on nasal calcitonin are conflicting in regard to bone loss prevention (27–30), and there are no studies on calcitonin in glucocorticoid-treated patients with fracture as an endpoint.

Analgesic Effects

Injectable and nasal salmon calcitonin may have an analgesic effect on the bone pain of acute vertebral fracture (31–37). The analgesic effect might be most apparent in the first weeks after vertebral fracture. The dosage of nasal calcitonin used varies from 200 to 400 IU daily. Calcitonin also appears to relieve bone pain in conditions associated with excessive bone resorption such as osteoporosis, Paget's disease, and tumor bony metastases (32). Salmon calcitonin, therefore, may have a potential role in reducing the pain of acute vertebral fracture, decreasing immobilization and reducing analgesic dependence.

Side Effects

Side effects with nasal calcitonin are known to be minimal. In the PROOF study, the only significant side effect was an increase in rhinitis. Headache frequency, however, actually decreased (11).

Resistance

As a biological agent, resistance to calcitonin in the form of antibodies (38) or down regulation (39) is of concern; however, the best way to identify patients who are resistant is not known at this time.

Administration and Clinical Recommendations

The recommended dosage of calcitonin nasal spray is 200 IU administered to one nostril each day, alternating between nostrils. There is no dosing restriction with regard to meals. In addition to calcitonin, patients should optimize calcium and Vitamin D intake (see Chapter 4). The medication should be refrigerated until opened, then kept at room temperature and covered to avoid evaporation and condensation.

Treatment with calcitonin may be considered in older women with osteoporosis who do not respond to other treatments or in whom other treatments are contraindicated.

Summary

Calcitonin is FDA approved for the treatment but not the prevention of postmenopausal osteoporosis. Nasal spray calcitonin is the most commonly used delivery system. Calcitonin is very safe. Its efficacy is considered less robust than either estrogen replacement therapy or a bisphosphonate such as alendronate. Calcitonin has been found to reduce risk of vertebral fracture by 36% in patients with prevalent vertebral fracture, similar to the effect of selective estrogen receptor modulators such as raloxifene (40). Calcitonin has not been found to significantly reduce risk of hip fracture.

Nasal spray calcitonin should also be considered one of the options for the treatment of the late menopausal patient with established osteoporosis who may not be tolerant of alendronate or risedronate. Other options include estrogen and raloxifene. It should also be considered as one of the options for initial treatment of the symptomatic patient with osteoporotic vertebral fracture because of its potential analgesic effect. Calcitonin, however, is not recommended for the prevention of osteoporosis in men or in women at the time of menopause due to the absence of data showing efficacy.

REFERENCES

1. **Azria M.** The Calcitonins: Physiology and Pharmacology. Basel: Karger: 1989.

2. **Azria M, Copp DH, Zanelli JM.** 25 years of salmon calcitonin: from synthesis to therapeutic use [Editorial]. Calcif Tissue Int. 1995;57:405–408.

3. **Chambers TJ, Moore A.** The sensitivity of isolated osteoclasts to morphological transformation by calcitonin. J Clin Endo Metab. 1983;57:819–824

4. **Mazzuoli G, Passeri M, Gennari C, et al.** Effects of salmon calcitonin in postmenopausal osteoporosis. A controlled double blind clinical study. Calcif Tissue Int. 1986;38:3–8.

5. **Agnusdei D, Gonelli S, Camporeale A, et al.** Clinical efficacy of treatment with salmon calcitonin, administered intranasally for 1 year, in stabilized postmenopausal osteoporosis. Minerva Endocrinol. 1989;14:169–176.

6. **Rico H, Revilla M, Hernandez E, et al.** Total and regional bone mineral content and fracture rate in postmenopausal osteoporosis treated with salmon calcitonin. A prospective study. Calcif Tissue Int. 1995;56:181–185.

7. **Mazzuoli GF, Tabolli S, Bigi F, et al.** Effects of salmon calcitonin on the bone loss induced by ovariectomy. Calcif Tissue Int. 1990;47:209–214.

8. **Meschia M, Brincat M, Barbaracini P, et al.** Effect of hormone replacement therapy and calcitonin on bone mass in postmenopausal women. Eur J Obstet Gynecol Reprod Biol. 1992;47:53–57.

9. **Kanis JA, Johnell O, Gulberg B, et al.** Evidence for efficacy of drugs affecting bone metabolism in preventing hip fracture. BMJ. 1992;305:1124–1128.

10. **Overgaard K, Hansen MA, Jensen SB, et al.** Effect of calcitonin given intranasally on bone mass and fracture rates in established osteoporosis. A dose response study. BMJ. 1992;305:556–561.

11. **Chesnut C, Silverman SL, Andriano K, et al for the PROOF Study Group.** A randomized trial of nasal spray calcitonin in postmenopausal women with established osteoporosis. The Prevent Recurrence of Osteoporotic Fractures Study. Am J Med. 2000;109:267–276

12. **Gennari C, Passeri M, Chierichetti SM, Piolini M.** Side effects of synthetic salmon and human calcitonin. Lancet. 1983;1:594–595.

13. **Overgaard K, Agnusdei D, Hansen M, et al.** Dose response bioactivity and bioavailability of salmon calcitonin in premenopausal and postmenopausal women. J Clin Endocrinol Metab. 1991;72:344–349.

14. **Reginster JY, Denis D, Albert A, et al.** 1 Year controlled randomized trial of prevention of early postmenopausal bone loss by intranasal calcitonin. Lancet. 1987;2:1481–1483.

15. **Overgaard K, Riis B, Christiansen C, et al.** Effect of calcitonin given intranasally on early postmenopausal bone loss. BMJ. 1989;299:477–479.

16. **Gennari C, Agnuddei D, Monatgnani M, et al.** An effective regimen of intranasal salmon calcitonin in early postmenopausal bone loss. Calcif Tissue Int. 1992;50:381–383.

17. **Overgaard K, Riis BJ, Christiansen C, et al.** Nasal calcitonin for treatment of established osteoporosis. Clin Endocrinol. 1989;30:435–442.

18. **Reginster JY, Denis D, Deroisy R, et al.** Long-term (3 years) prevention of trabecular postmenopausal bone loss with low dose intermittent nasal salmon calcitonin. J Bone Miner Res. 1994;9:69–73.

19. **Reginster Y, Meurmans L, Deroisy R, et al.** A 5-year controlled randomized study of prevention of postmenopausal trabecular bone loss with nasal salmon calcitonin and calcium. Eur J Clin Invest. 1994;24:565–569.

20. **Ellerington MC, Hillard TC, Whitcroft SIJ, et al.** Intranasal salmon calcitonin for the prevention and treatment of postmenopausal osteoporosis. Calcif Tissue Int. 1996;59:6–11.

21. **Flicker L, Hopper JL, Larkins RG, et al.** Nandrolone decanoate and intranasal calcitonin as therapy in established osteoporosis. Osteoporosis Int. 1997;7:29–35.

22. **Downs RW, Bell NH, Ettinger MP, et al.** Comparison of alendronate and intranasal calcitonin for treatment of osteoporosis in postmenopausal women. J Clin Endocrinol Metab. 2000;85:1783–1788.

23. **Campodarve I, Drinkwater BL, Insogna KL, et al.** Intranasal salmon calcitonin 50-200 IU does not prevent bone loss in early postmenopausal women (Abstr). An Med Interna. 1994;9(Suppl 1):S391.

24. Physicians' Desk Reference: Miacalcin. 55th ed. 2001:2194.

25. **Ringe JD, Welzel D.** Salmon calcitonin in the therapy of corticosteroid induced osteoporosis. Eur J Clin Pharmacol. 1987;33:35–39.

26. **Lunego M, Picado C, Del Rio L, et al.** Treatment of steroid induced osteopenia with calcitonin in corticosteroid dependent asthma. A one-year follow-up study. Am Rev Resp Dis. 1990;142:104–107.

27. **Luengo M, Pons F, Martinez de Osaba MJ, Picado C.** Prevention of further bone mass loss by nasal calcitonin in patients on long term glucocorticoid therapy for asthma. A two-year follow-up study. Thorax. 1994;49:1099–1102

28. **Sambrook P, Birmingham J, Kelly P, et al.** Prevention of corticosteroid osteoporosis: a comparison of calcium, calcitriol, and calcitonin. N Engl J Med. 328:1747–1752.

29. **Adachi JD, Bensen WG, Bell MJ, et al.** Salmon calcitonin nasal spray in the prevention of corticosteroid induced osteoporosis. Br J Rheumatol. 1997;36a:255–259.

30. **Healey JH, Paget SA, Williams-Russo P, et al.** A randomized controlled trial of salmon calcitonin to prevent bone loss in corticosteroid treated temporal arteritis and polymyalgia rheumatica. Calcif Tissue Int. 1996;58:73–80

31. **Lyritis GP, Paspati I, Karachalios T, et al.** Pain relief from nasal salmon calcitonin in osteoporotic vertebral crush fractures. A double blind placebo controlled study. Acta Orthop Scand. 1997;68(Suppl 275):112–114.

32. **Pontiroli AE, Pajetta E, Scaglia L, et al.** Analgesic effect of intranasal and intramuscular salmon calcitonin in postmenopausal osteoporosis. A double blind, double placebo study. Aging Clin Exp Res. 1994;6:459–463.

33. **Mannarini M, Fincato G, Galimberti S, et al.** Analgesic effect of salmon calcitonin suppositories in patients with bone pain. Curr Ther Res. 1994;55:1079–1083.

34. **Lyritis GP, Tsakalakos N, Magiasis B, et al.** Analgesic effect of salmon calcitonin in osteoporotic vertebral fractures. A double blind placebo controlled clinical study. Calcif Tissue Int. 1991;49:369–372.

35. **Gennari C, Agnusdei D, Gonelli S, Camporeale A.** Symptomatic treatment of osteoporosis: the pain model. Rev Clin Esp. 1991;188(Suppl 1):60–62.

36. **Pun KK, Chan LW.** Analgesic effect of intranasal salmon calcitonin in the treatment of osteoporotic vertebral fractures. Clin Therapeutics. 1989;11:205–209.

37. **Martin MI, Goicoechea C, Ormazabal MJ, Alfaro MJ.** Effect of the intraperitoneal administration of salmon calcitonin on the actions of opioid agonists. Gen Pharmacol. 1995;26:1695–1699.

38. **Reginster JY, Gennari C, Mautalen C, et al.** Influence of specific anti-salmon calcitonin antibodies on biological effectiveness of nasal calcitonin in Paget's disease of bone. Scand J Rheumatol. 1990;19:83–86.

39. **Takahashi S, Goldring S, Katz M, et al.** Downregulation of calcitonin receptor mRNA expression by calcitonin during human osteoclast-like cell differentiation. J Clin Invest. 1995;95:167–171.

40. **Ettinger B, Black DM, Mutlak BH, et al.** Reduction of vertebral fracture risk in postmenopausal women with osteoporosis treated with raloxifene: results from a 3-year randomized clinical trial. Multiple Outcomes of Raloxifene Evaluation (MORE) Investigators. JAMA. 1999;282:637–645.

Chapter 11

Anabolic Agents

ROBERT LINDSAY, MBChB, PhD

Key Points

- Randomized trials have shown that parathyroid hormone (PTH) by daily injection induces bone formation, increases bone mineral density of the spine, and reduces the risk of vertebral and nonvertebral fractures.

- PTH may be valuable for patients with severe osteoporosis; patients being considered for PTH should be referred to specialists who have experience with PTH therapy.

- Sodium fluoride is not approved for the treatment of osteoporosis. It stimulates trabecular bone formation and increases bone density, but the bone that is formed has a different mechanical structure. Randomized trials have drawn different conclusions about whether low-dose fluoride decreases or has no effect on the risk of spine fractures. There is concern that fluoride may increase nonvertebral and hip fracture risk.

- Other potential bone-forming agents, including growth hormone, anabolic steroids, and statins, are not yet of proven value.

All of the agents currently available for the treatment of osteoporosis work by decreasing bone remodeling rates. These drugs, known generically as antiresorptives, only produce small increases in bone mass, and the best of these agents reduce risk of fracture by no more than 50%. Agents that are anabolic to the skeleton and stimulate osteoblast activity, number, or lifespan can increase bone mass more dramatically than can antiresorptive agents. It is hoped that larger bone mineral density (BMD) increases produced by these agents will translate into a more pronounced reduction in risk of fracture. Possible candidates have included parathyroid hormone (PTH), fluoride, growth hormone/IGFs, anabolic steroids, and statins. These agents are reviewed in the sections that follow. At this time, clinical trial data supporting a true anabolic skeletal effect, with resultant increase in bone strength, are available only for PTH.

Parathyroid Hormone

The parathyroid gland responds to low serum calcium levels by increasing synthesis and secretion of PTH. PTH increases bone remodeling and renal synthesis of $1,25(OH)_2D$ and reduces urine calcium excretion. In primary hyperparathyroidism, in which a parathyroid adenoma is the most common cause, sustained excess PTH production produces hypercalcemia by exaggeration of these physiological mechanisms. Whereas exogenously delivered PTH can increase bone mass, primary hyperparathyroidism may lead to a decrease in bone mass, at least in the cortical skeleton. This difference may be caused by intermittent PTH elevations in the former case and relatively constant elevation in the latter case (1).

Clinical trials of PTH are summarized in Table 11-1. The first 3-year randomized study evaluated the effects of 1-34hPTH and hormone replacement therapy (HRT) compared with HRT alone in women with osteoporosis (5,6). 1-34hPTH was delivered as a single, daily, subcutaneous injection of 400 U (approximately 25 µg). Bone density increased in the spine by almost 14% (by dual energy x-ray absorptiometry [DXA]) in the PTH + HRT group, and a smaller but statistically significant increase occurred at the hip (4%) and in total body bone mass (4%). These increases in mass were accompanied by marked increments in biochemical markers of remodeling. Moreover, there was a dramatic and statistically significant reduction in vertebral fractures in the PTH + HRT group compared with the HRT-alone group (6). In a study of similar design and size, even greater increases in vertebral bone mass were seen in the PTH + HRT group over a 2-year period (10). In another trial, PTH alone (administered in a cyclic regimen, 1 week every 3 months) was compared with PTH followed by calcitonin administration (4). Both groups had a similar increase in bone mass at the spine and hip.

Trials confirm that PTH as a single agent improves bone mass in patients with osteoporosis. For example, in 217 women with postmenopausal osteoporosis, using the intact 1-84PTH peptide over 1 year (7,12), bone density increased in a dose-related fashion in the spine but not at other skeletal sites, and total body bone mass declined slightly, particularly at the highest dose. No fracture data were obtained. In a larger phase 3 study of 1637 postmenopausal women with osteoporosis, 1-34hPTH was given at one of two doses (20 or 40 µg/day subcutaneously) for 19 months (8). Significant increases in bone mass in the spine were seen, and by 18 months smaller increments in bone mass were evident at other skeletal sites, with an accompanying increase in total body bone mass. This study showed a 65% reduction in vertebral fractures, and a smaller, significant decline in peripheral fractures (40%). The most common side effects were hypercalcemia and an increase in urine calcium, but no renal stones occurred. Other side effects included headache, nausea (associated with hypercalcemia), and local irritation at the site of injection.

Administration of high doses of 1-34hPTH to rats for 60% or more of their lifespan produces osteosarcomas in up to 50% of animals. However, this is not thought to have relevance for the clinical use of PTH in the treatment of patients with osteoporosis.

PTH has been effective over 12 months in preventing bone loss in premenopausal women being treated at the same time with gonadotropin-releasing hormone (GnRH) for endometriosis (2,3). PTH has also been tested in a small study of men with osteoporosis in whom average spine BMD increase was 13.5% over 18 months (11).

PTH has also been used in a controlled clinical trial in patients on glucocorticoid therapy for rheumatologic conditions, again in conjunction with HRT (9). In this study, changes in bone mass were very similar to those seen when PTH was administered to postmenopausal women with primary osteoporosis on HRT, but there were too few fractures to see a significant difference between the groups.

PTH must be delivered by daily injection. Less frequent injections or alternate delivery mechanisms are options that are currently under investigation. The optimum duration of treatment with PTH is not clear. In the study of longest duration published thus far, vertebral bone mass continued to increase during the entire 3 years of treatment. Increases in bone mass at non-spine skeletal sites are not noted until the second year of PTH administration. Thus, 1 to 2 years of treatment may be required. The influence of a co-administered antiresorptive agent and the fate of newly synthesized bone after discontinuing PTH are unknown. In animals, bone mass falls when PTH is stopped, but that process can be inhibited by the use of antiresorptive medications (1). In one human trial, bone mass increments induced by PTH were maintained with HRT, and in another study, a further increase in bone mass was seen when a bisphosphonate was started after 1 year's treatment with PTH alone (6,12).

Table 11-1 Clinical Trials of PTH Administration

Author	Subjects	Age (Yr)	Intervention	BMD Results	Fractures
Finkelstein et al, 1994, 1998 (2,3)	40 premenopausal women with endometriosis treated with GnRH	Range, 21–43	hPTH (1–34) 40 mg/day with GnRH ($n = 20$) vs GnRH alone over 1 year	• Lumbar spine ↑ 8% vs cont PTH group • Lat spine ↑ 15% vs cont PTH group • PTH group no change hip vs 5% loss cont	Not done
Hodsman et al, 1997 (4)	20 postmenopausal women with osteoporosis and vertebral compression	Mean, 67 ± 8	hPTH (1–34) 800 IU/day 1 month of every 3 vs PTH + calcitonin 75 IU/day for 6 wk of every 3 months over 2 yr	• PTH and PTH + CT groups ↑ BMD 8%–10% in spine • NSC in either group in hip	No non-PTH control group
Lindsay et al, 1997 (5) and Cosman et al, 2001 (6)	50 postmenopausal women with osteoporosis, all treated with HRT for ≥ 1 yr	Mean, 59.5	hPTH (1–34) 25 µg/day + HRT vs HRT alone over 3 yr	• PTH + HRT ↑ spine BMD 14% vs HRT alone • PTH + HRT ↑ hip BMD 4% vs HRT alone • PTH + HRT ↑ TBBM 4% vs HRT alone	70%–100% ↓ vertebral fractures ($P < 0.05$)
Lindsay et al, 1998 (7)	217 postmenopausal women with osteoporosis	Range, 50–75; mean, 64.5	hPTH (1–84) 50, 75, or 100 µg/day vs pbo over 1 yr	• PTH ↑ spine BMD 3%, 5%, or 7% • No change in hip • TBBM ↓ 1% in 100 µg group	Not reported

Study	Population	Age	Treatment	BMD Results	Fracture Results
Neer et al, 2001 (8)	1637 postmenopausal women with osteoporosis	Mean, 69 ± 7	hPTH (1–34) 20 µg/day vs hPTH (1-34) 40 µg/day vs pbo over 21 months	• ↑ Spine BMD 9% • ↑ Hip BMD 3% (compared with placebo)	65% ↓ vertebral fractures 35% ↓ nonspine Both ($P < 0.05$)
Lane et al, 1998 (9)	51 postmenopausal women with glucocorticoid-induced osteoporosis, all on HRT	Range, 50–82; mean, 60 (HRT) and 65 (PTH + HRT)	hPTH (1–34) 25 mg/day + Premarin vs Premarin over 1 yr	• ↑ Spine BMD 9.8% • ↑ Hip 1.5% (NS)	Only 1 fracture (HRT group)
Roe et al, 1999 (10)	74 postmenopausal women with primary osteoporosis, all on HRT	>5 yr post-menopause	hPTH (1–34) 400 IU daily + HRT vs HRT alone over 2 yr	• ↑ AP Spine 28.3% • ↑ FN 10.8% (completers only)	Not reported
Kurland et al, 2000 (11)	23 men with primary osteoporosis	Range, 30–68	hPTH 25 µg/day vs pbo for 1.5 yr	• ↑ 13.5% spine BMD • ↑ 3% hip BMD	Not reported

BMD = bone mineral density; FN = femoral neck; HRT = hormone replacement therapy; NS = not significant; PTH = parathyroid hormone.

Clinical Recommendations

In general, PTH should not be used to treat patients who have low BMD alone. If PTH becomes an available treatment for osteoporosis, it might be offered most appropriately to postmenopausal women who present with osteoporotic fractures, particularly those of the spine, to build bone mass rapidly, perhaps over a 1- to 2-year treatment period. It might also be indicated for patients who remain at high fracture risk after 1 to 2 years of antiresorptive therapy, including patients who fracture or continue to lose bone (more than 5% at one or more sites, over 2 measurements) while on a potent antiresorptive agent. PTH may be used as a single agent or concurrently with antiresorptive agents. However, after completion of a course of PTH, it will probably be necessary to continue or initiate antiresorptive therapy. PTH also might represent an option for men with severe osteoporosis who have ongoing bone loss (more than 5% per year at one or more sites) or ongoing vertebral fractures while on bisphosphonate therapy; however, no anti-fracture efficacy has yet been established in this group. When PTH is approved, primary care physicians should probably refer patients to specialists in osteoporosis for consideration of PTH treatment.

Fluoride

Fluoride is not currently approved by the Food and Drug Administration for treatment of osteoporosis. The usual intake of fluoride is 0.3 to 0.5 mg/day in the absence of fluoridation of drinking water. An additional 1 mg/day can be obtained when fluoride is added to drinking water at 1 part per million. These low doses of fluoride are thought to be beneficial to teeth. Fluoride is well absorbed across the intestine (more than 90%), and approximately 50% of the absorbed amount is deposited into the skeleton, replacing hydroxyl groups on the apatite crystals. High fluoride intake, such as historically seen in the Punjab or in industrial fluoride workers, profoundly affects bone and teeth. An intake of just 2 to 4 mg/day will produce mottled teeth in children, and doubling of that intake produces radiographic osteoporosis. Excessive intakes (more than 20 mg fluoride ion) over long periods can produce crippling fluorosis, with fractures, exostoses, and accompanying neurologic complications, osteoarthritis, and calcium deposits in soft tissues, particularly the ligaments.

Several controlled clinical trials summarized in Table 11-2 (13–19) confirmed that fluoride can increase bone mass, especially in the spine. The size of the increase is comparable to that seen with PTH and greater than that seen with standard antiresorptive treatment. Despite the increased bone mass, however, fluoride does not significantly reduce fractures (Fig. 11-1) (19) because the ingestion of relatively high doses of fluoride probably results in poor quality bone. Fluoride is incorporated into the crystal in place of the hydroxyl group in hydroxyapatite. Crystal size and conformation are changed, both of which could adversely affect skeletal strength. In addition, the new bone is formed initially as woven bone (found only in the fetus) and not the normal lamellar bone usually synthesized in adults. Finally, impaired mineralization, especially evident when fluoride is not accompanied by calcium supplementation, will compound the problem. Slow-release sodium fluoride at a lower dose (50 mg/d) appears to be associated with reduction in vertebral fracture occurrence in one study, but confirmation of these results is not yet available.

Growth Hormone and the Insulin-Like Growth Factor System

Growth hormone (GH) deficiency is associated with a decrease in bone mass and an increased risk of fractures (20,21). In adults, treatment of growth hormone deficiency leads to increases in bone mass, reductions in body fat, and improved lean body mass. Because there is a decline in circulating insulin-like growth factor (IGF-1) with age postulated to be caused by declining secretion of GH, GH or IGF-1 might be useful in the treatment of osteoporosis. The use of GH leads to increases in circulating IGF-1, as expected, and bone turnover is increased by GH and secretagogues. However, the studies published thus far do not support a role for GH or IGF-1 as effective treatments for osteoporosis (20–22).

Short-term trials of growth hormone and agents that stimulate GH secretion have found small increments in lean body mass and decreased fat mass but little or no increase in BMD. Furthermore, any small increments in BMD may be the result of the increased lean body mass, rather than a true change in BMD. Side effects of GH may also limit the ability to give therapeutic doses; these side effects include fluid retention with secondary carpal tunnel syndrome, arthralgias, and myalgias. There are no fracture data for GH use in osteoporosis.

Anabolic Steroids

The class of steroids referred to as anabolic steroids generally comprises derivatives of male sex hormones and includes androgenic progestins (e.g., Norethindrone, Norgestrel). Androgens and anabolic steroids are not approved for the treatment of osteoporosis in the United States. The illicit use of such agents by young athletes and the subsequent controls on their prescription limited their general use and probably also their clinical evaluation. Moreover,

Table 11-2   Characteristics of Fluoride Trials

Author	Sample Size	Age (yr)	Inclusion Criteria	Vertebral Fracture Definition	BMD Measurement Sites	Treatment Arms	Control Arms	Study Duration (yr)
Christiansen, 1980	127 (25/102) 49 (24/25)	50 50	Postmenopausal (6 mo to 3 yr)		Forearm	1. NaF, 9 mg F + Ca 500 mg 2. NaF, 9 mg + Ca 500 mg + Vit D	1. Ca 500 mg 2. Ca 500 mg + Vit D	2
Gambacciani, 1995	60 (30/30)	52	T score < 1 SD of normal women		Lumbar; total body	MFP, 30 mg F + Ca 500 mg	Ca 500 mg	2
Grove, 1981	28 (14/14)	74	≥ 1 vertebral fractures		Forearm	Na, 9 mg F + Ca 500 mg + Vit D 5000 IU	Ca 500 mg + Vit D 500 IU	0.25
Hansson, 1987(13)	50 (25/25) 50 (25/25)	65 66	1–3 vertebral fractures		Lumbar	1. NaF, 4.5 mg F + Ca 1000 mg 2. NaF, 13.6 mg F + Ca 1000 mg	1. Ca 2000 mg 2. Ca 2000 mg	3
Kleerekoper, 1991 (14)*	84 (46/38)	67	≥ 1 vertebral fractures of contiguous vertebral wedge deformity	15% DVH	Radial midshaft	NaF, 34 mg F + Ca 1500 mg	Ca 1500 mg	4
Meunier, 1998	219 (73/146) 214 (68/146) 213 (67/146)	66 66 66	1–4 vertebral fractures, low lumbar BMD, T score > 5 SD	25% DVH	Lumbar; femoral neck	1. NaF, 22.6 mg F + Ca 1000 mg + Vit D 800 IU 2. NaF, 19.8 mg F + Ca 1000 mg + Vit D 800 IU 3. NaF, 26.4 mg F + Ca 1000 mg + Vit D 800 IU	1. Ca 1000 mg 2. Ca 1000 mg 3. Ca 1000 mg	2

Study	N (T/C)	Age	Inclusion criteria	DVH	Measurement sites	Treatment	Supplement	Years
Pak, 1995 (15)[†]	110 (54/56)	68	≥ 1 vertebral fracture and low lumbar BMD 50% of 30-year-old women	20% DVH	Lumbar: femoral neck; radial shaft	SR NaF, 27.5 mg F + Ca 400 mg	Ca 400 mg	4
Reginster, 1998 (16)[†]	164 (84/80)	63	T score < 2.50	20% DVH	Lumbar: total hip	MFP, 20 mg F + Ca 500 mg	Ca 500 mg	4
Riggs, 1983 (17)[†]	165 (61/104)	64	Osteopenia or 1–3 vertebral fractures	15% DVH		NaF, 27.5 mg F + Vit D	Vit D	4
Riggs, 1990 (18)	202 (101/101)	68	Osteopenia or 1–3 vertebral fractures and lumbar BMD < normal range for postmenopausal women	15% DVH	Lumbar: femoral neck; intertrochanter; radial shaft	NaF, 41.25 mg F + Ca 1500 mg	Ca 1500 mg	4
Sebet, 1991[‡]	76 (35/41)	60	T score < 2.5 and no vertebral fracture	25% DVH	Lumbar	MFP, 26.4 + Ca 500 mg	Ca 500 mg	2

* Study in which physical exercise was one of the interventions in both groups of treatment.
[†] Study in which hormone replacement therapy was given to a certain proportion of women in each treatment group.
[‡] Study including males.
Ca = calcium; DVH = decrease in vertebral height; F = doses of fluoride are given as elemental fluoride doses; MFP = monofluorophosphate; NaF = sodium fluoride; SR = slow released; Vit D = vitamin D.
All trials were randomized controlled trials with parallel group design.
Adapted from Haguenauer D, Welch V, Shea B, et al. Fluoride for the treatment of postmenopausal osteoporotic fractures. A meta-analysis. Osteoporos Int. 2000;11:727–738.

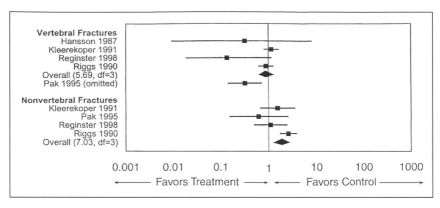

Figure 11-1   Meta-analysis of fluoride trials (19) showing relative risk of vertebral or nonvertebral fractures after 4 years of treatment with fluoride or placebo.

use of androgens in women is limited by androgenic side effects. Only a few small, controlled trials have been published, none with adequate data about fracture outcomes (23,24). In general, these agents seem to produce increments in bone mass similar to those seen with estrogens or other antiresorptive agents. Increases in bone mass may be exaggerated by the increased lean body mass induced by anabolic steroids. Addition of androgen (methyl testosterone) to estrogen produced a similar fall in biochemical markers of bone resorption, but maintained bone formation markers at pretreatment levels, suggesting that it might create positive balance within each remodeling cycle (25). Two studies have suggested that the increment in BMD is greater with the androgen/estrogen combination than with estrogen alone (26,27). The extraskeletal effects of androgen/estrogen combinations are dependent on the specific androgen preparation and dose, and may include potential beneficial effects on libido but potential detrimental effects on liver function and lipoproteins. At this time, it would not be reasonable to recommend estrogen/testosterone combinations for their effects on bone.

Statins

Recent animal studies also suggest that certain statin drugs might have bone-forming potential. Furthermore, three separate observational studies have suggested that statin use may be associated with a reduction in fracture occurrence (28–30). Two other studies suggest that statin use also results in higher bone mass (31,32). However, not all the observational data are positive (33,34), and, in lieu of any rigorous clinical trial evidence, statins should currently not be prescribed for osteoporosis prevention or treatment.

Summary

Agents that stimulate the formation of new bone hold the promise of the cure for osteoporosis. Several of the agents over the last decade that were hoped to achieve this goal have failed. To effect a cure for osteoporosis requires an increase in bone mass with correction of the accompanying architectural changes that are characteristic of osteoporotic bone. This requires not only thickening and strengthening remaining trabeculae but also initiating the building of new trabecular plates and restoring trabecular interconnections. Parathyroid hormone (20 µg/day subcutaneously) holds the promise of accomplishing many of these objectives.

REFERENCES

1. **Dempster DW, Cosman F, Parisien M, et al.** Anabolic actions of parathyroid hormone bone. Endocrine Rev. 1993;14:690–703.

2. **Finkelstein JS, Klibanski A, Schaefer EH, et al.** Parathyroid hormone for the prevention of bone loss induced by estrogen deficiency. N Engl J Med. 1994;331: 1618–1623.

3. **Finkelstein JS, Klibanski A, Arnold AL, et al.** Prevention of estrogen deficiency-related bone loss with human parathyroid hormone. A randomized controlled trial. JAMA. 1998;280:1067–1073.

4. **Hodsman AS, Fraher LJ, Watson AT, et al.** A randomized controlled trial to compare the efficacy of cyclical parathyroid hormone and sequential calcitonin to improve bone mass in postmenopausal women with osteoporosis. J Clin Endocrinol Metab. 1997;82:620–628.

5. **Lindsay R, Nieves J, Formica C, et al.** Randomized controlled study of effect of parathyroid hormone on vertebral-bone mass and fracture incidence among postmenopausal women on estrogen with osteoporosis. Lancet. 1997;350:550–555.

6. **Cosman F, Nieves J, Woelfert L, et al.** Parathyroid hormone added to established hormone therapy: effects on vertebral fracture and maintenance of bone mass after PTH withdrawal. J Bone Min Res. 2001;16:925–931.

7. **Lindsay R, Hodsman A, Genant H, et al, for the PTH Working Group.** A randomized controlled multi-center study of 1-84 hPTH for treatment of postmenopausal osteoporosis. ASBMR-IBMS Second Joint Meeting. 1998;1109.

8. **Neer RM, Arnaud CD, Zanchetta JR, et al.** Effect of parathyroid hormone (1-34) on fractures and bone mineral density in postmenopausal women with osteoporosis. N Engl J Med. 2001;344:1434–1441.

9. **Lane NE, Sanchez S, Modin G, et al.** Parathyroid hormone treatment can reverse corticosteroid-induced osteoporosis. Results of a randomized controlled clinical. J Clin Invest. 1998;102:1627–1633.

10. **Roe EB, Sanchez SD, DelPuerto A, et al.** Parathyroid hormone 1-34 (hPTH 1-34) and estrogen produce dramatic bone density increases in postmenopausal osteoporosis. Results from a placebo-controlled randomized trial. J Bone Miner Res. 1999;14(Suppl 1):S137.

11. **Kurland ES, Cosman F, McMahon DJ, et al.** Parathyroid hormone as a therapy for idiopathic osteoporosis in men: effects on bone mineral density and bone markers. J Clin Endocrinol Metab. 2000;85:3069-3076.

12. **Rittmaster RS, Bolognese M, Ettinger MP, et al.** Enhancement of bone mass in osteoporotic women with parathyroid hormone followed by alendronate. J Clin Endocrinol Metab. 2000;85:2129-2134.

13. **Hansson T, Roos B.** The effect of fluoride and calcium on spinal bone mineral content. A controlled, prospective (3 years) study. Calcif Tissue Int. 1987;40:315-317.

14. **Kleerekoper M, Peterson EJ, Nelson D et al.** A randomized trial of sodium fluoride as a treatment for postmenopausal osteoporosis. Osteoporos Int. 1991;1:155-161.

15. **Pak CY, Sakhae K, Adams-Huet B, et al.** Treatment of postmenopausal osteoporosis with slow-release sodium fluoride: Final report of a randomized controlled trial. Ann Intern Med. 1995;123:401-408.

16. **Reginster JY, Meurmans L, Zegels B, et al.** The effect of sodium monofluorophosphate plus calcium on vertebral fracture rate in postmenopausal women with moderate osteoporosis. A randomized controlled clinical trial. Ann Intern Med. 1998;129:1-8.

17. **Riggs BL.** Treatment of osteoporosis with sodium fluoride: an appraisal. Bone Miner Res. 1983;8:366-393.

18. **Riggs BL, Hodgson PF, O'Fallon WM, et al.** Effect of fluoride treatment on the fracture rate in postmenopausal women with osteoporosis. N Engl J Med. 1990;322: 802-809.

19. **Haguenauer D, Welch V, Shea B, et al.** Fluoride for the treatment of postmenopausal osteoporotic fractures: a meta-analysis. Osteoporos Int. 2000;11:727-738.

20. **Ohlsson C, Bengtsson B-A, Isaksson OGP, et al.** Growth hormone and bone. Endo Rev. 1998;19:55-79.

21. **Marcus R.** Recombinant human growth hormone as potential therapy for osteoporosis. Baillières Clin Endocrinol Metab. 1998;12:251-260.

22. **Sääf M, Hilding A, Thorén, et al.** Growth hormone treatment of osteoporotic postmenopausal women. A one-year placebo-controlled study. Eur J Endocrinol. 1999;140: 390-399.

23. **Chestnut C, Ivey JL, Gruber HE.** Stanozolol in postmenopausal osteoporosis therapeutic efficacy and possible mechanism of action. Metabolism. 1983;32:571-580.

24. **Christiansen CC.** Androgens and androgenic progestins. In: Marcus R, Feldman D, Kelsey J (eds). Osteoporosis. San Diego: Academic Press. 1996;1279-1292.

25. **Raisz LG, Wiita B, Artis A, et al.** Comparison of the effects of estrogen alone and estrogen plus androgen on biochemical markers of bone formation and resorption in postmenopausal women. J Clin Endocrinol Metab. 1996;81:37-43.

26. **Barrett-Connor E, Young R, Notelovitz M, et al.** A two-year, double-blind comparison of estrogen-androgen and conjugated estrogens in surgically menopausal women: effects on bone mineral density, symptoms and lipid profiles. J Reprod Med. 1999;44:1012-1020.

27. **Davis SR, McCloud P, Strauss BJG, Burger H.** Testosterone enhances estradiol's effects on postmenopausal bone density and sexuality. Maturitas. 1995;21:227-236.

28. **Wang PG, Solomon DH, Mogun H, Ivorn J.** HMG-CoA reductase inhibitors and the risk of hip fracture in elderly patients. JAMA. 2000;283:3211-3216.

29. **Meier CR, Schlinenger RS, Kraenzlin ME, et al.** HMG-CoA reductase inhibitors and the risk of fractures. JAMA. 2000;283:3205-3210.

30. **Chan KA, Andrade SE, Boles M, et al.** Inhibitors of hydroxymethylglutaryl-coenzyme: a reductase and risk of fracture among older women. Lancet. 2000;355: 2185–2188.

31. **Chung Y-S, Lee M-D, Lee S-K, et al.** HMG-GA reductase inhibitors increase BMD in type 2 diabetes mellitus patients. J Clin Endocrinol Metab. 2000;85:1137–1142.

32. **Edwards CJ, Hart DJ, Spector TD.** Oral statins and increased bone mineral density in postmenopausal women. Lancet. 2000;555:2218.

33. **LaCroix AZ, Cauley JA, Jackson R, et al.** Does statin use reduce risk of fracture in postmenopausal women? Results from the Women's Health Initiative Observational Study (WHI-OS). ASBMR 22nd Annual Meeting Abstract S155.

34. **Van Staa TP, Wegman SLJ, deVries F, et al.** Use of statins and risk of fractures. ASBMR 22nd Annual Meeting, Abstract S155.

CHAPTER 12

Glucocorticoid-Induced Osteoporosis

IAN R. REID, MD

FIONA WU

Key Points

- Glucocorticoids cause a decrease in bone mass and an increase in fracture risk, particularly during the first few months of therapy.

- Bisphosphonates have been shown to increase bone density and reduce fracture rates.

- Vitamin D metabolites may have a role as second-line therapy in patients who cannot take other agents.

- Parathyroid hormone increases bone formation, which is impaired in patients receiving treatment with steroids, and can substantially increase bone density. It may be a valuable option for patients with severe glucocorticoid osteoporosis.

- Studies of intranasal calcitonin for the treatment of steroid-induced osteoporosis have been conflicting; therefore, this agent is not recommended for prevention or treatment of osteoporosis in patients receiving glucocorticoids.

Patients using glucocorticoids are at increased risk of developing osteoporosis (1). Glucocorticoids have direct negative effects on bone cells and calcium metabolism. Patients who require glucocorticoids may have other risk factors for osteoporosis, such as inactivity, poor nutrition, and decreased circulating sex hormones. Because there are now effective therapies for preventing glucocorticoid-induced bone loss and fractures, assessment of risk of fractures and selective treatment to decrease risk is an essential part of good care for those receiving glucocorticoids. In this chapter, the mechanisms by which glucocorticoids contribute to bone loss are reviewed, and the therapies available for preventing bone loss and fracture in these patients are considered.

Pathogenesis

Glucocorticoids cause bone loss through many mechanisms. These include: reducing the absorption of calcium from the gut, increasing urinary losses of calcium by decreasing its renal tubular reabsorption, and reducing the production of androgens in both the testis and the adrenals. Glucocorticoids have variable effects on osteoclast number and activity. However, probably their most important effect is on the osteoblast. They decrease the number of osteoblasts, both by decreasing their proliferation and by increasing death (apoptosis) of osteoblasts and osteocytes. The production of the principal proteins of bone matrix by the surviving osteoblasts is also substantially reduced. The net effect of this is a dramatic reduction in bone formation rate (2).

Effects on Bone Density

Use of oral glucocorticoids is associated with a decrease in bone mass, greatest in the first few months of therapy. The losses may be considerable, but the degree of loss measured depends, to some extent, on the method used to estimate the loss. For example, bone biopsies show decreases in trabecular bone volume of almost 30% after 6 months of treatment with prednisone 10 to 25 mg/day, whereas studies using quantitative computed tomography (QCT) (3) demonstrate an average loss of 8% of trabecular bone density and 2% of cortical bone density after 20 weeks of prednisone 7.5 mg/day. Rates of loss may decrease after 6 to 12 months, but still remain two to three times higher in steroid-users than in control subjects after 5 years of use (4). Regardless of the method of measurement, bone density remains normally distributed with a standard deviation similar to that in normal subjects. This indicates that bone loss is fairly uniform between subjects and suggests that most patients are susceptible to the effects of steroids (5).

Bone density during steroid treatment is related to factors that influence pre-treatment bone density, such as body weight and age, the duration of steroid treatment, and the average dose of these drugs (1). The bone loss induced by glucocorticoids can be reversed after the withdrawal of these drugs, the period required for the restoration of bone density being approximately equal to the period of treatment (3). Alternate-day administration of glucocorticoids does not diminish bone loss. Cross-sectional studies have indicated that bone density is reduced in those using inhaled glucocorticoids; however, this may be due to past steroid use or to the underlying disease. The few randomized prospective studies have not found reductions in bone mass, although the studies have not been designed to assess the effects of high doses of inhaled steroids.

Effects on Fracture Incidence

A recent large retrospective cohort study has demonstrated that there is a rapid increase in fracture risk, with significant increases in the risk of nonvertebral fractures becoming apparent in the first 3 months of steroid use and an equally abrupt decline after cessation of treatment (1). Because glucocorticoids have the strongest effect on trabecular bone, fractures are most common in regions of the skeleton that are predominantly trabecular, such as the vertebral bodies and ribs. Hip and forearm fractures are also more common (1). Approximately one third of patients suffer vertebral fractures after 5 to 10 years of glucocorticoid treatment, although this can be much higher in older patients. Approximately 20% of older men (mean age 60 years) and postmenopausal women had vertebral fractures during the first year of steroid treatment in the placebo arms of two recent clinical trials of therapies for the prevention of steroid-induced osteoporosis, although no fractures occurred in premenopausal women (6,7). Fracture risk is related to the glucocorticoid dose (Table 12-1), the duration of its use, and the patient's age, body weight (inversely), and gender (increased risk in women).

Table 12-1   Effect of Glucocorticoid Dose on Risk of Fractures

Fracture Site	Prednisolone Dose		
	<2.5 mg/day	2.5–7.5 mg/day	>7.5 mg/day
Distal radius	1.10 (0.96–1.25)	1.04 (0.93–1.17)	1.19 (1.02–1.39)
Hip	0.99 (0.82–1.20)	1.77 (1.55–2.02)	2.27 (1.94–2.66)
Vertebra	1.55 (1.20–2.01)	2.59 (2.16–3.10)	5.18 (4.25–6.31)

Data are relative risks (95% confidence intervals) for fracture in glucocorticoid users, based on data in the United Kingdom General Practice Database. (From van Staa TP, Leufkens HGM, Abenhaim L, et al. Use of oral corticosteroids and risk of fractures. J Bone Miner Res. 2000;15:993–1000.)

Interventions to Increase Bone Mass

Studies about steroid osteoporosis have been considerably fewer and smaller than those in postmenopausal osteoporosis, so evidence for the anti-fracture efficacy of most agents is absent (Table 12-2). Some studies have assessed therapies at the time of first use of steroids and others in those already having had long-term steroid treatment. In general, efficacy of most agents has been similar in both situations.

Calcium and Vitamin D

Two randomized controlled trials of calcium and vitamin D combinations have recently been reported. Buckley and colleagues studied patients with rheumatoid arthritis who were receiving low-dose prednisone and were randomized to receive placebo or calcium 500 mg/day plus vitamin D 500 IU/day over 2 years (9). Those receiving calcium and vitamin D increased bone mass 5% compared with those receiving placebo. Because the vitamin D status of the study subjects was not assessed, it is not clear how much of this effect was due to treatment of vitamin D deficiency. In contrast, Adachi and colleagues (10) failed to show any benefit on lumbar spine bone density from the use of calciferol 50,000 U/wk plus calcium 1000 mg/day in a randomized, controlled

Table 12-2   Quality of Evidence for the Efficacy of Interventions in Glucocorticoid Osteoporosis

Intervention	Spine BMD	Hip BMD	Vertebral Fracture	Nonvertebral Fracture
Calcium	—	—	—	—
Calcium + Vit D	C	C	—	—
HRT	B	D	—	—
Testosterone	B	—	—	—
Etidronate	A	A	B	—
Alendronate	A	A	B	—
Risedronate	A	A	A	—
Calcitriol	C	—	—	—
Alfacalcidol	A	C	—	—
Fluoride	B	—	—	—
Calcitonin	B	—	—	—

A, positive evidence from one or more, adequately powered, randomized, controlled trials; B, positive evidence from smaller nondefinitive randomized, controlled trials; C, inconsistent results from randomized controlled trials; D, positive results from observational studies.
— Efficacy not established.

trial over 3 years. Thus, the case for either calcium or vitamin D in the management of steroid osteoporosis is not compelling.

Nevertheless, it is reasonable to provide calcium supplementation to those whose dietary intake is less than 1 to 1.5 g/day (i.e., 4 to 6 servings of dairy products) and in whom there are not contraindications (e.g., renal calculi). There is increasing evidence of deleterious effects on the skeleton of vitamin D deficiency in the frail elderly population, and this is relevant in frail, steroid-treated patients who are seldom outdoors. Therefore, it is reasonable to measure serum 25-hydroxyvitamin D in patients who are taking steroids or planning to take steroids chronically and to prescribe vitamin D (i.e., calciferol) to those with levels below 50 nmol/L. Supplemental calciferol should be given in doses of 500 to 1000 U/day or 20,000 to 50,000 U/month.

Bisphosphonates

The efficacy of the bisphosphonates was first demonstrated in a study of oral pamidronate in the treatment of steroid osteoporosis (Table 12-3) (11). This preparation is not widely available, but pamidronate infusions (30 mg) every 3 months appear to be comparably effective (12). Several trials have shown that cyclic etidronate is an effective therapy in steroid-treated subjects. For example, a large, randomized, controlled trial demonstrated prevention of bone loss at both the lumbar spine and the proximal femur in patients recently started on steroid treatment (8). Furthermore, it suggested that etidronate use was associated with reduction in height loss and a 50% reduction in vertebral fracture rates, although this was only statistically significant among the postmenopausal women. This treatment has high patient acceptability because medication is only taken for 2 weeks every 3 months.

Similarly, Saag and colleagues found that 1 year of alendronate 5 or 10 mg a day increased bone mass and prevented bone loss throughout the skeleton of patients taking corticosteroids, irrespective of the duration of previous steroid use (13). Vertebral fracture rates were reduced by about half in those on alendronate, although, again, this was only statistically significant among the postmenopausal women.

Risedronate also improves bone density to a degree that is comparable to the increases seen with etidronate and alendronate (8,14). Pooled data from patients on long-term steroids, treated with either 2.5 mg of risedronate or 5.0 mg of risedronate, showed a 70% reduction in vertebral fractures in the first year of treatment.

Of the various agents studied in steroid-treated subjects, the bisphosphonates have produced the most consistently positive results on bone density and the only evidence of reduced fracture rates. They can be used in most patient groups, including young adults, although safety data in children are

Table 12-3   Randomized Placebo-Controlled Trials of Bisphosphonates in Glucocorticoid-Induced Osteoporosis

Study	No. Commencing Study	Mean Age (Range) and Gender	Subject Characteristics†	Active Interventions	Follow-Up	Between-Group Differences in Spinal BMD	Between-Group Differences in BMD at Other Sites	Fractures
						Results**		
Reid, 1988 (11)	40	50 yr; 19 m, 10 prem, 6 post	• Resp, CTD, GI • Prior steroids: 5.8 yr • Dose during study: 13.7 mg/d	• APD 150 mg/d po • Calcium 1 g/d (all patients)	1 yr	+28.4%*	Metacarpal cortical area +2.4%*	
Herrala, 1998 (40)	74	57 yr (39–73); 33 m, 11 prem, 30 post	• Resp • Prior steroid: 8.1 yr • Dose during study: 8.3 mg/d	CLN: 800 mg, 1600 mg, 2400 mg daily po	1 yr	• 800 mg: +0.6% (NS) • 1600 mg: +3.1%* • 2400 mg: +3.5%*	Femoral neck for 2400 mg group only +4.0%*	
Adachi, 1997 (35)	141	61 yr (19–87); 54 m, 17 prem, 70 post	• Resp, rheum, immun • Prior steroids: <3 mo • Dose: 22 mg/d (baseline), 11 mg/d (1 yr)	Cyclic ETD††	1 yr	+3.7%*	• Trochanter +4.1%* • Femoral neck and radius NS	• New vertebral fx: ETD 9%, Pbo 15%, RR: 0.6 NS • New vertebral fx in postmenopausal women: ETD 3%, Pbo 22%, RR: 0.15*
Geusens, 1998 (39)		64 yr; 37 post	• Rheum, GI, sarcoidosis • Prior steroids: variable • Dose during study: 5.8 mg	• Cyclic ETD	2 yr	+9.3%*	Proximal femur NS	

Study	N	Demographics	Condition / Steroid	Treatment	Duration	BMD change	Outcomes
Pitt, 1998 (41)	49	59 yr; 19 m, 6 prem, 24 post	• Resp, PMR, CTD • Prior steroid: 8.5 yr • Dose during study: 7.4 mg/d	• Cyclic ETD • Calciferol 400 IU/d all patients during ETD/pbo-free weeks	2 yr	+4.5%*	Proximal femur, NS
Roux, 1998 (42)	117	59 yr; 42 m, 18 prem, 57 post	• Rheum, vasc, CTD, resp • Prior steroid: < 3 mo • Dose during study: 11.0 mg/d	• Cyclic ETD	1 yr	+3.1%*	Proximal femur
Cortet, 1999 (43)	83	62 yr; 28 m, 9 prem, 46 post	• Rheum, vasc • Prior steroid: < 3 mo • Dose during study: 9.5 mg/d	• Cyclic ETD	1 yr	+2.8%*	• Proximal femur NS
Saag, 1998 (13)	477	55 yr (17–83); 141 m, 104 prem, 232 post	• Rheum, vasc, resp, renal, derm, GI • Prior steroids: variable • Dose during study: 10.0 mg/d (median)	• ALN 5 or 10 mg daily po • Calcium 0.8–1.0 g/d and calciferol 250–500 IU/d (all patients)	1 yr	• 5 mg: +2.5%* • 10 mg: +3.3%*	• Sig at proximal femur for both ALN groups (+2–3%) • Sig in total body for 10 mg ALN group only (+0.7%) • New vertebral fx: ALN (combined) 2.3%, pbo 3.7%; RR: 0.6 NS • New vertebral fx in postmenopausal women: ALN (combined) 4.4%, pbo 13.0%; RR: 0.3*
Cohen, 1999 (8)	228	60 yr (18–85); 77 m, 46 prem, 105 post	• Rheum, resp, derm • Prior steroids: < 3 mo • Dose during study: 11.1 mg/d	• RSN 2.5 or 5 mg daily po • Calcium 500 mg/d (all patients)	1 yr	2.5 mg: +3.0%* 5 mg: +3.8%*	• Sig at trochanter for both RSN groups (+3–5%) • NS at radius for either RSN group • New vertebral fx: 5 mg ALN 5.7%, pbo 17.3%; RR: 0.3 NS (P = 0.07)

Cont'd

Table 12-3   Randomized Placebo-Controlled Trials of Bisphosphonates in Glucocorticoid-Induced Osteoporosis (Cont'd.)

Study	No. Commencing Study	Mean Age (Range) and Gender	Subject Characteristics[†]	Active Interventions	Follow-Up	Results[**]		Fractures
						Between-Group Differences in Spinal BMD	Between-Group Differences in BMD at Other Sites	
Reid 2000 (14)	290	59 yr (18–85); 109 m, 25 prem, 156 post	• Rheum, vasc, resp, derm • Prior steroid: 4.9 yr • Dose during study: 13.4 mg/d	• RSN 2.5 or 5 mg daily po • Calcium 1g/d and calciferol 400 IU/d (all patients)	1 yr	• 2.5 mg: +1.2% NS • 5 mg: +2.7%*	• Sig at proximal femur for 5 mg RNS group only (~+2%) • NS at radius for either RSN group	• New vertebral fx: RSN (combined), 5%, pbo 15%; RR: 0.3*

* $P < 0.05$.

† Underlying diagnosis, duration of steroid exposure prior to entry (mean), dose of steroid (in mg /day prednisone equivalent) during study period or as stated.

** BMD measured using dual-photon or dual energy x-ray absorptometry, except in Reid's 1988 study (11) in which quantitative computed tomography was used to measure spinal density. Positive differences denoted by "+" signs indicate changes in favor of the active intervention groups.

†† Cyclic etidronate regimen: 400 mg/d orally for 2 weeks in a 13-week cycle, with calcium supplementation (500–1000 mg/d) continuously or during the etidronate-free weeks. Control group received cyclical placebo and calcium.

KEY—m, male; prem, premenopausal women; post, postmenopausal women; resp, respiratory diseases; CTD, connective tissue diseases; GI, gastrointestinal diseases; rheum, rheumatic diseases; immun, immunological diseases; PMR, polymyalgia rheumatica; vasc, vasculitis; derm, dermatological diseases; pbo, placebo; APD, pamidronate; ETD, etidronate; ALN, alendronate; CLN, clodronate; RSN, risedronate; BMD, bone mineral density; NS, not significant; Sig, significant; RR, relative risk.

scant, and there are no data regarding the use of bisphosphonates in pregnant and lactating women.

Sex Hormones

Estrogen (in women) and testosterone (in men) have been used for a number of years in steroid-treated patients as a treatment for co-existing sex hormone deficiency. Non-randomized cohort studies have found beneficial effects of hormone replacement therapy (HRT) on spinal bone density in steroid-treated postmenopausal women, the benefits being comparable to those observed in other postmenopausal women (15,16). One randomized controlled trial of HRT in 42 postmenopausal women on steroids reported a 3.8% increase in spinal bone mineral density (BMD) at 2 years compared with a loss of 0.9% in those receiving calcium alone (between-groups difference, P less than 0.05) (17). A randomized, controlled, cross-over study of 15 steroid-treated asthmatic men showed a 5% increase in spinal BMD during 1 year of monthly depot injections of testosterone esters, with no change in the control period (18). This study also demonstrated that testosterone blocked the increase in fat mass and the loss of lean mass that occurred during the control period. Although these studies are small, they demonstrate changes in bone density that are comparable to those seen with either bisphosphonates in steroid users or with sex hormone replacement in patients not using steroids. There have been no trials of the effect of hormone therapy on risk of fractures in patients receiving steroids.

Anabolic steroids are androgens modified to reduce their virilizing effects. They have also been used for treating steroid-induced osteoporosis although they are not approved for this use in the United States. They seem to have little place in the management of men, in whom they are likely to further reduce testosterone levels. Testosterone is a better choice in men with low testosterone levels. The use of anabolic steroids in women has been associated with beneficial effects on bone mass. For example, Adami found between-groups differences in forearm bone density of 12% to 16% over 18 months in a randomized controlled trial of nandrolone decanoate (50 mg intramuscularly every 3 weeks) in 35 women (19). However, doses that improve bone mass also have virilizing side effects in almost one half of treated patients. Of these, deepening of the voice is of particular concern, because it is often irreversible.

Vitamin D Metabolites

The rationale for the use of vitamin D metabolites to treat osteoporosis is mixed because these agents increase both intestinal calcium absorption and bone resorption, the former being advantageous and the latter potentially hazardous. These agents also carry a small risk of hypercalcemia. The balance of potential benefits and risks may be different for different agents, dosages, and patient populations.

Calcitriol has been assessed in several randomized, controlled trials of steroid-induced osteoporosis. Dykman and colleagues (20) found no difference between calcitriol 0.4 µg/day and placebo in their effects on forearm bone density. Sambrook and others (21) reported a 1-year study in which patients starting glucocorticoid therapy were randomly assigned to receive calcium, calcium plus calcitriol (mean dose 0.6 µg/day), or these two agents combined with calcitonin (Table 12-4). Bone losses from the lumbar spine were 4.3%, 1.3%, and 0.2% in the respective groups. There was a similar, nonsignificant trend in distal radial bone loss, but no evidence of reduced bone loss in the proximal femur (3% in all groups). A large trial over 3 years in cardiac transplant patients showed no effect on lumbar spine density from calcitriol 0.25 µg/day (22). A trial comparing the use of calcitriol 0.5 µg/day with hormone replacement therapy in hypogonadal young women with systemic lupus erythematosus, found progressive bone loss in those taking the vitamin D analogue in comparison with increases in density in those receiving hormones (between-groups difference at the spine of 3.7% at 2 years) (23). There was also a significant difference between groups at the distal radius.

Studies of alfacalcidiol have more consistently demonstrated an attenuation of bone loss in patients with steroid-induced osteoporosis. For example, alfacalcidol has been shown to slow but not completely prevent femoral neck and lumbar spine bone loss after cardiac transplantation (24). A similar attenuation of lumbar spine bone loss has been reported in a predominantly nontransplant population with the use of alfacalcidol 1 µg/day (25); femoral bone density was not measured in this study. In a population of patients with established steroid-induced osteoporosis, all of whom received calcium supplements, Ringe has shown a beneficial effect of alfacalcidol 1 µg/day in comparison with calciferol (2.5% between-groups difference in lumbar spine density at 3 years) (26).

Therefore, the effects of vitamin D metabolites are inconsistent. Even in the positive studies, their effects tend to be less than those of bisphosphonates, and there have been no trials large enough to assess the effect of vitamin D metabolites on risk of fractures in steroid-treated patients. The best use of vitamin D metabolites may be as adjunctive therapy with either sex hormone replacement or a bisphosphonate in patients with severe osteoporosis, as has been shown to be beneficial in postmenopausal osteoporosis. Vitamin D metabolites may also have a role as a second-line therapy in patients for whom other agents are not acceptable. Serum calcium concentrations should be monitored monthly for the first 3 months of treatment, more frequently if higher doses are being used.

Table 12-4   Randomized Controlled Trials of Vitamin D Metabolites in Glucocorticoid-Induced Osteoporosis

Study	N*	Mean Age and Gender	Subject Characteristics	Intervention	Duration (yr)	Spine BMD
Sambrook, 1993 (21)	63	51 F:M = 49:14	Mostly rheumatologic conditions; Previous steroids: < 1 mo; Mean dose: 13.5 mg/dy	Calcitriol 0.6 µg/d; Both groups took calcium, 1 g/d	1	Control: −4.3%; Calcitriol: −1.3%†; No effect at hip or forearm
Stempfle, 1999 (22)	101	51 F:M = 21:111	3-yr post heart transplant; Previous steroids: 3 yr; Mean dose: ?	Calcitriol, 0.25 µg/d; Both groups took calcium 1 g/d plus sex steroids if hypogonadal	3	Control: +6.1%; Calcitriol: +5.7%
Reginster, 1999 (25)	107	57 F:M = 89:56	Mostly rheumatologic conditions; Previous steroids: < 1 mo; Mean dose: ~25 mg/d	Alfacalcidol 1 µg/d; Both groups took calcium 400 mg/d	1	Control: −5.7%; Alfacalcidol: +0.4%†
Ringe, 1999 (26)	85	61 F:M = 55:30	Respiratory and rheumatologic conditions; Previous steroids: 5 yr; Mean dose: 10 mg/d	Alfacalcidol 1 µg/d or calciferol 1000 IU/d; Both groups took calcium 500 mg/d	3	Control: −0.5%; Alfacalcidol: +2.0%†; No effect at hip

* Number providing bone mineral density (BMD) data.
† Between-groups difference, $P < 0.05$.

Fluoride

There is evidence from randomized, controlled trials that fluoride increases spinal bone density in steroid-treated subjects (27–30). However, its anti-fracture efficacy remains to be established, and it should not be used as a first-line agent in steroid osteoporosis. Its cautious use (sodium fluoride 40 mg/day) may be appropriate as an adjunctive therapy in patients with ongoing bone loss (>5% per year at one or more sites) or fractures, despite use of bisphosphonates and/or hormone replacement therapy (31). High doses of fluoride or use for more than 2 to 3 years can cause osteomalacia.

Calcitonin

There have been several randomized, controlled trials of calcitonin in patients receiving treatment with glucocorticoids. Rizzato (32) found that injections of salmon calcitonin (100 IU every 1 to 2 days) prevented bone loss over a 15-month period, whereas vertebral bone mass declined 14% in the control group. Using a similar regimen, Luengo (33) found a 6.5% difference between treatment groups over 12 months. However, calcitonin injections generally have poor acceptability to patients. Studies of intranasal calcitonin for the treatment of steroid-induced osteoporosis are conflicting. A small study by Montemurro demonstrated prevention of vertebral cancellous bone loss with a mixture of intranasal and intramuscular calcitonin, whereas the control group lost 14% of BMD over 1 year (34). However, a larger study by Adachi reported an approximately 1% difference from placebo in spine bone density with calcitonin nasal spray, and there was no effect at the hip or in the total body (35). There have been no studies about the effect of calcitonin on the risk of fractures in patients taking steroids. Until more consistent evidence of efficacy is available, intranasal calcitonin would seem to have little place in the management of steroid osteoporosis.

Parathyroid Hormone

Parathyroid hormone has theoretical appeal in steroid osteoporosis because it increases bone formation, which is impaired in steroid-treated patients. Similar to trials in postmenopausal osteoporosis, 1 year of treatment with parathyroid hormone in combination with HRT has been demonstrated to produce substantial increases in spinal bone density (11%, compared with 0% control) (36). Increases in hip density of about 5% above baseline were seen after an additional year off therapy. Parathyroid hormone could be considered for patients with severe osteoporosis or for those who continue to have ongoing bone loss (more than 5% per year at one or more sites) or fractures in spite of receiving an antiresorptive agent.

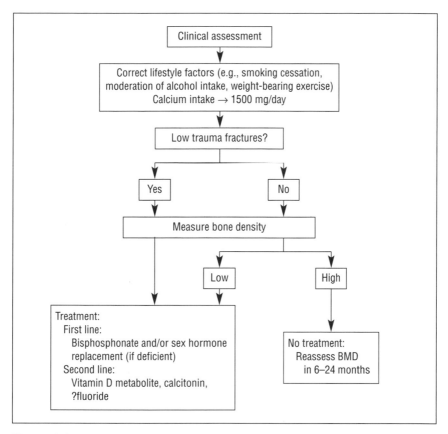

Figure 12-1   Flow chart for the evaluation and treatment of osteoporosis in patients receiving glucocorticoid therapy.

Clinical Recommendations

All patients should be encouraged to optimize diet and risk factors (e.g., cease smoking, drink only moderate amounts of alcohol, engage in weight-bearing exercise) (Fig. 12-1). Also, all patients should have BMD testing, and if the T score is less than –2.0 to –1.5 at the spine or hip, or the patient has a history of low-trauma fractures, pharmacologic therapy should be started (consider treatment at higher BMD with older patients, who are already at risk for age-related bone loss). Note that the T score threshold for intervention is different than that for postmenopausal osteoporosis. This is because rates of bone loss are greater in steroid-treated subjects, particularly in those just starting therapy and in those taking higher steroid doses (e.g., prednisone >10 mg/day), and because the risk of fractures appears to rise within 3 months after starting steroids. The need for ongoing prophylaxis after steroids have been discontinued should be judged by the same standards as for other individuals not taking steroids; that is, on the basis of bone density, age, fracture history, and other clinical risk factors.

When bone density at the hip and spine is near the treatment threshold (e.g., –1.5 to –2.0), intervention with a single agent is appropriate, the evidence being the strongest for one of the bisphosphonates. In hypogonadal subjects, one should also consider sex hormone replacement. Because the therapeutic efficacy of these agents on bone density is probably comparable (although there are no data regarding the anti-fracture efficacy of sex hormone replacement), the choice is based to some extent on a consideration of the patient's other medical problems, possible side-effects, and the cost of the treatment. Patients with marked bone loss, (e.g., T scores less than or equal to –4), or those with ongoing bone loss or fractures despite the use of a single agent, should be referred to a specialist in osteoporosis for consideration of PTH or additional therapies.

REFERENCES

1. **van Staa TP, Leufkens HGM, Abenhaim L, et al.** Use of oral corticosteroids and risk of fractures. J Bone Miner Res. 2000;15:993–1000.

2. **Reid IR.** Glucocorticoid osteoporosis: mechanisms and management. Eur J Endocrinol. 1997;137:209–217.

3. **Laan RFJM, Vanriel PLCM, Vandeputte LBA, et al.** Low-dose prednisone induces rapid reversible axial bone loss in patients with rheumatoid arthritis. A randomized, controlled study. Ann Intern Med. 1993;119:963–968.

4. **Saito JK, Davis JW, Wasnich RD, Ross PD.** Users of low-dose glucocorticoids have increased bone loss rates. A longitudinal study. Calcif Tissue Int. 1995;57:115–119.

5. **Reid IR.** Glucocorticoid-induced osteoporosis: assessment and treatment. J Clin Densitom. 1998;1:65–73.

6. **Lipworth BJ.** Systemic adverse effects of inhaled corticosteroid therapy. A systematic review and meta-analysis. Arch Intern Med. 1999;159:941–955.

7. **Adachi JD, Bensen WG, Brown J, et al.** Intermittent etidronate therapy to prevent corticosteroid-induced osteoporosis. N Engl J Med. 1997;337:382–387.

8. **Cohen S, Levy RM, Keller M, et al.** Risedronate therapy prevents corticosteroid-induced bone loss. A twelve-month, multicenter, randomized, double-blind, placebo-controlled, parallel-group study. Arthritis Rheum. 1999;42:2309–2318.

9. **Buckley LM, Leib ES, Cartularo KS, et al.** Calcium and vitamin D-3 supplementation prevents bone loss in the spine secondary to low-dose corticosteroids in patients with rheumatoid arthritis. A randomized, double-blind, placebo-controlled trial. Ann Intern Med. 1996;125:961–968.

10. **Adachi JD, Bensen WG, Bianchi F, et al.** Vitamin D and calcium in the prevention of corticosteroid induced osteoporosis. A 3-year follow-up. J Rheumatol. 1996;23: 995–1000.

11. **Reid IR, King AR, Alexander CJ, Ibbertson HK.** Prevention of steroid-induced osteoporosis with (3-amino-1-hydroxypropylidene)-1,1-bisphosphonate (APD). Lancet. 1988;1:143–146.

12. **Boutsen Y, Jamart J, Esselinckx W, et al.** Primary prevention of glucocorticoid-induced osteoporosis with intermittent intravenous pamidronate. A randomized trial. Calcif Tissue Int. 1997;61:266–271.

13. **Saag KG, Emkey R, Schnitzer TJ, et al.** Alendronate for the prevention and treatment of glucocorticoid-induced osteoporosis. N Engl J Med. 1998;339:292–299.

14. **Reid DM, Hughes RA, Laan RFJM, et al.** Efficacy and safety of daily risedronate in the treatment of corticosteroid-induced osteoporosis in men and women. A randomized trial. J Bone Miner Res. 2000;15:1006–1013.

15. **Lukert BP, Johnson BE, Robinson RG.** Estrogen and progesterone replacement therapy reduces glucocorticoid-induced bone loss. J Bone Miner Res. 1992;7:1063–1069.

16. **Grey AB, Cundy TF, Reid IR.** Continuous combined oestrogen/progestin therapy is well tolerated and increases bone density at the hip and spine in post-menopausal osteoporosis. Clin Endocrinol. 1994;40:671–677.

17. **Hall GM, Daniels M, Doyle DV, Spector TD.** Effect of hormone replacement therapy on bone mass in rheumatoid arthritis patients treated with and without steroids. Arthritis Rheum. 1994;37:1499–1505.

18. **Reid IR, Wattie DJ, Evans MC, Stapleton JP.** Testosterone therapy in glucocorticoid-treated men. Arch Intern Med. 1996;156:1173–1177.

19. **Adami S, Fossaluzza V, Rossini M, et al.** The prevention of corticosteroid-induced osteoporosis with nandrolone decanoate. Bone Miner. 1991;15:72–81.

20. **Dykman TR, Haralson KM, Gluck OS, et al.** Effect of oral 1,25-dihydroxy-vitamin D and calcium on glucocorticoid-induced osteopenia in patients with rheumatic diseases. Arthritis Rheum. 1984;27:1336–1343.

21. **Sambrook P, Birmingham J, Kelly P, et al.** Prevention of corticosteroid osteoporosis: a comparison of calcium, calcitriol, and calcitonin. N Engl J Med. 1993;328: 1747–1752.

22. **Stempfle HU, Werner C, Echtler S, et al.** Prevention of osteoporosis after cardiac transplantation. A prospective, longitudinal, randomized, double-blind trial with calcitriol. Transplantation. 1999;68:523–530.

23. **Kung AWC, Chan TM, Lau CS, et al.** Osteopenia in young hypogonadal women with systemic lupus erythematosus receiving chronic steroid therapy. A randomized controlled trial comparing calcitriol and hormonal replacement therapy. Rheumatology. 1999;38:1239–1244.

24. **Van Cleemput J, Daenen W, Geusens P, et al.** Prevention of bone loss in cardiac transplant recipients: a comparison of biphosphonates and vitamin D. Transplantation. 1996;61:1495–1499.

25. **Reginster JY, Kuntz D, Verdickt W, et al.** Prophylactic use of alfacalcidol in corticosteroid-induced osteoporosis. Osteoporos Int. 1999;9:75–81.

26. **Ringe JD, Coster A, Meng T, et al.** Treatment of glucocorticoid-induced osteoporosis with alfacalcidol/calcium versus vitamin D/calcium. Calcif Tissue Int. 1999;65: 337–340.

27. **Bayley TA, Muller C, Harrison J.** The long-term treatment of steroid osteoporosis with fluoride. J Bone Miner Res. 1990;5(Suppl 1):S157–S161.

28. **Rizzoli R, Chevalley T, Slosman DO, Bonjour JP.** Sodium monofluorophosphate increases vertebral bone mineral density in patients with corticosteroid-induced osteoporosis. Osteoporos Int. 1995;5:39–46.

29. **Guaydier-Souquieres G, Kotzki PO, Sabatier JP, et al.** In corticosteroid-treated respiratory diseases, monofluorophosphate increases lumbar bone density. A double-masked randomized study. Osteoporos Int. 1996;6:171–177.

30. **Lems WF, Jacobs WG, Bijlsma JWJ, et al.** Effect of sodium fluoride on the prevention of corticosteroid-induced osteoporosis. Osteoporos Int.1997;7:575–582.

31. **Lems WF, Jacobs JWG, Bijlsma JWJ, et al.** Is addition of sodium fluoride to cyclical etidronate beneficial in the treatment of corticosteroid induced osteoporosis? Ann Rheum Dis. 1997;56:357–363.

32. **Rizzato G, Tosi G, Schiraldi G, et al.** Bone protection with salmon calcitonin (sCT) in the long-term steroid therapy of chronic sarcoidosis. Sarcoidosis. 1988;5:99–103.

33. **Luengo M, Picado C, Del Rio L, et al.** Treatment of steroid-induced osteopenia with calcitonin in corticosteroid-dependent asthma. A one-year follow-up study. Am Rev Respir Dis. 1990;142:104–107.

34. **Montemurro L, Schiraldi G, Fraioli P, et al.** Prevention of corticosteroid-induced osteoporosis with salmon calcitonin in sarcoid patients. Calcif Tissue Int. 1991;49: 71–76.

35. **Adachi JD, Bensen WG, Bell MJ, et al.** Salmon calcitonin nasal spray in the prevention of corticosteroid-induced osteoporosis. Br J Rheumatol. 1997;36:255–259.

36. **Lane NE, Sanchez S, Modlin GW, et al.** Parathyroid hormone treatment can reverse corticosteroid-induced osteoporosis. Results of a randomized controlled clinical trial. J Clin Invest. 1998;102:1627–1633.

37. **Selby PL, Halsey JP, Adams KRH, et al.** Corticosteroids do not alter the threshold for vertebral fracture. J Bone Miner Res. 2000;15:952–956.

38. **Eddy DM, Johnston CC, Cummings SR, et al.** Osteoporosis: review of the evidence for prevention, diagnosis, and treatment and cost-effectiveness analysis. Osteoporos Int. 1998;8(Suppl 4):1–88.

39. **Geusens P, Dequeker J, Vanhoof J, et al.** Cyclical etidronate increases bone density in the spine and hip of postmenopausal women receiving long term corticosteroid treatment. A double blind, randomised placebo controlled study. Ann Rheum Dis. 1998;57:724–727.

40. **Herrala J, Puolijoki H, Liippo K, et al.** Clodronate is effective in preventing corticosteroid-induced bone loss among asthmatic patients. Bone. 1998;22:577–582.

41. **Pitt P, Li F, Todd P, et al.** A double blind placebo controlled study to determine the effects of intermittent cyclical etidronate on bone mineral density in patients on long term oral corticosteroid treatment. Thorax. 1998;53:351–356.

42. **Roux C, Oriente P, Laan R, et al.** Randomized trial of effect of cyclical etidronate in the prevention of corticosteroid-induced bone loss. J Clin Endocrinol Metab. 1998; 83:1128–1133.

43. **Cortet B, Hachulla E, Barton I, et al.** Evaluation of the efficacy of etidronate therapy in preventing glucocorticoid-induced bone loss in patients with inflammatory rheumatic diseases. A randomized study. Rev Rhum Engl Ed. 1999;66:214–219.

Clinical Cases

CHAPTER 13

Clinical Cases

SOPHIE A. JAMAL, MD

CASE 1   POSTMENOPAUSAL WOMAN WITH A HISTORY OF BREAST CANCER
WHO HAS HAD A VERTEBRAL FRACTURE

Mrs. W is a 68-year-old woman who presents with sudden-onset lower thoracic back pain that developed while she was lifting groceries. Three years ago she had estrogen receptor positive breast cancer that was treated with lumpectomy, radiation, and tamoxifen. Her only medication is tamoxifen 20 mg a day. She has no prior history of fractures and no risk factors for osteoporosis other than age and menopausal status. She has felt well without constitutional symptoms or pain until this acute episode. Physical examination is normal with the exception of tenderness at the T12 area. Specifically, there is no change in height or weight compared with previous examinations, and a neurologic exam is normal. Complete blood count (CBC) and serum calcium are normal. Lateral radiographs of the thoracic and lumbar spine demonstrate a vertebral compression fracture at T12. Bone mineral density (BMD) testing finds that the T score at L2–L4 is –2.7 and the T score at the femoral neck is –3.0.

How Are Metastases Caused by Breast Cancer Distinguished from an Osteoporotic Compression Fracture?

Table 13-1 lists the causes of acute vertebral fracture in more than 300 patients admitted to the hospital at the Cleveland Clinic, a tertiary referral center, from 1982 to 1986 (1). However, cancers and other causes of fracture, besides osteoporosis, will be much less common in ambulatory patients in primary care practice.

In this patient, it is important to differentiate between two causes of vertebral compression fractures, osteoporosis and metastatic cancer (in this case,

Table 13-1   Causes of Vertebral Compression Fractures in Patients Admitted to the Cleveland Clinic Hospital

Causes of Vertebral Compression Fracture	Number of Patients (%)
Osteoporosis	249 (78)
Metastatic neoplasms	51 (16)
Multiple myeloma	12 (4)
Vertebral osteomyelitis	6 (2)
Radiation therapy	1 (.3)
Total	319

Data from McHenry MC, et al. Vertebral osteomyelitis presenting as spinal compression fracture. Six patients with underlying osteoporosis. Arch Intern Med. 1988;148:417–423.

breast). The distinction is often difficult, but clues can be derived from the epidemiology, clinical history, radiographic features, and biochemical tests. In addition, consultation with an oncologist may be helpful.

Osteoporotic vertebral collapse most commonly involves the midthoracic area (T7–T8) and the thoracolumbar junction (T12 to L1). This is illustrated in Figure 13-1. In contrast, fractures of the upper thoracic spine (T2 to T6) are somewhat more likely to be caused by metastatic disease (2). Other radiological investigations that may help distinguish metastatic disease from osteoporosis include radionuclide bone scan (which may indicate the presence of other lesions and uptake outside of the vertebral bodies making metastatic disease more likely), computed tomography (CT) scan (which may demonstrate associated soft-tissue masses), and magnetic resonance imaging (MRI) scanning. In most cases, MRI scanning accurately distinguishes benign from malignant disease and can also distinguish among other etiologies of vertebral fracture. However, it cannot distinguish between traumatic and osteoporotic fractures, and it cannot be used to assess spine BMD. Many experts would consider MRI scanning in patients with laboratory abnormalities, T scores greater than −2.5, and in patients who have fractures in multiple sites or unusual locations. Note that BMD testing cannot determine the cause of vertebral fractures. However, it may be helpful in ruling out osteoporosis patients with normal BMD (T score greater than −1.0) because vertebral fractures caused by osteoporosis are very uncommon in women with BMD above −1.0.

No studies have addressed what laboratory tests should be ordered when investigating a patient with acute vertebral fracture (see Chapter 3). In this case, tests (serum calcium and CBC) were ordered that, if abnormal, would substantially increase the likelihood that the fracture is caused by metastatic disease. The fact that these tests are normal makes it somewhat less likely that Mrs. W's fracture is caused by metastatic breast cancer.

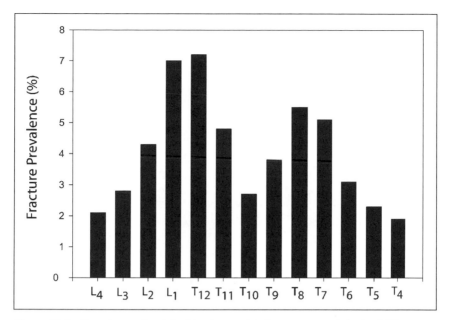

Figure 13-1 Prevalence of vertebral fractures related to osteoporosis in the 6479 women participating in the Fracture Intervention Trial. (Modified from Nevitt MC, et al. Association of prevalent vertebral fractures, bone density, and alendronate treatment with incident vertebral fractures: effect of number and spinal location of fractures. The Fracture Intervention Trial Research Group. Bone. 1999;25:613–619.)

Multiple myeloma should be considered as a cause of acute compression fractures if there is any other evidence to support that diagnosis, such as anemia, hypercalcemia, proteinuria, elevated total protein, or a patchy appearance of bone on x-ray. If any of these clues are present, a serum protein electrophoresis should be ordered because 85% of patients with multiple myeloma have a monoclonal spike on serum protein electrophoresis. For patients with more than one clinical finding typical of myeloma, an immuno-electrophoresis may be needed to confirm the diagnosis. In Mrs. W, multiple myeloma causing the vertebral compression fracture is extremely unlikely because the disease is rare and there is no evidence to suggest the diagnosis. Note that alkaline phosphatase might be elevated in Mrs. W. Although elevated alkaline phosphatase may be found in patients who have metastatic bone disease, alkaline phosphatase is also a non-specific indicator of a healing fracture and may remain elevated for up to 3 months. Thus, this test has little value in ruling out secondary causes of vertebral fracture.

Mrs. W's bone scan showed localized uptake at T12. Metastases often occur in several skeletal sites; the fact that the scan was positive only at one site implies that metastatic disease is less likely. In combination with the low BMD, the radiological appearance of the fracture, the normal blood tests, and the lack of other symptoms related to the progression of breast cancer, the most likely diagnosis by far is osteoporotic compression fracture.

Should This Patient Have Bone Density Testing?

Yes. BMD testing may help establish the etiology of fracture. A normal BMD (T score greater than −1.0) would substantially increase the chance that the fracture is caused by metastatic disease. In this case, BMD testing is not necessary to determine whether drug treatment for osteoporosis should be initiated. The presence of a vertebral fracture in a postmenopausal woman indicates such a high risk of subsequent fractures (about a 4-fold increased risk of spine fractures and a 2-fold increased risk of hip fractures) that it would be cost-effective to initiate drug treatment to prevent fracture regardless of BMD results (see Chapter 1). Note that patients with breast cancer may be at increased risk for osteoporotic fracture, likely caused by some of the treatments they receive for this condition. A recent case-control study found that compared with women without breast cancer, women with non-metastatic breast cancer have a 5-fold increased risk of osteoporotic vertebral fracture, and women with breast cancer and soft-tissue metastases (without evidence of skeletal metastases) have a 20-fold higher incidence of osteoporotic vertebral fracture (3).

Management of Acute Compression Fracture

Although there is no good study of the natural history of acute vertebral compression fracture, it is said that acute pain caused by fracture usually resolves in most cases within 10 weeks. Indeed, if the pain worsened in Mrs. W during the next month, this would increase the chance that the fracture is caused by metastatic disease. Occasionally, some women with mid-thoracic wedge fractures develop chronic pain as a result of changes in spinal shape. The pain caused by an osteoporotic compression fracture can be severe and disabling. About three quarters of these women have back pain that limits their activities for at least a week (4).

There are no randomized trials on the management of vertebral fractures. Acute fractures are likely best managed with analgesics (nonsteroidal anti-inflammatories such as acetaminophen) and early mobilization. If this is not sufficient, use of a soft brace may help. Muscle spasm also often accompanies acute vertebral compression fracture and can be treated effectively with heat and muscle relaxants. Constipation, which often occurs as a result of paralytic ileus after acute vertebral compression, should be treated symptomatically to avoid worsening of back pain. In addition, randomized blinded trials have demonstrated that calcitonin, either subcutaneously in doses of 50 to 100 IU per day or nasally in doses of 200 IU per day within 2 weeks of the fracture helps to reduce the duration of pain and the need for narcotics (see Chapter 10). Analgesics, bracing, and calcitonin may be required for up to 3 months.

Other treatments that are currently being studied to decrease the pain associated with vertebral fractures include percutaneous injection of artificial cement (polymethymethacrylate) into the vertebral body. Among 29 patients treated with this technique, 26 reported significant pain relief immediately after treatment (5). However, results from randomized controlled trials and data concerning the safety of this agent are lacking.

Treatment for Osteoporosis

Mrs. W should be advised about appropriate intakes of calcium (1200 mg/d) and vitamin D (400–800 IU/d). In addition, drug treatment should be instituted to decrease the risk of future fractures for all women with vertebral fractures. Mrs. W is taking tamoxifen. This drug, which has antiestrogen effects on the breast, has estrogen-like effects on the bone; however, effects on the risk of vertebral fracture are unknown (see Chapter 5).

Adding a bisphosphonate, such as alendronate, etidronate, or risedronate, to Mrs. W's regimen will increase BMD by about 3% to 4% over 2 years (see Chpater 9) (6). Note that while the bisphosphonate clodronate has been found to decrease the risk of bone metastases caused by breast cancer, this has not been shown for other bisphosphonates (6,7). Should Mrs. W be unable to tolerate a bisphosphonate, intranasal salmon calcitonin in doses of 200 IU may be used. However, calcitonin is less effective than alendronate at reducing the risk of vertebral and nonvertebral fractures, and the value of calcitonin in combination with tamoxifen has not been studied.

Given this woman's history of breast cancer, she should avoid estrogen therapy because it is contraindicated with tamoxifen and may increase her risk of recurrent breast cancer. Raloxifene is not recommended because it has not been studied as a treatment in women with breast cancer.

CASE SUMMARY

Mrs. W's vertebral fracture is likely caused by osteoporosis. This is supported by the clinical history, the radiographic features of the fracture, and the biochemical tests. Mrs. W was given treatment for the pain related to her vertebral fracture (acetaminophen 650 mg four times a day and nasal calcitonin 200 IU once daily), and she was started on alendronate 70 mg weekly for treatment of her osteoporosis with instructions to take it in the morning with a full glass of water and to avoid lying down or eating for 30 minutes. She will be seen in 1 month to re-evaluate her pain and to confirm that she is tolerating the alendronate.

CASE 2   51-YEAR-OLD WOMAN WITH AMENORRHEA AND HOT FLUSHES CONCERNED ABOUT DEVELOPING OSTEOPOROSIS

Mrs. J is a 51-year-old white woman with hot flushes and amenorrhea for the past year. She is otherwise well. She is not using any medication, and she neither drinks nor smokes. Mrs. J has not experienced height loss or fractures. Her mother has had height loss and a Dowager's hump, and Mrs. J is concerned about developing osteoporosis. She has no personal or family history of breast cancer or cardiovascular disease. Physical examination is normal.

Is This Patient at Risk for Osteoporosis?

Yes. Mrs. J is in her early postmenopausal years, a period of accelerated bone loss. Rates of postmenopausal bone loss vary between individuals. Further, within individuals rates of loss vary by skeletal sites. Typically, women who have natural menopause lose 1% to 3% of bone annually in the first 2 or 3 years after menopause. In contrast, women who undergo oophorectomy lose bone more rapidly: up to 5% in the first year (9).

Estrogen deficiency is the primary cause of postmenopausal bone loss (10). Postmenopausal women who are thin and smoke are at greatest risk for rapid loss (11–14). Note that calcium intake, physical activity, and alcohol consumption have not been associated with bone loss during this early postmenopausal period (15).

Having a mother with height loss may increase Mrs. J's risk of developing osteoporosis. However, it is important to note that only half the height loss that occurs with aging is attributable to vertebral fractures. There is no evidence that a maternal history of a Dowager's hump increases the risk of osteoporosis. Furthermore, a maternal history of hip fracture is a stronger risk factor for osteoporosis than a maternal history of vertebral fracture.

Would Fracture Risk Differ If This Patient Had a Different Racial Background?

African-American and Mexican-American women have about one third the risk of hip and vertebral fracture of white women (15,16). In African-American women, this difference is primarily caused by greater peak bone mass. African-American women may also have slower rates of postmenopausal bone loss than white women (17). The reasons for lower rates of hip and vertebral fracture in Mexican-American women have not been identified. Asian women living in the United States have a similar rate of hip fracture as white women. Differences in other fracture rates remain undefined.

These data suggest that as a group postmenopausal African-American and Mexican-American women are less likely to develop osteoporotic fractures compared to white women. However, there have not been studies that allow the determination of fracture risk from specific levels of BMD in these patients.

How Should This Patient Be Managed?

It is very important to distinguish between two therapeutic goals: the symptomatic relief of hot flushes and the prevention of chronic diseases such as osteoporosis. Clinicians and patients need to consider these goals separately when deciding upon a management plan.

Symptomatic Relief of Hot Flushes

Estrogen is the most appropriate therapy for the relief of hot flushes (8). For patients with an intact uterus, a progestin should also be prescribed. Chapter 6 reviews the commonly prescribed estrogens and progestins. If estrogen is being prescribed for hot flushes, it only needs to be taken for a short time. For example, a woman may choose to stop estrogen at 12 months and, if symptoms return, resume the estrogen and taper. Alternatively, a woman may choose to taper the estrogen. A reasonable schedule of tapering is to reduce or eliminate one dose per week every week or two, depending on symptoms.

Several other options are available for patients who do not wish to take estrogen. These include progestins and SSRI antidepressants (for example, Effexor) that small randomized trials have found to be effective, and Black cohosh, phytoestrogens, clonidine, and vitamin E capsules. The effectiveness of these agents relative to estrogen is unknown. The recommended dose and the efficacy for each agent are reviewed in Table 13-2.

Prevention and Treatment of Osteoporosis

The second therapeutic goal is the prevention of chronic diseases, specifically osteoporosis. All women should be given advice regarding calcium and vitamin D intake, exercise, and BMD testing, and pharmacologic therapy should be considered in specific patients.

Perimenopausal and postmenopausal women should take at least 1200 mg of calcium and 400 to 800 IU of vitamin D a day (see Chapter 4). Patients should also be advised to engage in regular exercise. A combination of weight-bearing high- or low-impact aerobic activity and muscle strengthening

Table 13-2   Alternative Agents for Relief of Hot Flushes

Agent	Dose	Efficacy in Relief of Hot Flushes
Progestins		
Transdermal progesterone cream	20 mg	Effective (19)
Medroxyprogesterone acetate	10 mg bid	Effective (20)
Megestrol acetate	20 mg bid	Likely effective (21)
SSRI antidepressants (Effexor)	37.5 mg od	Effective
Black cohosh	2 tablets daily	Possibly effective (22)
Phytoestrogens	Supplement diet with phytoestrogen foods	Possibly weakly effective (23)
Clonidine	0.05 mg bid, can increase to 0.2 mg bid	Efficiency uncertain (24); side effects common
Vitamin E capsules	800 IU/day	Efficacy uncertain (25)

(approximately 30 minutes, three times a week) is ideal (see Chapter 5). Note that these measures slow but do not prevent early postmenopausal bone loss.

Women who are concerned about the risk of developing osteoporosis and who are trying to make a decision regarding treatment should be offered BMD testing. BMD testing may serve several purposes. First, it will provide information regarding the risk of developing an osteoporotic fracture, a risk that cannot be elucidated by history alone (26). Second, it may help the patient make a decision about therapy (27). Third, it may increase the chance that women will follow through to begin and continue treatment (28). Physicians and patients should also consider BMD testing for women who are concerned about the risk of developing osteoporosis and have decided to start treatment. In this situation, baseline BMD testing before initiating treatment could be used to assess response to treatment (see Case 6).

It may be worthwhile to offer pharmacologic therapy to women with T scores below –2.0 at the femoral neck if other risk factors are present (personal history of fracture as an adult, history of fracture in first-degree relative, current cigarette smoking, and low body weight) and in women with T scores at the femoral neck below –2.5 regardless of risk factors. Drugs that could be used include hormone replacement therapy, bisphosphonates, or raloxifene. All of these medications require long-term use to prevent osteoporotic fracture. The benefits and risks of each of these medications are reviewed in their specific chapters. For Mrs. J, who has hot flushes and is concerned about developing osteoporosis, hormone replacement therapy is the most appropriate choice.

CASE SUMMARY

Mrs. J has decided to use estrogen for relief of her hot flushes. In addition, because she was concerned about her risk for developing osteoporosis, she was advised to take appropriate amounts of calcium and vitamin D and exercise regularly. BMD testing was obtained to evaluate risk for osteoporotic fracture and to facilitate decision making regarding therapy. Mrs. J had a T score of –2.0 at the spine and –1.5 at the femoral neck. Because she was going to take hormone replacement therapy for relief of hot flushes, she was advised to continue this for a year. She will be telephoned in 1 month to confirm that she is tolerating the medication, then seen in 1 year to assess her hot flushes and to consider whether to continue hormone replacement therapy for prevention of osteoporosis.

CASE 3   53-YEAR-OLD MAN WITH AN ATRAUMATIC WRIST FRACTURE

Mr. R is a 53-year-old man seen annually for routine medical assessment. Over the past year, he has been generally well. However, last month he slipped and fractured his wrist. Mr. R has smoked 1 package of cigarettes a day for 30 years. He drank 4 to 6 glasses of vodka a day for 20 years but stopped 6 months ago. He has never used steroids or other medications. He has no complaints of sexual dysfunction, height loss, or other low trauma fractures. His mother and sister have been diagnosed with osteoporosis. Physical examination is normal.

What is Meant by "Osteoporosis" in a Man?

Currently, there is no standard definition of osteoporosis for men. Women who have a vertebral fracture are, almost by definition, believed to have severe osteoporosis. In contrast, many men with vertebral fractures are thought to have them caused by trauma. Thus, it cannot be readily assumed that men with vertebral fractures have osteoporosis. Furthermore, although BMD testing in women can be used to define osteoporosis (a T score of equal to or lesser than –2.5 at either the hip or the spine compared with young women), the T score that defines osteoporosis among men is controversial. We suggest using a T score of equal to or less than –2.5 compared with young men. Although some still advocate using female T scores to define osteoporosis in men, this is problematic for two reasons: it would underestimate the expected prevalence of osteoporosis in men (29), and, because men may fracture at higher female T scores than women (approximately –2.0 for men compared with –2.5 for women), it would result in different fracture thresholds for men and women (30). Note that most manufacturers use male reference ranges to report T scores for men.

Is Osteoporosis in a Man Cause for Concern?

The estimated lifetime risk of any fracture is almost 40% in white women and 13% in white men aged 50 years and older (31). However, approximately 20% of all osteoporotic fractures occur in men (32). Furthermore, data from the European Vertebral Osteoporosis Study (EVOS) demonstrated that the prevalence of radiographic vertebral fractures is similar in men (233 out of 1098 men) and women (288 out of 2088 women) (33). Although the importance of radiographic fractures on the quality of life is well documented in women, similar data are not currently available for men.

What Are the Risk Factors for Osteoporotic Fractures in Men?

As in women, the two primary risk factors for osteoporotic fractures in men are probably low BMD and falls (or "diseases that increase the risk of injurious falls") (34,35). Additionally, men who have a hip fracture may suffer from other diseases. Table 13-3 lists the factors in the history and physical that should be considered having been associated with hip fractures in a case-control study of about 500 men (34). Note that while many other factors have

Table 13-3   Clinical Approach to the Evaluation of Male Osteoporosis

History	Physical Examination
Inquire about	*Inspect for*
Thyroid surgery	Stigmata of chronic alcohol abuse
Gastric surgery	Cushingoid appearance
Pernicious anemia	Thoracic kyphosis
Diarrhea	*Measure*
Chronic bronchitis	Height
Weight loss	Weight
Physical activity	*Assess*
History of falls	Visual acuity
Neurologic conditions (Parkinson's, hemiplegia)	Balance
Presence of vertigo/dizziness	
Current and past use of alcohol (and amount)	
Current smoking	
Current and past use of steroids	
History of low-trauma fractures, back pain, height loss	
Family history of osteoporosis/fractures	
Changes in shaving habits, hair growth, sexual function, problems with fertility, galactorrhea	

been purported to be associated with an increased risk of hip fracture in the medical literature (for example, hypogonadism, hyperthyroidism, chronic use of anticonvulsants, and multiple myeloma), these factors appear to have relatively little influence on the occurrence of hip fractures in the community.

How Should Osteoporosis in Men Be Evaluated?

Few data are available on the evaluation and diagnosis of osteoporosis in men. Men in whom osteoporosis is suspected (for example, men who have had a fracture as an adult, men with medical conditions, or men using medications associated with an increased risk of fracture) should have BMD testing. If the T score at the hip or spine is equal to or less than –2.5, a history and physical examination directed at identifying the cause of osteoporosis should be performed.

Laboratory testing can also be done to rule out more common causes of secondary osteoporosis. A reasonable initial evaluation might include the following tests: serum calcium, alkaline phosphatase, parathyroid hormone, creatinine, liver enzymes, free testosterone, TSH, CBC, and 24-hour urine for calcium and creatinine. Other tests that could be ordered based on clinical suspicion of disease are 24-hour urine monitoring for cortisol (Cushing's disease), serum prolactin (hypogonadism), IgG gliadin antibodies celiac disease), and serum protein electrophoresis (multiple myeloma) (see Chapter 3).

Several studies have found that serum estradiol is more strongly correlated with BMD than testosterone in men (36,37). Further, low serum estradiol may be a risk factor for future hip fracture in elderly men (38). However, there is no evidence that estrogen replacement therapy is an effective treatment for men with osteoporosis and low estradiol levels. Thus, measuring estradiol levels is not currently suggested.

If the history, physical examination, and laboratory testing fail to reveal the cause of osteoporosis, empiric therapy (see below) and close follow-up (office visits every 6 months and yearly BMD testing) can be considered. Men with substantial bone loss (cumulative loss of at least 5% of BMD at one or more sites during two separate measures) or those with at least two vertebral fractures during treatment should be referred to a specialist in bone disease.

How Should Osteoporosis in Men Be Treated?

All men should be advised to take in calcium and vitamin D (1000 to 1200 mg of calcium and 400 to 800 IU of vitamin D, depending on age) and to regularly participate in weight-bearing physical activity.

In addition, treatment with either alendronate or risedronate is possible. A recent 2-year placebo-controlled randomized trial in men with osteoporosis, some of whom had low testosterone levels, demonstrated that 10 mg of alendronate increased BMD and reduced the incidence of vertebral fractures compared with placebo (39). Indeed, alendronate has just recently been approved for the treatment of male osteoporosis (see Chapter 9). Risedronate has not been extensively studied in men with osteoporosis but is likely to have a similar efficacy in men as in women (40).

Calcitonin could be used in men who do not tolerate bisphosphonates. A small non-randomized study demonstrated that 100 IU of subcutaneous calcitonin three times a week increased BMD by about 3% at the hip and spine (41).

If a cause of osteoporosis is identified, specific treatments should be directed towards the cause. For example, men with steroid-induced osteoporosis should be treated with a bisphosphonate, and men with alcoholism should be advised to abstain from alcohol. The use of testosterone therapy should be limited to men with low levels of free testosterone who have no contraindications to the use of this medication (for example, prostatic hypertrophy or prostate cancer). Note that data to support the use of testosterone therapy in men with hypogonadism are limited; there are only a few small studies with short follow-up and BMD assessment, as opposed to documented reduction in fracture risk (42–44).

CASE SUMMARY

BMD testing obtained in Mr. R revealed a T score of –2.6 at the lumbar spine and a T score of –3.4 at the femoral neck. Laboratory tests were within the normal range. Mr. R's low bone mass is highly likely to be attributable to his excessive alcohol intake, smoking, and family history of osteoporosis. Mr. R was advised to stop smoking and counseled to remain abstinent from alcohol. Additionally, given Mr. R's low bone density and history of low-trauma fracture, he was given a prescription for alendronate 70 mg weekly. He will be seen in 4 weeks to confirm that he is tolerating the medication.

CASE 4   25-YEAR-OLD WOMAN WHOSE MOTHER HAS HAD A HIP FRACTURE CAUSED BY OSTEOPOROSIS INQUIRES ABOUT HER RISK

Miss R is a 25-year-old woman who presents for advice about preventing osteoporosis. This visit was prompted by her 65-year-old mother's recent hip fracture. Miss R began menstruating at age 13 and had regular menstrual cycles until age 19 but has not menstruated since. At age 19, she began exercising 2 hours daily and initiated a calorie-restricted diet; her weight decreased from 120 to 105 pounds, where it has stayed since. She has smoked 15 cigarettes a day for the last 9 years and dislikes dairy products, calcium supplements, and alcohol. She does not use medications currently but took the oral contraceptive pill for 3 years, from age 16 to 19. Miss R states that, until adolescence, she had a good calcium intake. She has always been physically active. She has had no fractures or back pain. Other than her mother, no family members have osteoporosis. On physical examination, Miss R weighs 105 pounds and is 5 feet, 4 inches tall. The remainder of the physical examination, including confrontational visual field testing and breast examination, is normal.

Is Osteoporosis in a Premenopausal Woman a Reasonable Concern?

Yes. Having a mother who has had an osteoporotic hip fracture doubles a daughter's risk of developing a hip fracture in later life (45). Thus, minimizing the risk of osteoporotic fracture should be a priority for Miss R. One way to reduce subsequent fracture risk is to maximize peak bone mass (the bone mass obtained at skeletal maturity). Bone density after menopause is determined by the balance between peak bone mass and subsequent rate and duration of bone loss. In healthy individuals, at least half of the peak bone mass is acquired during the second decade of life; thus the earlier health prevention measures are undertaken, the more likely they are to have impact in later life.

Peak bone mass is largely determined by genetic factors, but achievement of peak bone mass can be limited by low levels of estrogen. Other potentially important factors include very low body weight, lack of physical activity, poor calcium intake, and smoking.

How Should This Patient Be Investigated?

Miss R gives a history of prolonged secondary amenorrhea, indicating decreased estrogen production. Common causes of secondary amenorrhea include hypothalamic dysfunction (excessive exercise, anorexia nervosa, chronic illness, treatment with gonadatropin-releasing hormone agonists), pituitary tumors (prolactinoma), and premature ovarian failure. The cause of amenorrhea can often be identified by history. Laboratory tests that may be helpful include serum prolactin, luteinizing hormone (LH), and follicle-stimulating hormone (FSH). If the cause of amenorrhea is not readily identified, referral to an endocrinologist should be considered. In Miss R, the most likely cause of amenorrhea is anorexia nervosa. Laboratory testing revealed a normal serum prolactin, and low levels of LH and FSH, consistent with this diagnosis.

Of note, Miss R used the oral contraceptive pill for 3 years. A review of the literature suggests that in otherwise healthy premenopausal women oral contraceptive use is associated with higher postmenopausal bone mass, but the effect is small and has little clinical significance (46–49). Use of an oral contraceptive has not been extensively studied in premenopausal women with estrogen deficiency.

Should Premenopausal Women Have Bone Mineral Density Testing?

Generally speaking, BMD testing should not be performed in healthy, menstruating, premenopausal women because it is highly unlikely that, given the limited options for premenopausal women, treatment decisions would be changed because of the results of densitometry. These women should be given nutritional and lifestyle counseling, which can be done without bone mass measurement.

BMD testing should be performed in all premenopausal women who are starting treatment with oral steroids (see Chapter 9). Among premenopausal women with amenorrhea, consider BMD testing if it will help the patient accept intervention.

What Treatment Should Be Offered?

All premenopausal women, regardless of age and risk for osteoporosis, should be advised about lifestyle and nutritional factors that influence bone mass. These factors and the specific recommendations are listed in Table 13-4. These recommendations are based primarily on clinical experience caused by a paucity of clinical trials in this area. See Chapter 4 for details regarding calcium intake and Chapter 5 for details regarding exercise.

Table 13-4   Nutritional and Lifestyle Factors That May Influence Peak Bone Mass and Treatment

Factor	Recommendations
Calcium intake	1200 mg/day If this requirement cannot be met by dietary calcium intake, recommend a calcium supplement
Exercise	Should be tailored to the patient's fitness level. Generally would suggest: • Mid-impact aerobics (e.g., squash, tennis, jogging) for 20 minutes 3 times per week • Weight training for back and hip muscle groups, 8 repetitions 3 times per week
Smoking	Stop smoking
Alcohol consumption	Identify and treat alcoholism

Among women with estrogen deficiency, specific treatment should be tailored to the cause of the deficiency. Controlled trials of agents such as bisphosphonates or calcitonin are lacking in premenopausal women. Miss R likely has low bone density secondary to anorexia nervosa. The goal of medical therapy in this condition is to increase weight and promote the return of spontaneous menses. Achievement of these goals effectively increases the bone mass in anorexic patients (50,51). Although calcium intake has not been shown to be correlated with bone mass in anorexic patients, it seems prudent to prescribe a daily intake of at least 1200 mg. Patients should be advised to continue with moderate levels of exercise, but more intense physical activity should be avoided because of the risk of pathologic fractures, slower weight gain, and prolonged ammenorrhea.

What About Estrogen Therapy?

Estrogen therapy is controversial. Only one randomized controlled trial has studied the effects of estrogen and progestin administration in 48 women with anorexia (52). The study concluded that, although there may be some gain in lumbar spine bone mass in patients with extremely low body weight, sex steroids cannot prevent bone loss in anorexia nervosa, possibly because the dose of estrogen, effective in treating postmenopausal women, is inadequate for a younger population and possibly because estrogen deficiency is only one of several factors contributing to the low bone mass observed in women with anorexia. Other factors may include malnutrition, low body mass, low levels of insulin-like growth factor-1, decreased androgen production, and elevated glucocorticoid levels (52). Further studies are needed to address these issues. Until that time, a treatment plan should emphasize weight gain (aim for a body mass index of equal to or greater than 19) with a spontaneous resumption of menses. One may consider using the oral contraceptive pill until adequate weight gain is achieved. Note that, in some cases, referral to an eating disorder clinic, if available, may also be helpful (Table 13-5).

What About Bisphosphonates?

Bisphosphonates are retained in the skeleton for decades, and the lack of evidence regarding the safety of very long-term exposure and use during pregnancy has led most experts to avoid bisphosphonate treatment in premenopausal women (see Chapter 9).

Treatments for other causes of estrogen deficiency leading to low bone mass are listed in Table 13-6. Although there are no randomized controlled trials to support the use of the oral contraceptive pill in these conditions, this may be a logical approach to consider while working to alleviate the underlying problem.

Table 13-5   Approach to the Diagnosis and Treatment of Low Bone Mass Caused by Anorexia Nervosa*

1. *Rule out other causes of estrogen deficiency*
   - Measure: LH, FSH, prolactin (levels of LH and FSH in anorexia nervosa patients can be normal or low; prolactin levels should be normal)

2. *Advise*
   - 1200 mg calcium
   - Increase caloric intake
   - Decrease exercise

3. *Consider*
   - Bone mineral density testing if it may help convince patient to accept treatment
   - Oral contraceptive use
   - Referral to an eating disorder clinic/specialist

Treatment goal: Resumption of menses (typically when body mass index (BMI) ≥ 19)

FSH, follicle-stimulating hormone; LH, luteinizing hormone.
* Treatments for other causes of estrogen deficiency leading to low bone mass are listed in Table 13-6. Although there are no randomized controlled trials to support the use of the oral contraceptive pill in these conditions, this may be a logical approach to consider while working to alleviate the underlying problem.

Table 13-6   Causes and Treatments for Low Bone Mass Caused by Estrogen Deficiency

Cause	Treatment
Excessive exercise	Reduce physical activity, consider OCP in the interim
Stress	Treat underlying problem, consider OCP in the interim
Chronic illness	Treat underlying problem, consider OCP in the interim
Use of GnRH agonists	Estrogen replacement therapy until menses resume
Pituitary tumors	Surgical or medical treatment of tumor to ensure menses resumes
Ovarian failure	Estrogen replacement therapy

GnRH = gonadotropin-releasing hormone, OCP = oral contraceptive pill.

CASE SUMMARY

Miss R probably has low bone density secondary to anorexia nervosa. This, in addition to her family history of osteoporosis, puts her at increased risk for future osteoporotic fractures. After discussion, Miss R was willing to limit her exercise to 1 hour a day, take in 1200 mg of calcium a day, and increase her caloric intake. She will be seen in 3 months. If her weight has not increased, treatment options include BMD testing (which may help to convince her to accept treatment), referral to an eating disorder clinic, and use of the oral contraceptive pill until a BMI of greater than 19 is achieved. When Miss R reaches a BMI of 19 or greater, the oral contraceptive pill should be stopped to assess for resumption of spontaneous menses.

CASE 5   73-YEAR-OLD WOMAN ADMITTED TO THE ORTHOPEDIC SERVICE WITH A HIP FRACTURE

Mrs. S, a 73-year-old woman, has been admitted to the orthopedic service with a right hip fracture after tripping over a rug at home. She smokes one pack of cigarettes a day and has done so for 50 years. She does not drink alcohol. She lives alone and spends most of her time watching television. Mrs. S broke her wrist 15 years ago, when she slipped on ice. She has no history of height loss. She knows of no family history of osteoporosis. Mrs. S last presented 6 months ago after she had had a fall at home. At that time she had no serious injuries, weighed 90 pounds, and was 5 feet, 1 inch tall.

How Important Are Hip Fractures?

One of every six white women will have a hip fracture during her lifetime (45). Hip fracture is a major cause of disability and premature death. For example, the average length of stay in an acute care hospital after a hip fracture is 3 weeks; about one third of patients must remain in long-term care institutions for at least 1 year, and about half return home but must depend on other people or devices for mobility. Furthermore, the occurrence of a hip fracture is associated with a 20% increase in mortality. Note that most deaths are not caused by the fracture itself but rather to conditions that are associated with both fracture and mortality, such as heart disease (53). Thus, the increased mortality associated with hip fractures is best addressed by treating the underlying disease. Hip fractures are also expensive; in 1995, the estimated annual cost of hip fracture in the United States was 13.8 billion dollars (54).

How Should This Patient Be Managed?

Short-term management includes surgical treatment for her hip fracture and rehabilitation. Optimizing nutrition, with the use of protein supplements, may also help recovery after a hip fracture (see Chapter 4). In the long term, the primary aim of treatment is to prevent further fractures. This should involve a multidisciplinary approach (described in detail later) with a focus on three components: first, identification and treatment of specific risk factors associated with an increased risk of fracture; second, treatment to reduce falls; and third, assessment and treatment of osteoporosis.

Ideally, one would like to prevent the occurrence of any fractures. Elderly patients, the group at greatest risk for fracture, should be carefully assessed to ensure that modifiable risk factors for fracture are eliminated. They should be asked about falls and be evaluated for osteoporosis with appropriate therapies instituted. Mrs. S had a wrist fracture and a history of falls that antedated her hip fracture. Fall-prevention techniques and treatment for osteoporosis at the time of her wrist fracture may have prevented her hip fracture. Now that she has had a hip fracture, her risk of breaking her other hip is substantially increased.

Physicians and surgeons who do not feel comfortable with the long-term management of patients with hip fractures should consult with an internist or endocrinologist who is an expert in the management of osteoporosis. This principle holds true for all patients with fractures.

Identification and Treatment of Risk Factors Associated with an Increased Risk of Fracture

The common risk factors for fracture are reviewed in Chapter 1. Generally speaking, any chronic condition that impairs mobility may increase fracture risk. Thus, these conditions should be identified and, if possible, treated. Patients should also be advised to maintain a healthy body weight because weight loss and low body weight increase the risk of fracture. Modifiable risk factors should also be examined (Table 13-7). Most increase fracture risk by increasing the propensity to fall or through an association with BMD.

Treatment to Reduce Falls

Falls are a significant cause of hip fracture. More than 90% of hip fractures occur after a fall (55). About 30% of persons older than age 65 years and 40% older than age 80 years fall each year, and 5% to 10% of falls result in fractures (56,57). Thus, prevention of falls should be a priority in the management of patients with previous hip fractures.

Table 13-7   Modifiable Risk Factors That Should Be Assessed in Patients with Fractures

- Impaired vision
- Physical inactivity
- Use of sedatives
- Low bone mineral density
- Hazards in the home (e.g., scatter rugs, slippery surfaces) that increase risk of falling
- Smoking
- Impaired mental status (depression)
- Low levels of 25-OH vitamin D

Patients who have had a hip fracture should receive a physical therapy referral for advice about continuing physical activity. Activity need not be strenuous. For example, an intervention consisting of gait-training, balance, and strengthening exercises, in addition to medication adjustment and behavioral instructions aimed at modifying risk factors for falls, has been shown to reduce the risk of falling among community-dwelling elderly people (58). A home assessment from an occupational therapist may also be beneficial to decrease the environmental home hazards that are associated with an increased risk of falling and to teach fall-prevention behaviors.

Modification of risk factors can have a significant impact on reducing the risk of future fractures. For example, it is estimated that an elderly woman who stops smoking can reduce her risk of hip fracture by about 40% (59). One should also consider the use of hip protectors, where available, to reduce the risk of fall-related fractures. A randomized controlled trial involving ambulatory, frail adults demonstrates that using external hip protectors reduced hip fractures by about 60% (60). Hip protectors can be used to prevent hip fractures in cases in which risk factors cannot be modified, or they can be combined with other strategies to prevent fall-related fractures (Figure 13-2).

Assessment and Treatment of Osteoporosis

Mrs. S has had low trauma fractures of the hip and the wrist. In the absence of underlying medical diseases, the most likely etiology of these fractures is

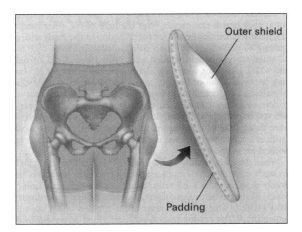

Figure 13-2 One type of hip protector. The outer shields are worn inside pockets of undergarment. (From Vogelsang H, Ferenci P, Resch H, et al. Prevention of bone mineral loss in patients with Crohn's disease by long-term oral vitamin D supplementation. Eur J Gastroenterol Hepatol. 1995;7:609–614; with permission.)

osteoporosis. In this case, BMD testing is unlikely to help in making the diagnosis and unlikely to influence initial treatment decisions. Although controversial, BMD testing could serve as a baseline by which to assess response to treatment, and it may be useful to order it for this purpose. BMD testing should be performed on the *nonfractured* hip as opposed to the lumbar spine. If not feasible, the heel or forearm should be measured with pDXA (see Chapter 2). Lumbar spine BMD in elderly patients may be difficult to interpret because of degenerative changes.

Nutritional Intervention

Unless contraindicated, patients who have had an osteoporotic fracture should be given calcium and vitamin D supplements to ensure they are receiving at least 1200 mg of calcium and 800 IU of vitamin D per day.

Pharmacologic Therapy

In general, most patients with hip fractures will have osteoporosis and a higher risk for future fractures and should usually receive pharmacologic therapy. The most appropriate agents are the bisphosphonates (either alendronate 10 mg/d or 70 mg/wk, or risedronate 5 mg/d). Randomized, double-blind, placebo-controlled trials have demonstrated that both these drugs can increase BMD and prevent fractures (vertebral and nonvertebral) in women with established osteoporosis (see Chapter 9) (61,62). Hormone replacement therapy is probably a second choice for women who cannot tolerate bisphosphonates.

CASE SUMMARY

Mrs. S smokes, is physically inactive, and has an increased propensity to fall. These risk factors for fractures can be modified. She was advised to stop smoking, and assessments from an occupational and physical therapist were obtained. In addition, Mrs. S had BMD testing that demonstrated a T score in her left hip of –3.5. She was advised to take appropriate amounts of calcium and vitamin D and started on risedronate 5 mg/d. She will be seen in follow-up in 3 months and have repeat BMD testing in 2 years.

CASE 6   POSTMENOPAUSAL WOMAN ON ALENDRONATE FOR 1 YEAR WITH A DECREASE IN BONE MINERAL DENSITY

Mrs. R is a 65-year-old postmenopausal woman who is being treated with alendronate 10 mg/d for osteoporosis. She is otherwise healthy, with no atraumatic fractures or height loss. Bone mineral density testing after 1 year of alendronate reveals a T score at the lumbar spine of –2.6 and a T score at the femoral neck of –2.8. Compared with her previous bone density, her bone mineral density is 3% lower at the hip and 5% lower at the spine. She wants to know if the treatment is helping her.

Has This Patient Really Lost Bone Mineral Density?

Mrs. R may have lost BMD despite prescription of an effective treatment. Alternatively, the observed decrease may not be real but rather caused by imprecision in measuring BMD. Imprecision can occur because of variability in the test or because of patient characteristics (such as positioning), but these variations are so small that they cannot be detected, and thus cannot be corrected by experienced densitometrists.

One study has demonstrated that women like Mrs. R who have lower BMD the first year of treatment with effective drugs usually have higher BMD the next year, even though no changes are made in their treatment (63). This is caused by "regression to the mean": unusual responses to treatment (such as loss of bone density while receiving an effective agent) are more likely caused by subtle errors in the measurement rather than by problems with the patient or the drug. Consequently, patients with such responses are likely to have more typical responses (higher BMD) if treatment is continued and the measurement is repeated (see Chapter 2).

If the Change in Bone Mineral Density Is Real, Why Did It Decline?

There are three possible explanations. First, Mrs. R may have been taking her alendronate improperly (with meals, beverages, or medications that interfere with its absorption) or not at all. Second, Mrs. R may have responded because she lost less bone density than she would have without treatment; in other words, the alendronate attenuated her bone loss, and she had an unrecognized response. Third, and least likely, Mrs. R may be resistant to the effects of alendronate. Resistance to this drug or other drugs used for the treatment of osteoporosis has not been documented.

The clinician should ask Mrs. R if she is taking her alendronate and how she is taking it. If she has adhered to the alendronate treatment and is taking it properly, the decrease in bone mass is most likely explained either by regression to the mean or by an unrecognized response to treatment. There is also evidence that although Mrs. R appears to be losing bone density, her risk of fractures is much lower than it would be if she were not taking alendronate.

Mrs. R should be advised to continue with the alendronate and be reassured that she is likely to have better results during the next year. Unfortunately, there are no data about the clinical meaning of changes in bone density after the first period of testing. In general, however, one expects smaller increases and a greater chance of apparent decreases in bone density after 2 or 3 years of treatment. This does not mean, however, that the treatment has stopped working.

How Often Should Bone Mineral Density Testing Be Performed?

BMD testing is typically used to monitor response to treatment or, in patients not receiving drug therapy, to determine if they are losing bone density at an unusually rapid rate. Currently, the optimum frequency with which to perform BMD testing is not known.

There are three principles to consider when deciding how frequently to measure BMD. First, most women gain bone density during the first year of treatment with hormone replacement therapy, alendronate, risedronate, or raloxifene. Second, large increases or decreases in BMD within a year of treatment are likely caused by measurement error (this is also true for monitoring over 2 years because the additional change in the second year is only about 1%). Third, use of BMD testing to reinforce adherence to therapy may have limited value because most problems with adherence occur within the first 3 months of starting treatment, long before BMD is useful enough to assess changes in bone density. If a physician and patient agree to monitor treatment with bone density measurements, BMD should be measured every 2 years, mainly because this is a frequency that will be paid for by Medicare.

Patients who are starting on corticosteroids are different: they may lose very large amounts of bone density (5% to 10%) in just the first few months. Thus, it may be worthwhile to measure bone density in these patients when steroids are started and again within 3 to 6 months (see Chapter 12).

When Should Treatment Be Changed?

It is sometimes said that a few patients who take effective drugs for osteoporosis fail to respond. Although some lose bone or suffer fractures, they may be having a better outcome than they would have had without treatment or on a different treatment. For example, a woman who loses 3% at the hip and 1% at the spine while taking alendronate may be losing much less than she would have without treatment. Even if there are nonresponders, there is no good way to identify a patient who is not responding to treatment and would benefit from changing treatment or adding another. Combining two antiresorptive drugs such as estrogen and bisphosphonate will decrease bone turnover and increase bone density a little more than will either agent taken separately. For example, a recent randomized controlled trial demonstrated that the addition of alendronate in women who are already receiving hormone replacement therapy was associated with a 2% increase in lumbar spine and hip trochanter

BMD at 1 year (64). The addition of hormone replacement therapy to ongoing alendronate therapy would likely have similar effects. Note that although the combination of raloxifene with other antiresorptives has not been studied, tamoxifen (an agent similar to raloxifene) in combination with the bisphosphonate clodronate has been found to be safe and more effective than tamoxifen alone at increasing BMD (65).

In the absence of evidence, the addition of a second treatment (estrogen to bisphosphonate or bisphosphonate to estrogen or raloxifene) can be considered if the patient suffers two vertebral fractures or has a total of 5% or more loss of BMD at one or more sites after two periods of measurement at either site.

CASE SUMMARY

Mrs. R has adhered to the alendronate therapy and is taking it properly. Thus, the decrease in bone mass is probably caused by regression to the mean. Whatever the case, her risk of fracture is probably much lower than it would be if she were not taking alendronate. Mrs. R was advised to continue with the alendronate with a change to 70 mg once weekly.

CASE 7   30-YEAR-OLD MAN WITH CROHN'S DISEASE HAVING A FLARE

Mr. R is a 30-year-old man with Crohn's disease involving the terminal ileum. He is currently experiencing a flare and has been taking prednisone 40 mg daily for the past 2 weeks. Since his diagnosis 5 years ago, he has experienced flares about twice yearly. Typically, flares require 40 mg of prednisone daily for 4 weeks that is subsequently tapered over 2 months. He has not had bowel surgery. His only other medication is Pentasa 4 g daily. He is not taking vitamin D or calcium supplements. He has no history of nephrolithiasis, height loss, fractures, or family history of osteoporosis. He does not smoke or drink. On physical examination, he does not appear Cushingnoid. He is six feet tall and weighs 150 pounds.

Are Patients with Crohn's Disease at Risk for Osteoporosis?

In case-control studies, more patients with inflammatory bowel disease (IBD, including ulcerative colitis and Crohn's disease) have reduced BMD compared with healthy controls. Approximately 5% to 30% of patients with IBD have osteoporosis (66,67). Longitudinal studies demonstrate rates of annual bone loss ranging from less than 1% to 6% (68,69).

A few prospective and cross-sectional studies have examined risk factors for rapid bone loss and low BMD. A high cumulative lifetime dose of steroids is the strongest and most consistent predictor. It is unclear whether patients with IBD are at risk for osteoporosis independent of steroid use. Two small studies demonstrated that, among newly diagnosed individuals, patients with Crohn's disease have lower BMD than do patients with ulcerative colitis (69,70). However, a larger study found no difference in BMD among newly diagnosed patients with IBD, patients with IBD who had never received steroids, and healthy controls (71).

In addition to corticosteroid use, other risk factors for low BMD among patients with IBD include female gender, low body weight, increased age, and, for women, smoking and menopause. Note that although low serum calcium and vitamin D levels, duration of disease, and bowel resections have been suggested as risk factors for osteoporosis, these factors have not been correlated with bone loss (in longitudinal studies) or bone density (in cross-sectional studies). Furthermore, although disease activity has been purported to play a role in the development of osteoporosis in IBD, a correlation between markers of disease activity and the development of osteoporosis has not been reported. Mr. R is at risk for low bone density and ongoing bone loss because of his high lifetime use of steroids and his low body weight.

How Should This Patient Be Managed?

Data on the management of osteoporosis among patients with IBD are limited. Accordingly, recommendations are based primarily on clinical experience. Management recommendations consist of three parts: 1) optimized nutrition and exercise in all patients, 2) bone mineral density testing in specific patients, and 3) pharmacologic treatment in selected patients.

Optimized Nutrition and Exercise
A randomized placebo-controlled trial of calcium supplementation among patients with IBD found no difference in BMD after 1 year of treatment with 1000 mg of calcium carbonate and 250 IU vitamin D (72). This study had limited generalization because all patients were receiving corticosteroids and a large number had osteopenia or osteoporosis at baseline. Until further studies are available, it is reasonable to ensure that patients with IBD have an adequate calcium intake (at least 1200 mg/d), with the exception of individuals with a past history of nephrolithiasis. For these patients, a 24-hour urine calcium level can be measured. Hypercalciuric patients should be treated with hydrochlorthiazide (starting at 25 mg/d) to reduce the risk of future stones and improve calcium balance. Note that the effects on BMD and fracture are not known. However, a recent randomized double-blind placebo-controlled trial in healthy older adults demonstrated that low-dose hydrochlorthiazide preserves BMD at the hip and spine (73).

One should also ensure adequate vitamin D intake (400 to 800 IU/d). A randomized placebo-controlled trial among patients with Crohn's disease found that 1000 IU of vitamin D daily prevented a 7% decrease in BMD over 1 year (74). Note that some patients with IBD, and Crohn's disease in particular, are at risk of developing vitamin D deficiency and osteomalacia (for example, patients with jejunal and ileal disease or resections, patients receiving treatment with cholestyramine, and patients with hepatobiliary complications). In these patients, measurement of serum 25-OH vitamin D is warranted. Adequate vitamin D replacement may reduce the osteomalacic component of the bone disease (75). In addition, all patients with IBD should be advised not to smoke and to exercise regularly.

Bone Mineral Density Testing in Specific Patients

Until studies demonstrate a clear association between IBD and osteoporosis independent of steroid use, BMD should only be measured in specific patient groups. Patients who should receive BMD testing include perimenopausal and postmenopausal women, patients who have had past prolonged treatment with steroids (7.5 mg or more of prednisone a day for 3 months or more), and those who are being started on steroids for what is anticipated to be prolonged treatment (3 months or more) or who are likely to have intermittent treatment with steroids in the future (see Chapter 12). Individual factors, such as malnutrition or history of fractures, may also guide BMD testing.

Pharmacologic Treatment

Pharmacologic treatment should be based on the results of BMD testing and considered for all patients with osteoporosis or osteopenia. Drugs to consider include the bisphosphonates (alendronate, etidronate, risedronate). Studies of steroid-induced osteoporosis, which have included patients with IBD, have demonstrated that bisphosphonates are safe and effective in these patients (76) (see Chapter 12). Note that because bisphosphonates are absorbed predominantly in the duodenum and jejunum, it is theoretically possible that patients with extensive disease in these regions may have impaired absorption.

In postmenopausal women, one could consider hormone replacement therapy. A 2-year nonrandomized trial of 47 postmenopausal women with IBD demonstrated that bone loss at the forearm and lumbar spine was prevented with conjugated estrogen and progesterone (77).

Case Summary

Mr. R was advised to take 1200 mg of calcium and 400 IU of vitamin D. Serum 25-OH vitamin D levels were normal. BMD testing revealed a T score of –2.3 at the femoral neck and –3.4 at the lumbar spine. Because of his steroid use and BMD results, Mr. R was started on risedronate 5 mg/d. He will be seen in 1 month.

REFERENCES

1. **McHenry MC, et al.** Vertebral osteomyelitis presenting as spinal compression fracture. Six patients with underlying osteoporosis. Arch Intern Med. 1988;148:417–423.

2. **Biyani A, et al.** Thoracic spine fractures in patients older than 50 years. Clin Orthop. 1996;328:190–193.

3. **Kanis JA, et al.** A high incidence of vertebral fracture in women with breast cancer. Br J Cancer. 1999;79:1179–1181.

4. **Nevitt MC, et al.** Effect of alendronate on limited-activity days and bed-disability days caused by back pain in postmenopausal women with existing vertebral fractures. Fracture Intervention Trial Research Group. Arch Intern Med. 2000;160:77–85.

5. **Jensen ME, et al.** Percutaneous polymethylmethacrylate vertebroplasty in the treatment of osteoporotic vertebral body compression fractures: technical aspects. Am J Neuroradiol. 1997;18:1897–1904.

6. **Saarto T, et al.** Clodronate improves bone mineral density in post-menopausal breast cancer patients treated with adjuvant antioestrogens. Br J Cancer. 1997;75:602–605.

7. **Diel IJ, et al.** Reduction in new metastases in breast cancer with adjuvant clodronate treatment. N Engl J Med. 1998;339:357–363.

8. **Nevitt MC, et al.** Association of prevalent vertebral fractures, bone density, and alendronate treatment with incident vertebral fractures: effect of number and spinal location of fractures. The Fracture Intervention Trial Research Group. Bone. 1999;25:613–619.

9. **Ettinger B, Genant HK, Cann CE.** Postmenopausal bone loss is prevented by treatment with low-dosage estrogen with calcium. Ann Intern Med. 1987;106:40–45.

10. **Slemenda C, et al.** Sex steroids and bone mass. A study of changes about the time of menopause. J Clin Invest. 1987;80:1261–1269.

11. **Reeve J, et al.** Determinants of the first decade of bone loss after menopause at spine, hip and radius. QJM. 1999;92:261–273.

12. **Ravn P, et al.** Low body mass index is an important risk factor for low bone mass and increased bone loss in early postmenopausal women. Early Postmenopausal Intervention Cohort (EPIC) study group. J Bone Miner Res. 1999;14:1622–1627.

13. **Sowers MR, et al.** Radial bone mineral density in pre- and perimenopausal women. A prospective study of rates and risk factors for loss. J Bone Miner Res. 1992;7:647–657.

14. **Young R, et al.** Rates of bone loss in peri- and postmenopausal women. A 4 year, prospective, population-based study. Clin Sci (Colch). 1996;91:307–312.

15. **Bauer RL, Deyo RA.** Low risk of vertebral fracture in Mexican American women. Arch Intern Med. 1987;147:1437–1439.

16. **Bauer RL.** Ethnic differences in hip fracture: a reduced incidence in Mexican Americans. Am J Epidemiol. 1988;127:145–149.

17. **Luckey MM, et al.** A prospective study of bone loss in African-American and white women. A clinical research center study. J Clin Endocrinol Metab. 1996;81:2948–2956.

18. **Coope J, Thomson JM, Poller L.** Effects of "natural oestrogen" replacement therapy on menopausal symptoms and blood clotting. BMJ. 1975;4:139–143.

19. **Leonetti HB, Longo S, Anasti JN.** Transdermal progesterone cream for vasomotor symptoms and postmenopausal bone loss. Obstet Gynecol. 1999;94:225–228.

20. **Albrecht BH, et al.** Objective evidence that placebo and oral medroxyprogesterone acetate therapy diminish menopausal vasomotor flushes. Am J Obstet Gynecol. 1981; 139:631–635.

21. **Erlik Y, et al.** Effect of megestrol acetate on flushing and bone metabolism in post-menopausal women. Maturitas. 1981;3:167–172.

22. **Liske E.** Therapeutic efficacy and safety of *Cimicifuga racemosa* for gynecologic disorders. Adv Therapy. 1998;15:43–51.

23. **Brzezinski A, et al.** Short-term effects of phytoestrogen-rich diet on postmenopausal women. Menopause. 1997;4:89–94.

24. **Laufer LR, et al.** Effect of clonidine on hot flashes in postmenopausal women. Obstet Gynecol. 1982;60:583–586.

25. **Barton DL, et al.** Prospective evaluation of vitamin E for hot flashes in breast cancer survivors. J Clin Oncol. 1998;16:495–500.

26. **Slemenda CW, et al.** Predictors of bone mass in perimenopausal women. A prospective study of clinical data using photon absorptiometry. Ann Intern Med. 1990;112: 96–101.

27. **Cummings SR, et al.** Should prescription of postmenopausal hormone therapy be based on the results of bone densitometry? Ann Intern Med. 1990;113:565–567.

28. **Rubin SM, Cummings SR.** Results of bone densitometry affect women's decisions about taking measures to prevent fractures. Ann Intern Med. 1992;116(Pt 1):990–995.

29. **Faulkner KG, Orwoll E.** Use of the WHO criterion in men: is –2.5 the right number? J Bone Miner Res. 2000;15(Suppl 1):S169.

30. **Cauley JA, et al.** Do men and women fracture at the same BMD level? J Bone Miner Res. 2000;15(Suppl):S144.

31. **Melton LJD, et al.** Perspective. How many women have osteoporosis? J Bone Miner Res. 1992;7:1005–1010.

32. **Anderson FH.** Osteoporosis in men. Int J Clin Pract. 1998;52:176–180.

33. **Lunt M, et al.** Bone density variation and its effects on risk of vertebral deformity in men and women studied in thirteen European centers. The EVOS Study. J Bone Miner Res. 1997;12:1883–1894.

34. **Poor G, et al.** Predictors of hip fractures in elderly men. J Bone Miner Res. 1995;10: 1900–1907.

35. **Ross PD.** Risk factors for osteoporotic fracture. Endocrinol Metab Clin North Am. 1998;27:289–301.

36. **Greendale GA, Edelstein S, Barrett-Connor E.** Endogenous sex steroids and bone mineral density in older women and men. The Rancho Bernardo Study. J Bone Miner Res. 1997;12:1833–1843.

37. **Slemenda CW, et al.** Sex steroids and bone mass in older men: positive associations with serum estrogens and negative associations with androgens. J Clin Invest. 1997; 100:1755–1759.

38. **Amin S, et al.** Serum estradiol and the risk for hip fractures in elderly men. J Bone Miner Res. 2000;15(Suppl):S159.

39. **Orwoll E, et al.** Alendronate for the treatment of osteoporosis in men. N Engl J Med. 2000;343:604–610.

40. **Harris ST, et al.** Effects of risedronate treatment on vertebral and nonvertebral fractures in women with postmenopausal osteoporosis. A randomized controlled trial. Vertebral Efficacy with Risedronate Therapy (VERT) Study Group. JAMA. 1999;282: 1344–1352.

41. **Erlacher L, et al.** Salmon calcitonin and calcium in the treatment of male osteoporosis: the effect on bone mineral density. Wien Klin Wochenschr. 1997;109:270–274.

42. **Anderson FH, Francis RM, Faulkner K.** Androgen supplementation in eugonadal men with osteoporosis: effects of 6 months of treatment on bone mineral density and cardiovascular risk factors. Bone. 1996;18:171–177.

43. **Katznelson L, et al.** Increase in bone density and lean body mass during testosterone administration in men with acquired hypogonadism. J Clin Endocrinol Metab. 1996; 81:4358–4365.

44. **Snyder PJ, et al.** Effect of testosterone treatment on bone mineral density in men over 65 years of age. J Clin Endocrinol Metab. 1999;84:1966–1972.

45. **Cummings SR, et al.** Risk factors for hip fracture in white women. Study of Osteoporotic Fractures Research Group. N Engl J Med. 1995;332:767–773.

46. **Kritz-Silverstein D, Barrett-Connor E.** Bone mineral density in postmenopausal women as determined by prior oral contraceptive use. Am J Public Health. 1993;83:100–102.

47. **Michaelsson K, et al.** Oral-contraceptive use and risk of hip fracture. A case-control study. Lancet. 1999;353:1481–1484.

48. **Sowers MR, Galuska DA.** Epidemiology of bone mass in premenopausal women. Epidemiol Rev. 1993;15:374–398.

49. **Tuppurainen M, et al.** The effect of previous oral contraceptive use on bone mineral density in perimenopausal women. Osteoporos Int. 1994;4:93–98.

50. **Bachrach LK, et al.** Recovery from osteopenia in adolescent girls with anorexia nervosa. J Clin Endocrinol Metab. 1991;72:602–606.

51. **Joyce JM, et al.** Osteoporosis in women with eating disorders: comparison of physical parameters, exercise, and menstrual status with SPA and DPA evaluation. J Nucl Med. 1990;31:325–331.

52. **Klibanski A, et al.** The effects of estrogen administration on trabecular bone loss in young women with anorexia nervosa. J Clin Endocrinol Metab. 1995;80:898–904.

53. **Browner WS, et al.** Mortality following fractures in older women. The study of osteoporotic fractures. Arch Intern Med. 1996;156:1521–1525.

54. **Ray NF, et al.** Medical expenditures for the treatment of osteoporotic fractures in the United States in 1995. Report from the National Osteoporosis Foundation. J Bone Miner Res. 1997;12:24–35.

55. **Grisso JA, et al.** Risk factors for falls as a cause of hip fracture in women. The Northeast Hip Fracture Study Group. N Engl J Med. 1991;324:1326–1331.

56. **Tinetti ME, Speechley M, Ginter SF.** Risk factors for falls among elderly persons living in the community. N Engl J Med. 1988;319:1701–1707.

57. **Nevitt MC.** Falls in the elderly: Risk factors and prevention. In: Masdeu JC, Sudarsky L, Wolfson (eds). Gait Disorders of Aging: Falls and Therapeutic Strategies. Philadelphia: Lippincott-Raven; 1987.

58. **Tinetti ME, et al.** A multifactorial intervention to reduce the risk of falling among elderly people living in the community. N Engl J Med. 1994;331:821–827.

59. **Cummings SR.** Treatable and untreatable risk factors for hip fracture. Bone. 1996; 18(Suppl 3):165S-167S.

60. **Kannus P, Parkkari J, Miemi S, et al.** Prevention of hip fracture in elderly people with use of a hip protector. N Engl J Med. 2000;343:1506–1513.

61. **Black DM, et al.** Randomised trial of effect of alendronate on risk of fracture in women with existing vertebral fractures. Fracture Intervention Trial Research Group. Lancet. 1996;348:1535–1541.

62. **Harris ST, et al.** Effects of risedronate treatment on vertebral and nonvertebral fractures in women with postmenopausal osteoporosis. A randomized controlled trial. Vertebral Efficacy with Risedronate Therapy (VERT) Study Group. JAMA. 1999;282:1344–1352.

63. **Cummings SR, et al.** Monitoring osteoporosis therapy with bone densitometry: misleading changes and regression to the mean. Fracture Intervention Trial Research Group. JAMA. 2000;283:1318–1321.

64. **Lindsay R, et al.** Addition of alendronate to ongoing hormone replacement therapy in the treatment of osteoporosis. A randomized, controlled clinical trial. J Clin Endocrinol Metab. 1999;84:3076–3081.

65. **Saarto T, et al.** Clodronate improves bone mineral density in post-menopausal breast cancer patients treated with adjuvant antioestrogens. Br J Cancer. 1997;75:602–605.

66. **Bjarnason I, Macpherson A, Mackintosh C, et al.** Reduced bone density in patients with inflammatory bowel disease. Gut. 1997;40:228–233.

67. **Valentine JF, Sninsky CA.** Prevention and treatment of osteoporosis in patients with inflammatory bowel disease. Am J Gastroenterol. 1999;94:878–883.

68. **Schulte C, Dignass AU, Mann K, Goebell H.** Bone loss in patients with inflammatory bowel disease is less than expected. A follow-up study. Scand J Gastroenterol. 1999; 34:696–702.

69. **Roux C, Abitbol V, Chaussade S, et al.** Bone loss in patients with inflammatory bowel disease: a prospective study. Osteoporos Int. 1995;5:156–160.

70. **Ghosh S, Cowen S, Hannan WJ, Ferguson A.** Low bone mineral density in Crohn's disease, but not in ulcerative colitis, at diagnosis. Gastroenterology. 1994;107:1031–1039.

71. **Silvennoinen JA, Karttunen TJ, Niemela SE, et al.** A controlled study of bone mineral density in patients with inflammatory bowel disease. Gut. 1995;37:71–76.

72. **Bernstein CN, Seeger LL, Anton PA, et al.** A randomized, placebo-controlled trial of calcium supplementation for decreased bone density in corticosteroid-using patients with inflammatory bowel disease. A pilot study. Aliment Pharmacol Ther. 1996; 10:777–786.

73. **LaCroix AZ, Ott SM, Ichikawa L, et al.** Low-dose hydrochlorothiazide and preservation of bone mineral density in older adults. A randomized, double-blind, placebo-controlled trial. Ann Intern Med. 2000;133:516–526.

74. **Vogelsang H, Ferenci P, Resch H, et al.** Prevention of bone mineral loss in patients with Crohn's disease by long-term oral vitamin D supplementation. Eur J Gastroenterol Hepatol. 1995;7:609–614.

75. **Driscoll RH, Jr., Meredith SC, Sitrin M, Rosenberg IH.** Vitamin D deficiency and bone disease in patients with Crohn's disease. Gastroenterology. 1982;83:1252–1258.

76. **Saag KG, Emkey R, Schnitzer TJ, et al.** Alendronate for the prevention and treatment of glucocorticoid-induced osteoporosis. Glucocorticoid-Induced Osteoporosis Intervention Study Group. N Engl J Med. 1998;339:292–299.

77. **Clements D, Compston JE, Evans WD, Rhodes J.** Hormone replacement therapy prevents bone loss in patients with inflammatory bowel disease. Gut. 1993;34:1543–1546.

Selection of Medications and Guidelines for Fracture Prevention

Selection of Medications and Guidelines for Fracture Prevention

FELICIA COSMAN, MD
SOPHIE A. JAMAL, MD
STEVEN R. CUMMINGS, MD

This chapter is a summary of the previous chapters and presents a practical approach to the prevention of fractures in practice. We start with the editors' Guidelines adapted from the 1998 National Osteoporosis Foundation (NOF) Guidelines (1), then provide a general strategy for prescription of medications for prevention of fractures, and end with some ideas for putting prevention into practice.

Recommendations for Prevention

The NOF sponsored a very rigorous process of review and analysis of evidence that included formal assessment of the cost-effectiveness of risk factor and bone density screening and treatment for prevention of fractures (2). Based on this process, the NOF developed a Physicians' Guide that also incorporated the views of experts about approaches to prevention. Two of the editors of this book (FC and SRC) participated in this process. These earlier guidelines established very important principles, such as screening of white women aged 65 or older and making decisions to start drug treatment based on the results of hip-bone density and risk factors. Specifically, the 1998 NOF Guidelines advocated pharmacologic therapy for postmenopausal women with a T score of –2.0 or below and –1.5 or below in postmenopausal women who had clinical risk factors.

273

Since the original Guidelines were developed, there have been a number of advances, many reviewed in this book. In particular, there is stronger evidence that women with osteoporosis benefit the most from one of several treatments for osteoporosis. Therefore, using the NOF Guidelines as a starting point, the authors have developed recommendations that reflect this new evidence. Similar treatment guidelines were also developed by the American Academy of Clinical Endocrinology in 2001.

Guidelines for Prevention of Fractures

General Recommendations

- Counsel all individuals on the risk of osteoporosis. Osteoporosis is a "silent" risk factor for fracture, just as hypertension is for stroke. From age 50 on, one out of two white women and one in eight men can expect to suffer a hip, forearm, or spine fracture.

- Advise all patients to obtain an adequate intake of dietary calcium (at least 1200 mg/day, including supplements if necessary). Advise all patients to obtain an adequate intake of vitamin D (at least 400 IU per day). In particular, all patients who are homebound or in long-term care should receive 800 IU/day of vitamin D.

- Recommend lifelong regular weight-bearing and muscle-strengthening exercise to reduce the risk of falls and fractures.

- Advise and help patients to quit smoking.

- Recognize and treat alcoholism.

Bone Mineral Density Testing

- Recommend bone mineral density (BMD) testing to all white women aged 65 and older, regardless of additional risk factors.

- In postmenopausal women under age 65, measure bone density in all postmenopausal white women who have had fractures and in other individuals with one or more risk factors. The principal risk factors are taking oral glucocorticoid therapy for more than 3 months, parental history of hip or confirmed spine fracture, weight less than 127 lbs, current cigarette smoking, and selected chronic diseases known to be associated with osteoporosis (see Chapter 3).

- There are currently no evidence-based guidelines for bone density testing in non-white women and men.

- It is clinically reasonable to perform bone density testing in non-white women and men who have significant risk factors for fracture, for example in people receiving long-term steroids or who have had atraumatic fractures.

Pharmacologic Treatment

- Recommend pharmacologic treatment for any individual with a hip or vertebral fracture or osteoporosis indicated by BMD testing (a T score of less than or equal to –2.5 at the femoral neck or lumbar spine).

- Consider pharmacologic prevention of osteoporosis for women with a T score at the hip or lumbar spine between –1.5 and –2.5, depending on number and strength of clinical risk factors; for women who have had a low trauma fracture; for women who are at high risk because of long-term oral steroid use; and for women who have other strong risk factors or chronic diseases that are known to increase the risk of fractures.

- Pharmacologic options approved by the US FDA for osteoporosis prevention or treatment include bisphosphonates (alendronate, risedronate), raloxifene, PTH, estrogen (hormone replacement therapy [HRT]), or calcitonin. A discussion of how to select medication for individual patients follows.

Note that these recommendations may not apply to countries outside of the United States, Canada, and Europe, where risk of fractures is lower, densitometry is less accessible, and treatments are more expensive in relation to the financial means of patients. In these circumstances, it is reasonable to reserve testing and treatment to patients who have more risk factors for fracture than these recommendations suggest for white women.

Selection of Treatment for Individual Patients

Pharmacologic intervention for management of osteoporosis must be tailored to individual patients according to the patient's age, fracture history, and the medication's effect on the risk for other diseases. Determining the optimal duration of treatment must also follow some of the same considerations. One approach is to use a medication only for the duration of time that clinical trials indicate efficacy and safety. For most agents, however, there are only data for up to 5 years. It is likely that effects against fracture might wane with time after discontinuation of the drug, making short-term treatment inadequate.

Another approach is to continue any therapy indefinitely. The problem with this, of course, is that patients might be subjected to long-term safety issues in addition to unknown long-term efficacy. Some data indicate a slightly lesser effect on fracture reduction between years 1 and 4 compared with effects against fracture during the first year of therapy. Beyond this time period, no good clinical trial data exist with fracture as the primary outcome. Furthermore, long-term safety might be an issue with agents such as the bisphosphonates, which accumulate in bone with a very long half-life (estimated at 10 years). The ability of the skeleton to remodel in response to fatigue damage after very long-term treatment is unknown. The third approach is to rotate agents to obtain an optimal efficacy and safety profile, a concept that can be termed *serial monotherapy*. Regardless of the approach, physicians should review treatment plans annually in light of new data and concepts about long-term prevention of fractures.

Women in the Early Menopausal Years (Late 40s to Early 50s)

For patients who are recently menopausal and having menopausal symptoms, estrogens are the most effective choice to relieve menopausal symptoms. Estrogen will also protect bone mass. However, if a woman takes estrogen for treatment of symptoms, it may be possible to taper and discontinue therapy within 6 months to a year. In a smaller group of women, more prolonged treatment might be necessary for relief of menopausal symptoms.

Asymptomatic patients who have osteoporosis should consider treatment to prevent fractures. For these patients, small clinical trials suggest that estrogen might reduce fracture risk in this age group. Patients making the choice regarding HRT for prevention of fractures must weigh the risks and benefits of estrogen for a variety of conditions including ischemic heart disease, venous thromboembolism, uterine and colon cancer, and the risk of breast cancer after long-term use. If a patient continues to use estrogen for potential prevention of fractures, it is wise to reconsider the risks and benefits of ongoing use of HRT every few years because the risk of breast cancer, particularly in thin women, appears to increase with duration of use beyond 5 to 10 years. The risk of estrogen alone, in the absence of progestin, may differ with regard to this outcome.

If a woman with osteoporosis elects to stop estrogen therapy, it is important to note that bone loss tends to ensue at a rapid rate upon estrogen withdrawal, and observational studies indicate that any protection against fracture largely disappears within a few years after stopping.

Women who choose to stop taking estrogen but have osteoporosis or a high enough risk of fractures to warrant drug therapy should consider alternative treatment such as bisphosphonate or raloxifene (see below).

Women in the Middle Menopausal Years
(Early 50s to Late 60s)

Estrogen is usually not needed for control of symptoms at this stage. If a woman has been taking estrogen for several years, it is wise to consider whether estrogen should be continued in view of data about the risks and potential benefits of long-term estrogen therapy.

If a woman has osteoporosis or risk of fractures that warrants drug therapy to prevent fractures, a bisphosphonate is a reasonable choice, especially if the patient has severe osteoporosis or additional risk factors for hip fracture. Bisphosphonates not only protect against vertebral and hip fracture but also against other types fractures that produce a substantial amount of morbidity and disability in this age group. The optimal duration of bisphosphonate therapy is unknown. The potential downsides of continuing bisphosphonates for a very long term are reviewed above. If started in these relatively young women and then discontinued after 5 years, it is unclear what fracture reduction effect will persist 10 to 20 years later.

Raloxifene is also a reasonable alternative for many women for the purpose of reducing the risk of vertebral fracture; it has the additional advantage of reducing the risk of breast cancer.

Women who have osteoporosis in this age group and who cannot take bisphosphonates or raloxifene, and cannot or have decided not to take estrogen, may benefit from intranasal calcitonin. However, calcitonin appears to be the weakest agent for improvement of bone density and prevention of fractures.

Late Menopausal Women (Middle or
Late 60s and Older)

Note that almost 50% of women who live to age 65 have bone density levels consistent with a diagnosis of osteoporosis. These women are at substantially increased risk for hip fracture as a function of both age and BMD. Because of the strength of clinical trial data that bisphosphonates effectively reduce the risk of hip and other fractures, this class of drugs is clearly the treatment of choice for women in this age group. It is reasonable to use alternative dosing strategies, such as 70 mg of alendronate once per week or 35 mg of risedronate once per week, in any patients who have difficulty with the daily regimen. Even considering the use of a once-weekly H_2 blocker or proton-pump inhibitor before a once-weekly regimen of bisphosphonate is reasonable in these women. If these strategies for bisphosphonate use fail, estrogen and raloxifene may be alternatives; however, evidence from trials confirming that they reduce the risk of hip fracture is lacking. Calcitonin, which appears to have the weakest effects, is another alternative.

Box 14-1   Prevention of Fractures in White Women

- For all: adequate calcium, vitamin D, and lifelong exercise

- Recommend BMD testing (preferably hip)
  —All white women ≥ age 65
  —50–65 with ≥ 1 risk factor for fracture*

- Recommend drug treatment† for women with
  —Vertebral or hip fracture
  —T score ≤ –2.5 at the hip (or spine)

- Consider drug tx if T score < –1.5 + risk factors

* Past fracture, parental or hip fracture, weight < 127 lbs, smoking, selected chronic diseases that increase fracture risk, current oral steroid treatment ≥ 3 months.
† Alendronate, risedronate, raloxifene, PTH, estrogen, or nasal calcitonin.

Combination Treatments

Trials have generally found that combinations of anti-resorptive drugs such as bisphosphonate and estrogen add a little BMD to what is achieved by a single drug. There is no evidence (and probably never will be) that combinations reduce fracture risk significantly more than the most effective drug alone. Because these agents seem to act mainly by reducing bone resorption, it is unlikely that there would be a substantial further reduction in fracture. Even if combinations decrease risk somewhat more than individual drugs, combination therapy adds cost and risk of side-effects and may increase the concern about the long-term effects of dramatic reductions in bone turnover. Therefore, combination therapies should be used very sparingly in managing patients with osteoporosis and should probably never be used simply for reducing the rate of bone loss in patients without osteoporosis.

An additional drug is sometimes added because a patient appears to have lost bone density during monitoring. This should prompt queries about adherence but not necessarily a change in treatment. It is important to recognize that decreases in bone density during treatment are common, even with effective drug treatments, and are usually followed by increases in bone density if the single treatment is continued (see Chapter 2). A second drug is sometimes added if a patient suffers a fracture during treatment. However, it is important to note that occurrence of a fracture does not mean that treatment is inadequate. Existing therapies only reduce fracture risk; they do not necessarily prevent all fractures. Fractures may continue with effective

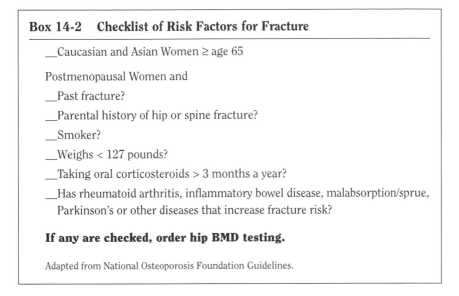

Box 14-2   Checklist of Risk Factors for Fracture

__Caucasian and Asian Women ≥ age 65

Postmenopausal Women and

__Past fracture?

__Parental history of hip or spine fracture?

__Smoker?

__Weighs < 127 pounds?

__Taking oral corticosteroids > 3 months a year?

__Has rheumatoid arthritis, inflammatory bowel disease, malabsorption/sprue, Parkinson's or other diseases that increase fracture risk?

If any are checked, order hip BMD testing.

Adapted from National Osteoporosis Foundation Guidelines.

treatment, and addition of a second drug cannot be expected to 'prevent' fractures or even improve the effectiveness of a treatment regimen.

Parathyroid hormone works by a different mechanism than do antiresorptive drugs. Addition of parathyroid hormone may be a valuable option to reduce fracture risk for patients with severe osteoporosis who continue to be at high risk despite antiresorptive therapy (see Chapter 11).

How to Put Prevention of Osteoporosis into Practice

Advances in the past decade have resulted in the ability of physicians to effectively prevent fractures. Prevention of osteoporosis and fractures should be part of the repertoire of all primary care providers, but the importance of osteoporosis may not come to mind during a short patient visit, especially with elderly patients who have many other problems that seem more urgent. However, it is worthwhile to take a few moments, with the help of office staff, to make a few simple arrangements that will make prevention of osteoporosis and fractures an easier and more integrated part of the primary care practice.

Provide Patients with Information

The NOF has excellent, colorful, and readable brochures that your patients will appreciate, which cover topics such as nutrition, exercise, and bone

---

Box 14-3   Scoring of Risk Factors for Fracture

Schedule BMD Testing if Score ≥ 6:

__5 points if patient is not black

__4 points if patient has rheumatoid arthritis

__4 points for a history of each fracture of the wrist, hip, or rib that occurred with minimal trauma after age 45 (maximum of 12 points)

__Add points equal to 3 times the first digit of age in years (e.g., patient aged 53 = 3 × 50 = 150)

__1 point if patient has never used estrogen

__Subtract weight in pounds and divide by 10 (truncated to integer) for final score

---

density testing. They can be conveniently ordered at the NOF Web site, www.nof.org.

Involve Office Staff

Office staff may aid in counseling patients about osteoporosis, bone density testing, and basic health information. For example, staff may quickly become familiar with guidelines for bone density testing and advice about calcium and exercise and could give this information to selected patients either routinely or at the doctor's request.

Add Screening for Fracture Risk and Prevention of Fractures to the Patient Screening Checklist

Many offices have checklists or systems for reminding patients, for example, to get periodic mammograms. Consider incorporating a checklist or system for patient reminders about fracture risk screenings. Several risk factor lists have been shown to have very high sensitivities for identifying patients with osteoporosis.

Make Referrals for Bone Mineral Density Testing Easy

Post the telephone number of a nearby facility that is experienced and reliable at testing BMD, particularly one that offers dual x-ray absorptiometry (3) testing of hip and spine. Make sure that referral or order slips for BMD testing are readily available in examination rooms or at the front desk.

A Final Word

Fractures are preventable but only if physicians take the first simple steps toward recognizing patients who are at risk and recommending effective treatments. It is hoped that the preceding chapters have provided the reader with the information necessary to screen and identify patients at risk for osteoporosis, and to effectively treat them, both preventively and symptomatically.

Boxes 14-1 to 14-3 summarize suggestions for prevention of fractures and risk factor information.

REFERENCES

1. **National Osteoporosis Foundation.** Physician's Guide to Prevention and Treatment of Osteoporosis. Belle Mead, NJ: Excerpta Medica; 1998.
2. Osteoporosis: Review of the Evidence for Prevention, Diagnosis, and Tretment, and Cost-Effectiveness Analysis. Status Report. Osteoporos Int. 1998;(Suppl 4):1–88.
3. **Cadarette SM, Jaglal SB, Murray TM, et al.** Evaluation of decision rules for referring women for bone densitometry by dual-energy x-ray absorptiometry. JAMA. 2001;286: 57–63.

Index

A

Absorptiometry, dual energy x-ray,
    55–56
Absorption of calcium, 86
Activity, physical. *See* Exercise
Age
    bone changes with, 11–12
    fracture risk related to, 39–40
Alcohol, 101–102
Alendronate
    for breast cancer patient, 245
    case study of, 260–263
    indications for, 182
    instructions about, 191–192
    studies of, 183–187
Alkaline phosphatase, 62
    in secondary osteoporosis, 76, 79
Amenorrhea, 246–249
Anabolic agent, 209–219
    fluoride, 214, 216–217
    growth hormone, 215
    insulin-like growth factor, 215
    parathyroid hormone and, 210–214
    statins, 218
    steroids, 215, 218
Analgesic effect of calcitonin, 204–205
Anorexia nervosa, 253–254
Antibody, endomysial, 81
Antiresorptive therapy, 70
Areal bone density, 31
Atraumatic wrist fracture, 249–252
Atrophy, vaginal, 140

B

Back pain, radiography for, 50
Biochemical marker, 60–71. *See also*
    Marker
Biologic variability in bone turnover
    markers, 69–71
Bisphosphonate, 181–193
    anorexia nervosa and, 255–256
    bone resorption markers and, 67–68
    for breast cancer patient, 245
    Crohn's disease and, 265

Bisphosphonate (*cont'd.*)
    glucocorticoid-induced osteoporosis
        and, 227–231
Black cohosh, 170–171
Bone
    biology of, 3–12
        age-related changes and, 11–12
        minerals in, 4
        protein in, 3–4
        remodeling in, 8–11
    exercise affecting, 110
    phytoestrogen and, 172, 174
    structure of, 5–7
Bone densitometry, 29–49. *See also*
    Densitometry
Bone density. *See* Bone mineral density
Bone loss
    age-related, 11–12
    bisphosphonates to prevent, 189
    marker of, 64–65
Bone mass
    in athlete, 112
    calcium and, 87–88
    definition of, 30, 31
    fracture risk and, 13
    genetics of, 16
    in nonathlete, 112–113
    peak, 253
    raloxifene and, 160
    risk for decrease in, 16–17
    tamoxifen and, 154
    vitamin D and, 95
Bone mineral content, 30, 31
Bone mineral density
    alendronate and, 260–263
    bisphosphonates and, 183, 189
    calcitonin and, 198, 201
    cancer and, 242
    definition of, 30, 31
    differences in, 32–33
    estrogen and, 128–133
    fracture risk related to, 38–40
    glucocorticoid-induced osteoporosis
        and, 224–225
    physical activity and, 113–117
    phytoestrogen and, 172
    protein and, 95, 98

Bone mineral density (*cont'd.*)
    risedronate and, 187–189
    secondary osteoporosis and, 42–43
    vitamin D and, 96
Bone turnover, markers of, 60–71. *See also* Marker
Bone ultrasound attenuation, 31
Boron, 101
Breast
    raloxifene and, 162–163
    tamoxifen and, 158
Breast cancer
    estrogen and, 142
    phytoestrogens and, 174
    vertebral fracture with, 241–246
Breast Cancer Prevention Trial, 157

C

Caffeine, 99
Calcitonin, 197–206
    bone resorption markers and, 67–68
    effects of, 204–205
    for glucocorticoid-induced
        osteoporosis, 204, 234
    injectable, 198–200
    as nasal spray, 201–204
    recommendations for, 205
Calcium, 86–94
    bone mass and, 87–88
    for breast cancer patient, 245
    estrogen and, 129
    glucocorticoid-induced osteoporosis
        and, 226–227
    hip fracture and, 260
    metabolism of, 86–87
    National Osteoporosis Foundation
        guidelines for, 274
    nutrients affecting, 87
    for premenopausal female, 254
    prevention of osteoporosis and, 19
    recommendations for, 88
    in secondary osteoporosis, 76, 77,
        78
    supplementation with, 88–94
    vitamin D and, 95, 97
Calcium carbonate, 89
Calcium citrate, 89, 93
Calcium hydroxyapatite, 4
Cardiovascular system, phytoestrogens
    and, 174–175

Celiac disease, secondary osteoporosis
    in, 81
Cell, bone, 5, 8
Central nervous system
    raloxifene and, 163
    tamoxifen and, 159
Child, calcium for, 87
Cholesterol
    estrogen and, 140–141
    tamoxifen and, 158–159
Clinical case, 241–266
    alendronate therapy, 260–263
    amenorrhea and hot flushes, 246–249
    atraumatic wrist fracture in male,
        249–252
    Crohn's disease, 263–266
    fracture risk, 252–257
    hip fracture, 257–260
    vertebral fracture with breast cancer,
        241–246
Clodronate, 182
Clomiphene, 152
Coefficient of variation, 31
collA2 gene, 4
Collagen
    in bone, 3–4
    crosslinks of, 62–63
Combination drug therapy, 278–279
Complete blood count, 76
Compression fracture. *See* Vertebral
    fracture
Computed tomography, quantitative, 30
Conjugated equine estrogen, 138, 139
Contraceptive, oral, 253–254
Cortical bone, 5–6
Cortisol, 80–81
Coumestan, 170
Creatinine, 77
Crohn's disease, 263–266
CTX, urine, 64, 65
Cushing's syndrome, 80–81

D

Densitometry, 29–49
    alendronate and, 262
    in breast cancer patient, 244
    clinical uses of, 37–43
        diagnosing osteoporosis, 40–42
        drug treatment and, 43
        fracture risk prediction, 37–40

Densitometry (*cont'd.*)
    clinical uses of (*cont'd.*)
        medical evaluation, 42–43
    in early postmenopausal patient, 248
    indications for, 43–44
    for monitoring, 46–49
    National Osteoporosis Foundation
        guidelines for, 274–275
    in premenopausal female, 254
    recommendations for, 280
    sites for, 44–46
    techniques used for, 33–37
    terminology of, 30–33
    ultrasound, 36–37, 46
        characteristics of, 36–37
Density, bone. *See* Bone mineral density
Deydroepiandrosterone (DHEA),
    169–170, 175–176
DHEAS, 175–176
Diet, 85–103. *See also* Nutrition
Drinking water, fluoride in, 101
Drug therapy
    combination, 278–279
    densitometry and, 43
    in early menopause, 276
    in middle menopause, 277
    National Osteoporosis Foundation
        recommendations for, 275
    for postmenopausal patient, 277–280
    for prevention of, 19–20
Dual energy x-ray absorptiometry
    of hip, 33–34
    peripheral, 35
    vertebral fracture and, 55–56

E

Education, patient
    about estrogen therapy, 145–146
    about osteoporosis, 279–280
Elderly
    exercise and, 120
    hip fracture in, 257–260
    hormone replacement therapy in,
        139
Electrophoresis, 76, 80
Endometrial cancer, 142–143
Endomysial antibody, 81
Endplate vertebral fracture, 51
Esophagitis, 191
Esterified estrogen, 143

Estradiol, 78
Estrogen, 127–146
    anorexia nervosa and, 255–256
    bone mineral density and,
        128–133
    bone resorption markers and, 67–68
    calcium supplements and, 129
    controlled trials of, 135–138
    FDA-approved, 134
    fracture prevention and, 138–139
    for hot flushes, 247
    osteoporotic fracture and, 129, 134
Estrogen-receptor modulator, selective,
    151–164
Estrogen-receptor positive breast
    cancer, 158
Ethnic differences, 20–21
Etidronate, 182
    for breast cancer patient, 245
    indications for, 182
    studies of, 183
Exercise, 109–122
    controlled trials of, 113–120
    Crohn's disease and, 264–265
    falls and fractures and, 117
    observational studies of, 111–113
    physiology of, 110–111
    for premenopausal female, 254
    prevention of osteoporosis and, 19
    recommendations for, 121–122
    vertebral fractures and, 117, 121

F

Fall
    physical activity and, 113
    treatment to reduce, 258–259
Fatigue damage to bone, 6
FDA-approved estrogen, 134
Female
    bone densitometry of, 43
    femoral T score of, 40
    fracture risk in, 13, 14
    postmenopausal. *See* Postmenopausal
        female
Femoral neck
    bone densitometry of, 44–45
    T score of, fracture risk and, 40
Flare of Crohn's disease, 263–266
Flow chart for glucocorticoid-induced
    osteoporosis, 235

Fluoride, 101, 214, 216–217
  for glucocorticoid-induced
    osteoporosis, 234
Food. *See* Nutrition
Food and Drug Administration,
    estrogens approved by, 134
Food group, 102
Fracture
  alendronate and, 187
  calcitonin and, 198, 201, 204
  consequences of, 18
  epidemiology of, 13–18
  estrogen and, 129, 134, 138–139
  hip
    case study of, 257–260
    importance of, 16
    in secondary osteoporosis, 73–74
  physical activity and, 113
  prevention and treatment of, 18–22
  risedronate and, 189, 190
  risk of, 13–18
    amenorrhea and, 246–249
    bone markers predicting, 65
    densitometry in assessment of,
      37–40
    screening for, 280
  tamoxifen and, 156, 157
  vertebral. *See* Vertebral fracture
  vitamin D and, 95, 97

G

Gastrointestinal system, alendronate
    affecting, 191
Gender, fracture risk related to, 13,
    17
Gene, *collA2*, 4
Genetics, bone mass and, 16
Geographic region, practice guidelines
    and, 20–21
Gla-protein, 62
Gliadin, 81
Glucocorticoid-induced osteoporosis,
    204, 223–236
  bisphosphonates for, 227–231
  bone density and, 224–225
  calcitonin for, 234
  calcium in, 226–227
  flow chart for, 235
  fluoride for, 234
  fracture and, 225

Glucocorticoid-induced osteoporosis
    (*cont'd.*)
  parathyroid hormone for, 234
  pathogenesis of, 224
  recommendations for, 235–236
  sex hormones and, 231
  vitamin D for, 226–227, 231–233
Gonadotropin, 78
Growth, bone changes in, 11
Growth hormone, 215

H

Hand
  radiograph of, 36
  wrist fracture in male and,
    249–252
Heart and Estrogen/Progestin
    Replacement Study, 138, 141
Heart disease, 140–141
Height, vertebral fracture and, 55
High-density lipoprotein
  estrogen and, 140–141
  tamoxifen and, 158–159
Hip
  bone densitometry of, 44–45
  dual energy x-ray absorptiometry of,
    33–34
Hip fracture
  case study of, 257–260
  importance of, 16, 257
  in secondary osteoporosis, 73–74
Histamine in mastocytosis, 81
Hormone
  growth, 215
  parathyroid, 210–214
    glucocorticoid-induced
      osteoporosis and, 234
    in secondary osteoporosis, 79–80
    vitamin D and, 94
  sex
    glucocorticoid-induced
      osteoporosis and, 231
    in secondary osteoporosis, 77–78
  testosterone, 76–78
Hormone replacement therapy,
    127–146. *See also* Estrogen
  parathyroid hormone and,
    210–211
  selective estrogen-receptor
    modulators and, 169

Hot flushes, amenorrhea with, 246–249
Hydroxyapatite, 181

I

Injectable calcitonin, 198–200
Insulin-like growth factor, 215
Ipriflavone, 172, 174
Isoflavone, 170

L

Lead in calcium supplement, 89
Lignan, 170
Lining cell, 5
Lipoprotein
    estrogen and, 140–141
    tamoxifen and, 158–159
Liver function test, 76
Long-term care, 44
Low-density lipoprotein
    estrogen and, 140–141
    tamoxifen and, 158–159

M

Magnesium, 100–101
Male
    alendronate for, 187
    bone densitometry of, 43
    fracture risk in, 13, 14
    wrist fracture in, 249–252
Marker, 60–71
    of bone formation, 62
    of bone remodeling, 60–62
    of bone resorption, 62–63
    fracture risk and, 65
    interpretation of, 63–64
    of postmenopausal bone loss, 64–65
    treatment response and, 65, 66, 67
Mass, bone. See Bone mass
Mastocytosis, 81
Matrix protein, 4
Menopause
    bone changes with, 11–12
    calcium loss in, 86–87
Metabolism
    of calcium, 86–87

Metabolism (*cont'd.*)
    phytoestrogen and, 172, 174
Metastasis, breast cancer, 241–246
Microdamage, 6, 31
Microfracture to bone, 31
Mineral, 4, 30
Mineral density, bone. See Bone mineral density
Mineralization, 4
Modulator, selective estrogen-receptor, 151–164
Monitoring
    bone markers for, 65, 67–69
    densitometry for, 46–49
Multiple myeloma
    protein electrophoresis for, 80
    vertebral fracture and, 243
Muscle, exercise affecting, 110–111

N

Nasal spray calcitonin, 201–204
National Osteoporosis Foundation guidelines, 273–275
Natural progesterone, 175
Nervous system
    raloxifene and, 163
    tamoxifen and, 159
Nitrogen-containing bisphosphonate, 182
Nitrogen-free bisphosphonate, 182
Non-collagen protein, 4
Non-white female, 43
Nutrition, 85–103
    alcohol and, 101–102
    boron and, 101
    caffeine and, 99
    calcium and, 86–94
        bone mass and, 87–88
        metabolism of, 86–87
        recommendations for, 88
        supplementation with, 88–94
    Crohn's disease and, 264–265
    fluoride and, 101
    food groups and, 102
    magnesium and, 100–101
    phosphorus and, 98
    protein and, 95, 98
    salt and, 98
    vitamin A and, 100
    vitamin C and, 100

Nutrition (*cont'd.*)
vitamin D and, 94–97
vitamin K and, 99–100
NXT, urine, 64, 65, 67

O

Oral contraceptive, 253–254
Osteoblast
estrogen receptors and, 171
in remodeling, 9–11
Osteocalcin, 62
Osteoclast, 8, 10–11
Osteocyte, 8
Osteon, 5
Osteopenia, 31
Osteoporosis
definition of, 31
densiometry in diagnosis of, 40–42
prevention and treatment of, 18–21

P

Pain, back, radiography for, 50
Parathyroid hormone, 210–214
glucocorticoid-induced osteoporosis
and, 234
in secondary osteoporosis, 79–80
vitamin D and, 94
Patient education, 279–280
about estrogen therapy, 145–146
Peripheral dual energy x-ray
absorptiometry, 35
Pharmacokinetics of bisphosphonates,
191–192
Phosphorus, 98
Physical activity, 109–122
controlled trials of, 113–120
Crohn's disease and, 264–265
in early postmenopausal patient,
247–248
falls and fractures and, 117
observational studies of, 111–113
physiology of, 110–111
for premenopausal female, 254
recommendations for, 121–122
vertebral fractures and, 117, 121
Phytoestrogen, 169–177
bone metabolism and, 172, 174
classification of, 170–171

Phytoestrogen (*cont'd.*)
mechanism of action, 171–172
skeletal effects of, 173
tissue-specific effects of, 174–175
Postmenopausal female
alendronate and, 184–186
alendronate for, 260–263
calcitonin and, 200, 202–203
calcium for, 88, 90–92
drug therapy recommendations for,
277–280
estrogen therapy for, 127–146. *See
also* Estrogen
exercise and, 113–116
fracture risk in, 246–247
marker of bone resorption in, 64–65
raloxifene in, 161–164
risedronate and, 189
tamoxifen and, 153–157
Premenopausal female
calcium for, 87–88
exercise and, 117, 118–119
osteoporosis risk in, 253
Prevention of osteoporosis, 18–21
Procollagen type I C propeptide, 62
Procollagen type I N propeptide, 62
Progesterone, natural, 175
Prolactin, 78
Protein
in bone, 3–4
calcium loss and, 86–87
dietary, 95, 98
excess, 102
Protein electrophoresis, 76, 80
Pyridinium crosslink of type I collagen,
62–63

Q

Quantitative computed tomography, 30
indications for, 36

R

Racial differences, in fracture risk,
246–247
Radiography
of hand, 36
of vertebral fracture
indications for, 49–51

Radiography (cont'd.)
    of vertebral fracture (cont'd.)
        interpretation of, 51–55
Raloxifene, 152
    bone resorption markers and,
        67–68
    breast and, 162–163
    central nervous system and, 163
    recommendations on, 163–164
    reproductive system and, 163
    skeletal effects of, 160, 161
    vascular disease and, 163
Remodeling, bone
    alendronate and, 191
    markers of, 60, 62
    normal, 7–11
Reproductive system
    raloxifene and, 163
    tamoxifen and, 159
Resistance, to calcitonin, 205
Resorption, bone, markers of, 60–63
Resveratrol, 170–171
Rib fracture, 73
Risedronate
    for breast cancer patient, 245
    indications for, 182
    instructions about, 191–192
    studies of, 187–190

S

Safety of calcium supplement, 88–89
Salmon calcitonin, 201–204
Salt, dietary, 98
Secondary amenorrhea, 253
Secondary osteoporosis, 20
    calcium homeostasis and, 78–80
    celiac disease and, 81
    Cushing's syndrome and, 80–81
    densitometry in diagnosis of, 42–43
    evaluation of, 71–73
    fracture in
        hip, 73–74
        rib and vertebral, 73
    low bone density and, 74–75
    mastocytosis and, 81
    multiple myeloma and, 80
    sex hormones and, 77–78
    testing for, 75–77
    thyroid-stimulating hormone and,
        80

Selective estrogen-receptor modulator
    (SERM), 151–164
    hormone replacement therapy and,
        169
    raloxifene, 161–164
    tamoxifen, 152–161
Serum calcium in secondary
    osteoporosis, 78
Sex hormone
    glucocorticoid-induced osteoporosis
        and, 231
    in secondary osteoporosis, 77–78
Single energy x-ray absorptiometry of, 34
Skeletal system
    ipriflavone and, 173
    raloxifene and, 160, 161
    tamoxifen effects on, 153–157
Sodium
    calcium loss and, 86
    salt intake and, 98
Spine
    imaging of, 49–56
        dual energy x-ray absorptiometry,
            34–35, 55–56
        fracture location and, 51
        interpretation of, 51–55
        when to take, 49–51
    vertebral fracture of. See Vertebral
        fracture
Statin, 218
Steroid, anabolic, 215, 218
Strength, exercise and, 110–111
Supplement
    calcium, 88–94, 129. See also
        Calcium
    vitamin K, 99–100

T

T score, 30–32
    bisphosphonates and, 192
    drug therapy and, 275
    in early postmenopausal patient, 248
    in secondary osteoporosis, 74
Tamoxifen, 152
    breast and, 158
    central nervous system and, 159
    recommendations for, 159, 161
    reproductive system and, 159
    skeletal effects of, 153–157
    vascular disease and, 158–159

Telopeptide of type I collagen, 62–63
Terminology in bone densitometry,
    30–33
Testosterone, 76, 77–78
Thyroid-stimulating hormone, 76,
    80
Tibolone, 152
Toremifene, 152
Trabecular bone
    density of, 31
    structure of, 5, 6

U

Ultrasound, necessity of, 46
Ultrasound attenuation, bone, 31
Ultrasound densitometry, 36–37
Urinary calcium
    protein and, 95
    in secondary osteoporosis, 77, 79
    sodium and, 86–87
Urine CTX, 64, 65
Urine NXT, 64, 65, 67

V

Vaginal atrophy, 140
Vaginal bleeding, 145
Variability, biologic, in bone turnover
    markers, 69–71
Vascular system
    phytoestrogens and, 174
    raloxifene and, 163
    tamoxifen and, 158–159
Vertebral fracture
    alendronate and, 187
    breast cancer with, 241–246
    exercise and, 117, 121
    radiography of
        indications for, 49–51
        interpretation of, 51–55
    raloxifene and, 161

Vertebral fracture (*cont'd.*)
    risk of, 15–16
    in secondary osteoporosis, 73
    types and location of, 51
Vitamin A, 100
Vitamin C, 100
Vitamin D, 94–97
    for glucocorticoid-induced
        osteoporosis, 226–227, 231–233
    for hip fracture, 260
    nutrition and, 94–97
    recommendations for, 87
    in secondary osteoporosis, 79
Vitamin K
    supplement of, 99–100
    warfarin and, 100
Volumetric bone density, 30, 31

W

Warfarin, vitamin K and, 100
Wedge fracture, 51
Weight, osteoporosis risk and, 252–253
Weight-bearing exercise, 122
White female, bone densitometry in, 44
Wrist fracture, 249–252

X

X-ray absorptiometry
    dual energy
        of hip, 33–34
        peripheral, 35
        spinal, 34–35, 55–56
        vertebral fracture and, 55–56
    single energy, 34

Z

Z score, 30–32
    in secondary osteoporosis, 74